I0042053

Frontiers in Anti-cancer Drug Discovery

(*Volume 12*)

Edited by

Atta-ur-Rahman, *FRS*
Kings College, University of Cambridge, Cambridge, UK

&

M. Iqbal Choudhary
H.E.J. Research Institute of Chemistry, International Center for Chemical and Biological Sciences, University of Karachi, Karachi, Pakistan

Frontiers in Anti-Cancer Drug Discovery

Volume # 12

Editors: Atta-ur-Rahman and M. Iqbal Choudhary

ISSN (Online): 1879-6656

ISSN (Print): 2451-8395

ISBN (Online): 978-981-14-8738-5

ISBN (Print): 978-981-14-8736-1

ISBN (Paperback): 978-981-14-8737-8

©2021, Bentham Books imprint.

Published by Bentham Science Publishers Pte. Ltd. Singapore. All Rights Reserved.

BENTHAM SCIENCE PUBLISHERS LTD.
End User License Agreement (for non-institutional, personal use)

This is an agreement between you and Bentham Science Publishers Ltd. Please read this License Agreement carefully before using the ebook/echapter/ejournal (**"Work"**). Your use of the Work constitutes your agreement to the terms and conditions set forth in this License Agreement. If you do not agree to these terms and conditions then you should not use the Work.

Bentham Science Publishers agrees to grant you a non-exclusive, non-transferable limited license to use the Work subject to and in accordance with the following terms and conditions. This License Agreement is for non-library, personal use only. For a library / institutional / multi user license in respect of the Work, please contact: permission@benthamscience.net.

Usage Rules:

1. All rights reserved: The Work is the subject of copyright and Bentham Science Publishers either owns the Work (and the copyright in it) or is licensed to distribute the Work. You shall not copy, reproduce, modify, remove, delete, augment, add to, publish, transmit, sell, resell, create derivative works from, or in any way exploit the Work or make the Work available for others to do any of the same, in any form or by any means, in whole or in part, in each case without the prior written permission of Bentham Science Publishers, unless stated otherwise in this License Agreement.
2. You may download a copy of the Work on one occasion to one personal computer (including tablet, laptop, desktop, or other such devices). You may make one back-up copy of the Work to avoid losing it.
3. The unauthorised use or distribution of copyrighted or other proprietary content is illegal and could subject you to liability for substantial money damages. You will be liable for any damage resulting from your misuse of the Work or any violation of this License Agreement, including any infringement by you of copyrights or proprietary rights.

Disclaimer:

Bentham Science Publishers does not guarantee that the information in the Work is error-free, or warrant that it will meet your requirements or that access to the Work will be uninterrupted or error-free. The Work is provided "as is" without warranty of any kind, either express or implied or statutory, including, without limitation, implied warranties of merchantability and fitness for a particular purpose. The entire risk as to the results and performance of the Work is assumed by you. No responsibility is assumed by Bentham Science Publishers, its staff, editors and/or authors for any injury and/or damage to persons or property as a matter of products liability, negligence or otherwise, or from any use or operation of any methods, products instruction, advertisements or ideas contained in the Work.

Limitation of Liability:

In no event will Bentham Science Publishers, its staff, editors and/or authors, be liable for any damages, including, without limitation, special, incidental and/or consequential damages and/or damages for lost data and/or profits arising out of (whether directly or indirectly) the use or inability to use the Work. The entire liability of Bentham Science Publishers shall be limited to the amount actually paid by you for the Work.

General:

1. Any dispute or claim arising out of or in connection with this License Agreement or the Work (including non-contractual disputes or claims) will be governed by and construed in accordance with the laws of Singapore. Each party agrees that the courts of the state of Singapore shall have exclusive jurisdiction to settle any dispute or claim arising out of or in connection with this License Agreement or the Work (including non-contractual disputes or claims).
2. Your rights under this License Agreement will automatically terminate without notice and without the

need for a court order if at any point you breach any terms of this License Agreement. In no event will any delay or failure by Bentham Science Publishers in enforcing your compliance with this License Agreement constitute a waiver of any of its rights.

3. You acknowledge that you have read this License Agreement, and agree to be bound by its terms and conditions. To the extent that any other terms and conditions presented on any website of Bentham Science Publishers conflict with, or are inconsistent with, the terms and conditions set out in this License Agreement, you acknowledge that the terms and conditions set out in this License Agreement shall prevail.

Bentham Science Publishers Pte. Ltd.
80 Robinson Road #02-00
Singapore 068898
Singapore
Email: subscriptions@benthamscience.net

BENTHAM SCIENCE

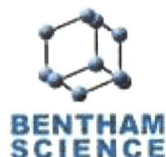

CONTENTS

PREFACE i

LIST OF CONTRIBUTORS iii

CHAPTER 1 CANNABINOID-BASED ANTI-CANCER STRATEGIES: SLOWLY
APPROACHING THE BEDSIDE 1
Paula Morales and Nadine Jagerovic
INTRODUCTION 1
PALLIATIVE EFFECTS 2
ANTITUMOR PROPERTIES 5
    ECS Regulation in Cancer Tissue 5
    Molecular Basis for Cannabinoid Antitumor Actions 7
        Antiproliferative and Pro-apoptotic Effects 7
        Effects on Tumor Invasion, Metastasis and Angiogenesis 9
    Towards Clinical Antitumor Application 9
ANTITUMOR CANNABINOIDS 11
    Endocannabinoids and Endocannabinoid-like Synthetic Derivatives 11
    Phytocannabinoids and Phytocannabinoid-like Synthetic Derivatives 14
    Synthetic Cannabinoids 17
        Aminoalkylindoles 17
        Arylpyrazoles 18
        Cannabinoid Quinones 19
        Other Antitumor Cannabinergic Ligands 20
CONCLUSION AND FUTURE PROSPECTS 21
CONSENT FOR PUBLICATION 22
CONFLICT OF INTEREST 22
ACKNOWLEDGEMENTS 22
REFERENCES 22

CHAPTER 2 THE BENEFICIAL EFFECTS OF TURMERIC AND ITS ACTIVE
CONSTITUENT IN CANCER TREATMENT: CURRENT AND FUTURE TRENDS 37
Giftson J. Senapathy, Blassan P. George and Heidi Abrahamse
INTRODUCTION 38
PHYTOCHEMISTRY OF CURCUMIN 40
STRUCTURE ACTIVITY RELATIONSHIP 41
PHARMACOLOGICAL PROPERTIES OF CURCUMIN 42
    Antioxidant and Prooxidant Nature of Curcumin 43
ANTICANCER ACTIVITY OF CURCUMIN 43
    Genitourinary Cancer 46
    Lung Cancer 46
    Breast Cancer 46
    Melanoma 47
    Ovarian Cancer 47
    Cervical Cancer 47
    Brain Tumor 48
    Prostate Cancer 48
    Head and Neck Cancer 48
    Gastro Intestinal Cancer 49
    Mode of Action of Curcumin 49
    Effect of Curcumin on Cancer Signaling Pathways 49
    Combination Therapies of Curcumin with other Drugs 52

  Curcumin Analogs and Cancer Stem Cells 53
 CHALLENGES IN TURMERIC AND CURCUMIN TREATMENTS 53
 FUTURE PROSPECTS 56
 CONCLUDING REMARKS 57
 CONSENT FOR PUBLICATION 57
 CONFLICT OF INTEREST 57
 ACKNOWLEDGEMENTS 57
 REFERENCES 58

CHAPTER 3 IMMUNOTHERAPY APPROACHES FOCUSING ON CANCER STEM CELLS 68
Marcela Rodrigues de Camargo, Rafael Carneiro Ortiz, Carolina Mendonça
Gorgulho, Vanessa Soares Lara and *Camila Oliveira Rodini*
 INTRODUCTION 68
 STEM CELLS 70
  Cancer Stem Cells 72
 CANCER IMMUNOTHERAPY 76
  Cancer Stem Cell-Based Immunotherapy 80
 CONCLUSION 87
 CONSENT FOR PUBLICATION 87
 CONFLICT OF INTEREST 88
 ACKNOWLEDGEMENTS 88
 LIST OF ABBREVIATION 88
 REFERENCES 89

CHAPTER 4 IMMUNOTHERAPY FOR THE TREATMENT OF HEPATOCELLULAR
CARCINOMA 101
Stepan M. Esagian, Ioannis A. Ziogas and *Georgios Tsoulfas*
 INTRODUCTION 101
  Epidemiology 101
  Management 102
   Early and Intermediate Hepatocellular Carcinoma 102
  Advanced Hepatocellular Carcinoma Management 102
   Sorafenib and Other Targeted Molecular Agents 102
  Immunotherapy 103
   History 103
   Immunotherapy in the Context of Hepatocellular Carcinoma 104
 MECHANISMS OF ACTION 104
  Immune Checkpoints and Cancer Immunoediting 104
  The PD-1/PD-L1 Pathway 105
  The CTLA-4 Pathway 105
  Combination to Enhance Anti-tumor Immune Responses 106
 FDA-APPROVED IMMUNOTHERAPY REGIMENS FOR HCC 107
  Single-agent Immune Checkpoint Inhibitors 107
   Nivolumab 107
   Pembrolizumab 110
  Double Immune Checkpoint Inhibitor Combination 112
   Nivolumab and Ipilimumab 112
  Immune Checkpoint Inhibitor and anti-VEGF Monoclonal Antibody Combination 113
   Atezolizumab and Bevacizumab 113
 NON-FDA APPROVED IMMUNOTHERAPY UNDER INVESTIGATION 116
  Single-agent Immune Checkpoint Inhibitors 116
   Tislelizumab 116

       Camrelizumab 118
       Durvalumab 119
       Tremelimumab 120
       Atezolizumab 120
    Immune Checkpoint Inhibitor and Tyrosine Kinase Inhibitor Combination 120
       Pembrolizumab and Lenvatinib 120
       Atezolizumab and Cabozantinib 121
       Avelumab and Axitinib 122
       Camrelizumab and Apatinib 122
    Immune Checkpoint Inhibitor and anti-VEGF Monoclonal Antibody Combination 124
       Durvalumab and Ramucirumab 124
    Double Immune Checkpoint Inhibitor Combination 124
       Tremelimumab and Durvalumab 124
    Immune Checkpoint Inhibitor and Locoregional Therapy Combination 125
       Tremelimumab and Ablation 125
  IMMUNOTHERAPY IN THE SETTING OF LIVER TRANSPLANTATION 127
  CONCLUSION 128
  CONSENT FOR PUBLICATION 128
  CONFLICT OF INTEREST 128
  ACKNOWLEDGEMENTS 128
  REFERENCES 128

**CHAPTER 5 ROLE OF BIOMARKERS IN DEVELOPING THERAPIES FOR
GLIOBLASTOMA MULTIFORME** 141
  Vijeta Prakash and *Reema Gabrani*
  INTRODUCTION 141
  BIOMARKERS IN MOLECULAR AND METABOLIC PATHWAYS 142
    Epidermal Growth Factor Receptor 143
    MGMT 144
    Tumor Protein p53 145
    Isocitrate Dehydrogenase 145
    Voltage-dependent Anion Channel 146
  MICRO RNA BIOMARKERS 147
  GBM CANCER STEM CELLS AS BIOMARKER BASED THERAPY 149
  IMAGING MODALITIES AS BIOMARKER 151
  IMMUNE CHECKPOINT AS BIOMARKER 152
    Programmed Cell Death Ligand 153
    CXCR4 153
    ADAMTSL4 153
    CAVIN1 154
    Heat Shock Protein-70 154
  CONCLUSION 154
  ABBREVIATIONS 155
  CONSENT FOR PUBLICATION 156
  CONFLICT OF INTEREST 156
  ACKNOWLEDGEMENTS 156
  REFERENCES 157

**CHAPTER 6 POLY (ADP-RIBOSE) POLYMERASES AS NEW DRUG TARGETS IN
CANCER TREATMENT** 164
  Fatih Tok and *Bedia Koçyiğit-Kaymakçıoğlu*
  INTRODUCTION 164

    Mechanisms of DNA Damage and Repair 165

    PARP Inhibitors and Their Mechanisms of Action 166

    Development and Clinical Trials of PARP Inhibitors in Cancer Treatment 169

    Recent Advances with PARP Inhibitor Research 173

CONCLUSION 187

CONSENT FOR PUBLICATION 188

CONFLICT OF INTEREST 188

ACKNOWLEDGEMENTS 188

REFERENCES 188

SUBJECT INDEX 196

PREFACE

Cancer has been the major reason of mortality and morbidity since ancient times. With increase in life expectancy and change in life style, the prevalence of cancers has increased exponentially. Molecular etiologies of cancers are often complex, but modern tools in molecular biology and pathology have been able to decipher them for the identification of many new targets for anti-cancer drug development. Cancer treatment also faces many challenges, such as heterogeneity, drug resistance, adverse effects of chemotherapy, and frequent relapses. The quantum of research in this field has been phenomenal in recent years, and keeping oneself abreast of recent developments is rather challenging. The book series *"Frontiers in Anti-cancer Drug Discovery"* is aimed to provide critical commentaries and updates on the most exciting developments in the multidisciplinary field of anti-cancer drug developments. The present volume 12 of the series has 6 (six) comprehensive reviews, contributed by leading practitioners in these fields. These reviews broadly cover various drug targets, therapeutic strategies as well as new classes of therapies for the prevention or treatment of diverse cancers.

The chapter by Morales and Jagerovic focusses on current developments in cannabinoid-based anticancer drugs. The review discusses how cannabinoids modulate tumor growth and induce autophagy-mediated apoptosis in diverse cancer models, apart from their classical use in the management of pain and adverse effects of chemotherapy. The second chapter by Abrahamse *et al* presents mounting evidence on the prevention, treatment and reversal of cancer developments with the wonder spice turmeric (*Curcuma longa*). The authors have discussed various aspects including pharmacokinetics, pre-clinical, and clinical evidences of the anti-oxidant, anti-inflammatory, and anti-cancer effects of curcumin, as well as the key constituent of turmeric. Immunotherapy for treatment of cancer has drawn major scientific attention in recent years. The potential of cancer stem cells (CSC) to target tumor mass has been the focus of a review by Camargo *et al*. Tsoulfas *et al* have critically reviewed the scientific literature on hepatocellular carcinoma (HCCS) and its immunotherapy. They discuss various classes of immune checkpoints inhibitors (ICIs, their limitation and advantages over other classes of drugs for the treatment of HCC. Cancer biomarkers play an important role in the diagnosis, prognosis and treatment monitoring. Prakash and Gabrani have reviewed the role and mechanism of biomarkers in developing therapies against glioblastoma multiforme (GBM). The potential of biomarkers as drug targets and development of effective and innovative therapies, based on biomarkers against GBM, has been comprehensively discussed. Tok and Kaymakcioglu have focused on the identification of poly(ADP-ribose) polymerases (PARP) as drug targets for anticancer drug development. PARP are important nuclear enzymes responsible for genomic repair, telomerase regulation, transcription and regulation of cell death. PARP inhibitors have been approved for the treatment of breast and ovarian cancers. We hope that these contributions will help readers in gaining a better understanding of this important subject.

We would to like to express our gratitude to all the authors of above cited review articles for their excellent contributions in this dynamic field of general and scientific interest. The efforts of the efficient team of Bentham Science Publishers for the timely production of the 12ᵗʰ volume, particularly of Ms. Fariya Zulfiqar (Manager Publications), and Mr. Mahmood Alam (Editorial Director) are gratefully acknowledged.

Atta-ur-Rahman, *FRS*
Kings College
University of Cambridge
Cambridge
UK

M. Iqbal Choudhary
H.E.J. Research Institute of Chemistry
International Center for Chemical and Biological Sciences
University of Karachi
Karachi, Pakistan

List of Contributors

Blassan P. George — Laser Research Centre, Faculty of Health Sciences, University of Johannesburg, P.O. Box 17011, Doornfontein 2028, South Africa

Bedia Koçyiğit-Kaymakçıoğlu — Department of Pharmaceutical Chemistry, Faculty of Pharmacy, Marmara University, Istanbul 34854, Turkey

Camila Oliveira Rodini — Department of Biological Sciences, Bauru School of Dentistry, University of São Paulo, Bauru, São Paulo, Brazil

Carolina Mendonça Gorgulho — ImmunoSurgery/Immunotherapy Unit, Champalimaud Foundation - Champalimaud Centre for the Unknown, Brasília Avenue, 1400-038 Lisbon, Portugal

Fatih Tok — Department of Pharmaceutical Chemistry, Faculty of Pharmacy, Marmara University, Istanbul 34854, Turkey

Georgios Tsoulfas — First Department of Surgery, Aristotle University of Thessaloniki, Thessaloniki, Greece

Giftson J. Senapathy — Laser Research Centre, Faculty of Health Sciences, University of Johannesburg, P.O. Box 17011, Doornfontein 2028, South Africa

Heidi Abrahamse — Laser Research Centre, Faculty of Health Sciences, University of Johannesburg, P.O. Box 17011, Doornfontein 2028, South Africa

Ioannis A. Ziogas — First Department of Surgery, Aristotle University of Thessaloniki, Thessaloniki, Greece

Marcela Rodrigues de Camargo — Department of Surgery, Stomatology, Pathology and Radiology. Bauru School of Dentistry, University of São Paulo, Bauru, São Paulo, Brazil

Nadine Jagerovic — Instituto de Química Médica, CSIC, Calle Juan de la Cierva, 3, 28006 Madrid, Spain

Paula Morales — Instituto de Química Médica, CSIC, Calle Juan de la Cierva, 3, 28006 Madrid, Spain

Rafael Carneiro Ortiz — Department of Biological Sciences, Bauru School of Dentistry, University of São Paulo, Bauru, São Paulo, Brazil

Reema Gabrani — Jaypee Institute of Information Technology, A-10, Sector-62, Noida, Uttar Pradesh 201309, India

Stepan M. Esagian — Faculty of Medicine, Democritus University of Thrace, Alexandroupoulis, Greece

Vanessa Soares Lara — Department of Surgery, Stomatology, Pathology and Radiology. Bauru School of Dentistry, University of São Paulo, Bauru, São Paulo, Brazil

Vijeta Prakash — Jaypee Institute of Information Technology, A-10, Sector-62, Noida, Uttar Pradesh 201309, India

CHAPTER 1

Cannabinoid-based Anti-cancer Strategies: Slowly Approaching the Bedside

Paula Morales[1,*] and **Nadine Jagerovic**[1,*]

[1] *Instituto de Química Médica, CSIC, Calle Juan de la Cierva, 3, 28006 Madrid, Spain*

Abstract: Modulation of the endocannabinoid system has emerged as a potential therapeutic strategy for the treatment of diverse types of cancer and related pathologies. Thus far, the use of specific cannabinoids has been primarily approved for the management of chemotherapy-induced side effects. Palliative actions of cannabinoids include the control of nausea and vomiting, pain alleviation and appetite stimulation. Moreover, a growing body of research has exposed the anticarcinogenic potential of cannabinoids. *In vitro* and *in vivo* studies have shown that endogenous, plant-derived and synthetic cannabinoids can effectively modulate tumor growth in diverse cancer models. Although this has not yet reached the bedside, ongoing clinical trials and research efforts may approach cannabinoid-based antitumor therapies to cancer patients in the near future.

So far, studies on cannabinoids as antitumor agents have been mainly focused on understanding the mechanism of action of well-known phytocannabinoids such as Δ^9-THC or CBD. However, novel cannabinoids with antitumor properties are also emerging in the literature. In this chapter, we aim to provide an updated overview of the therapeutic potential of cannabinoids in cancer. We will comprehensively summarize the diverse cannabinoid structures exerting antitumor properties analyzing the molecular basis of these actions. Recent and ongoing clinical trials will be considered to provide a deeper insight into the current scenario of cannabinoids in oncology.

Keywords: Apoptosis, Cancer, Cannabinoids, CB_1R, CB_2R, Chemotherapy, Clinical trials, Endocannabinoid system, GPR55, Palliative effects.

INTRODUCTION

Despite the progress made in treating many types of cancer, effective therapies are still lacking for some of them, including pancreatic, liver and glioblastoma. Chemotherapy remains one of the principal options for cancer treatment.

---

* **Corresponding authors Nadine Jagerovic and Paula Morales:** Instituto de Química Médica, CSIC, Calle Juan de la Cierva, 3, 28006 Madrid, Spain; Tel: +345 622 900; E-mails: nadine@iqm.csic.es (NJ) and paula.morales@iqm.csic.es (PM).

Atta-ur-Rahman & M. Iqbal Choudhary (Eds.)
All rights reserved-© 2021 Bentham Science Publishers

However, improving the aggressive current chemotherapies is still challenging nowadays. Identifying and validating new biological targets involved in cancer cell survival, growth, and metastasis is a widely used approach in anti-cancer drug discovery. In this context, the endocannabinoid system (ECS) emerges as a promising anticancer target [1 - 11]. Thus, understanding the antitumor mechanism of action of the two main components of the plant *Cannabis Sativa*, (-)Δ^9-tetrahydrocannabinol (THC) and cannabidiol (CBD), has been so far the main concern. These phytocannabinoids modulate ECS that was discovered in the '90s following the identification of two G-protein coupled receptors (GPCRs), CB_1 and CB_2 cannabinoid receptors (CB_1R and CB_2R), endogenous ligands named endocannabinoids along with their metabolic enzymes [12 - 16]. N-arachidonoy--ethanolamine (AEA) and 2-arachidonoylglycerol (2-AG) are the two main endocannabinoids and fatty acid amide hydrolase (FAAH), monoacylglycerol lipase (MAGL), N-acyl-phosphatidylethanolamine-hydrolysing phospholipase D (NAPE-PLD), and sn-1-specific diacylglycerol lipase-α and -β (DGLα; DGLβ) are their anabolic and catabolic related enzymes [17]. CB_1R and CB_2R are widely expressed in the human body. CB_1R is one of the most abundant GPCRs in the brain especially expressed in the cortex, basal nuclei, hippocampus, and cerebellum. CB_1R is also present in peripheral organs (liver, kidney, heart, adipose tissue, muscle, lung, pancreas), and immune cells (monocytes and macrophages). CB_2R is present in the brain but to a much less extent than CB_1R. However, its expression in the immune system is predominant (lymphocytes, natural killer cells, macrophages, and neutrophils). The phytocannabinoid THC acts on both receptors, CB_1R and CB_2R, CB_1R activation in the brain being responsible for its psychotropic effects. The non-psychoactive CBD has been reported to modulate these receptors through allosterism mechanisms with evidence as negative allosteric modulator (NAM) of THC and 2-AG at CB_1R [18] and positive allosteric modulation and partial agonist at CB_2R [19, 20]. CBD has also been shown to modulate CB_1R-CB_2R heteromers [21]. Under different physiopathological processes, the mechanism of action of CBD and THC can engage other diverse biological targets such as enzymes, transporters, GPCRs, nuclear and ionotropic receptors, most of them related to ECS [22]. These two phytocannabinoids have been the most explored cannabinoids as antitumor agents. Few synthetic cannabinoids with anticancer properties have been reported in the literature [23]. In this chapter, a general perspective on the potential of cannabinoids in cancer pathology is provided.

PALLIATIVE EFFECTS

Cannabis has been proposed to improve quality of life during cancer chemotherapy by reducing unwanted effects such as nausea, vomiting, lack of appetite and pain [24 - 29]. Dronabinol (THC; Marinol®) and nabilone (Cesamet®)

were approved by the US Food and Drug Administration (FDA) for the management of chemotherapy-induced nausea and vomiting (CINV) in the mid '80s [30 - 32]. However, the major limitations of the use of these potent CB_1R agonists are their CNS side-effects at high doses, the unpredictable gastrointestinal absorption when use orally, and a delayed onset of action. Thus, in western countries, dronabinol or nabilone are currently prescribed to cancer chemotherapy patients who failed to respond to conventional treatments [25, 33, 34]. Diverse randomized controlled trials studying oral formulations of cannabinoids (dronabinol and nabilone) for the prophylaxis of CINV evidence a cannabinoid efficacy superior to conventional and new generation of antiemetic drugs, such as ondansetran, a serotonin ($5HT_3$) antagonist, or aprepitant, a neurokin-1 inhibitor [25, 26]. However, a great percentage of patients experienced dysphoria, euphoria, and sedation. The presence of side-effects and the lack of sufficient medical data slow their general use in clinical practice. More recently, clinical trials using CBD/THC extracts for the prevention of CINV are showing improved efficacy and psychotropic effects [35, 36]. The presence of CBD is suggested to improve tolerance and efficacy. The role of CB_1R and/or CB_2R in the antiemetic actions of cannabinoids is still elusive [37]. Studies realized in a shrew model of emesis revealed that CB_2R may not have a role in vomiting as does CB_1R due to a low level of expression in the emetic loci [37].

Cannabis and THC have led to increasing appetite, mostly in noncancerous contexts thus far. For instance, THC is widely used for AIDS-related cachexia. By activating CB_1R, THC can increase appetite and promote weight gain. Studies assessing the effects of cannabinoids in cancer patients have also shown to have a potential stimulatory effect on appetite and food intake [28]. However, only a few randomized controlled trials have been reported so far, the safety issue remaining the bottom line [38]. Nevertheless, considering that cancer cachexia (CCA) is frequently undertreated or treated by progestogens that only increase adipose tissue, cannabinoids could be an interesting alternative. For instance, a randomized double blind with 78 patients with anorexia associated with advanced lung cancer has been realized to support the nabilone effect on the attenuation of anorexia, nutritional status and quality of life (ClinicalTrials.gov Identifier: NCT02802540). Another clinical assay (Phase 3) is currently in process for assessing safety and efficacy of inhaled synthetic THC/CBD for improving physical functioning and for modulating cachexia progression in patients with advanced cancer and associated cachexia (ClinicalTrials.gov Identifier: NCT04001010).

The management of cancer pain continues to be elusive since conventional treatment for moderate-to-severe conditions requires the use of opioids. The effectiveness of cannabinoids in alleviating cancer-related pain has been evidenced in different animal models [25, 27 - 29, 39]. For instance, in platinum antitumor-induced models of neuropathic pain, the CB_1R/CB_2R agonist WIN55,212–2 and THC, the CB_2 agonist JWH-133, and CBD [40, 41]. Cannabinoids have also showed efficacy for cancer pain management in other models including paclitaxel, and vincristine-evoked neuropathies [27, 42, 43]. Both CB_1R and CB_2R have been shown to be implicated in analgesia and anti-inflammatory processes. Nevertheless, the etiology of cancer-related pain is so complex that the predominance of one mechanism of action over the other may depend on the type, location, and severity of the cancer. In this context, the use of CB_1R peripherally-restricted cannabinoids represents an interesting approach. The synthetic peripherally restricted cannabinoid PrNMI suppresses chemotherapy-induced peripheral neuropathy pain in a rat model of cisplatin-induced neuropathy without appreciable CNS side effects or tolerance to repetitive administration [44]. This effect was demonstrated to be primarily mediated by CB_1R and not CB_2R activation. Nevertheless, selective CB_2R activation has been shown to be an efficient target for pain generated by bone tumors and metastases [45]. In a murine model of bone cancer pain that mimics metastatic bone cancer pain in humans, 2-AG reduced mechanical hyperalgesia evoked by the growth of a fibrosarcoma tumor in and around the calcaneus bone with an efficacy comparable to that of morphine [46]. This effect was shown to be mediated by activation of peripheral CB_2R but not CB_1R. Only few randomized trials focused on the analgesic effects of cannabinoids for cancer pain have been conducted so far [47]. They support that cannabinoids are effective adjuvants for cancer pain. However, it seems that cannabinoid treatment at safe low and medium doses does not completely substitute opioid therapy. Although, Sativex® (Combined 1:1 THC/CBD; also named Nabidiolex and Nabiximol) is prescribed in several countries as an adjunctive analgesic treatment [48] for adult patients with advanced cancer, unfortunately limited data do not allow confirming efficacy, safety, and utility of cannabinoids in the management of cancer pain. Nevertheless, recent clinical trials could support evidence for cannabinoids as analgesics for cancer patients. For instance, THC and CBD are currently in Phase 2 for taxane-induced peripheral neuropathy that affects a significant number of women undergoing breast cancer treatment (ClinicalTrials.gov Identifier: NCT03782402). Another Phase 2 clinical trial uses CBD for the prevention of chemotherapy-induced peripheral neuropathy in patients receiving oxaliplatin or paclitaxel based chemotherapy (ClinicalTrials.gov Identifier: NCT04582591).

The use of cannabinoids to address other injuries caused by chemotherapeutic agents are explored such doxorubicin-induced cardiomyopathy and cisplatin-induced nephrotoxicity for which CBD showed protecting properties [49, 50].

In general, lack of large clinical trials, heterogeneous conditions and schedule 1 classification of cannabis and cannabinoids exclude cannabinoid treatments as a regular option for palliative management in cancer patients. Cannabis-based drugs are prescribed for patients who failed to respond to conventional treatments.

Another aspect that needs to be taking into account is the use of cannabis plant products available in state-regulated markets. Clinical evidence is urgently needed to be able to advise patients on which cannabis-based products to take, or to avoid, in managing cancer-related symptoms. Clinical trials are currently set up to determine which cannabis extract combination (THC/CBD) is most effective at treating cancer related symptoms (ClinicalTrials.gov Identifier: NCT03948074 and NCT03617692).

ANTITUMOR PROPERTIES

Cannabis and cannabinoids have been primarily used for palliative purposes in cancer patients. In recent years, they have been proposed as anticancer agents [1 - 11]. In fact, antitumor effects of cannabinoids have been reported in numerous *in vitro* and *in vivo* models of cancer [10, 51, 52]. Four decades ago, one of the first evidences has been reported in mice model in which Lewis lung adenocarcinoma growth was retarded by the oral administration of THC, Δ^8-THC and cannabinol [53]. Unfortunately, these first findings did not get further consequences until the discovery of the ECS three decades ago. Starting in the late '90s, an emerging body of investigation points to the antitumor properties of cannabinoids. Cannabinoids have been shown to reduce tumor growth and progression on a wide range of cancer cells, in culture and in nude mice tumor xenografts, including lung carcinomas, gliomas, thyroid epithelial cancer, skin carcinomas, and lymphomas among others [11, 52, 54 - 59]. The mechanisms of action through which cannabinoids impact cancer cell cycle and survival are quite complex and their characterization remains incomplete. Moreover, the role played by the ECS in cell proliferation, arrest cell cycle, apoptosis, autophagy, cancer cell vascular adhesiveness, invasiveness, and metastasis formation depends on the cancer type and tissue. Thus, the cell signaling pathways implicated in these processes may differ depending on specific cancers and/or experimental models. In this sense, efforts at pre-clinical stage have being done to elucidate these mechanisms [51]. Unfortunately, only few clinical trials have been realized so far.

ECS Regulation in Cancer Tissue

The antitumor activity displayed by cannabis-related drugs suggests that the ECS contributes not only to the basic cell functions but also to cancer on-set and development. The ECS is upregulated in malignant compared with non-tumor tissue [52, 54, 60, 61] being tumor type-specific [10, 61].

Increase in CB_2R expression has been observed in distinct types of tumors, such as glioblastoma [62], estrogen receptor-negative breast tumors [63], bladder cancer [64, 65], colon cancer progression [66], and in diverse breast tumors [67, 68], whereas elevated levels of CB_1R has been detected in other cancers such as gastric carcinoma [69], rhabdomyosarcoma [70], melanoma [71], and colorectal cancer [66, 72]. These observations do not exclude the participation of both receptors CB_1R and CB_2R. Their increased expression has been reported in hepatocellular carcinoma [73], mantle cell lymphoma [74], acute myeloid leukemia [75], malignant astrocytomas [76], and human pancreatic cancer [55].

Significant high levels of endocannabinoids have also be detected in tumor cells including glioblastoma, meningioma, pituitary adenoma, prostate and colon carcinoma, and endometrial sarcoma [11, 77 - 80]. As well, high levels of endocannabinoid degradation enzymes FAAH [79, 81] and MAGL [64, 80] have been detected in aggressive human cancer cells and primary tumors. Hence, inhibition of FAAH [81, 82] and MAGL [64, 80, 83] has been suggested as therapeutic strategies for tumor defense.

Due to the fact that dysregulation of the ECS plays an important role in the physiopathology of cancer, an aspect that needs to be explored and taken into account is a possible tumor-promoting effect under certain conditions as it has been reported in few studies [76, 84]. It has been suggested that over-activation of ECS could induce tumorigenesis [61] and could be responsible to tumor aggressiveness [79, 80]. Responding to these hypotheses, it has been proposed a biphasic action on CBRs with pro-proliferative activity at low concentrations of endocannabinoids and antiproliferative and pro-apoptotic effects at high doses of exogenous cannabinoids [11].

The intervention of the ECS-related orphan receptor GPR55 has been proposed in the proliferative effect of THC on diverse cancer cell lines. Effectively, GPR55 has been reported *in vitro* and *in vivo* to be upregulated in cancer cell lines including gliomas, breast adenocarcinoma and squamous skin cell carcinoma [85 - 88]. In a model of colitis-associated colorectal cancer, GPR55$^{-/-}$ mice developed less and smaller tumors than their wild-type [89]. Thus, antagonizing GPR55 has emerged as a promising therapeutic target in oncology as well as a new cancer biomarker with possible prognostic value [90]. Studies on GPCRs dimers reveal that GPR55-CB_2R heterodimers are expressed in cancer cells and human tumors representing new potential therapeutic targets [91, 92].

The transient receptor potential vanilloid 1 (TRPV1) channel has emerged in the ECS as an ionotropic cannabinoid receptor [93]. Experimental findings indicate that TRPV1 may mediate endocannabinoid action in cancer processes. TRPV1 activation by the endocannabinoid AEA induces apoptosis in human glioma cells [94] and interferes with endometrial cancer cell death [95]. TRPV1, along with CB_2R, is also involved in the modulation of human breast carcinoma growth by the phytocannabinoid CBD [96].

Several studies have shown that peroxisome proliferator activated receptors PPARγ and PPARα, well-known transcriptional effectors involved in regulating biological processes including cell growth, differentiation and apoptosis, can mediate the antitumor activity of cannabinoids in an independent manner or *via* CB_1R and/or CB_2R [97].

Cannabis- and cannabinoid-based drugs have a remarkable therapeutic potential in controlling cancer processes through different elements of the extended ECS. Nevertheless, further research is required for understanding the role plays by the ECS in these processes.

Molecular Basis for Cannabinoid Antitumor Actions

Significant evidence supports the cellular pathways involved in cell proliferation and survival triggered after CB_1R and CB_2R activation. These signaling pathways involved key mediator factors important at least for four mechanisms: direct inhibition of transformed-cell growth through the suppression of mitogenic signal, induction of apoptosis, inhibition of tumor angiogenesis and metastasis.

Antiproliferative and Pro-apoptotic Effects

At the subcellular level, various signaling pathways are associated with cannabinoid-induced cancer cell death through apoptosis and/or inhibition of cancer cell proliferation (Fig. **1**) [98]. Activation of either CB_1R or CB_2R induces *de novo* synthesis of sphingolipid ceramide, a key regulator of programmed cell death. The synthesis of pro-apoptotic ceramide occurs in the endoplasmic reticular (ER) *via* activation of the enzyme ceramide synthase. Further insight into the specific signalling events downstream of ceramide indicates a main mechanism of cannabinoid-induced cell death with some variations inherent to different types of cancer cells [98]. The main pathway demonstrated in glioma, pancreatic, and hepatic cancer cells, and melanoma cells is the p8/TRIB3–mediated autophagy pathway [55, 72, 99, 100]. Up-regulation of the stress-regulated protein p8 together with several of its downstream targets such as the endoplasmic reticulum (ER) stress-related transcription factors ATF4 and CHOP, and the pseudokinase tribbles-homologue 3 (TRIB3) are involved in the control of tumorigenesis and tumor progression by cannabinoids [54, 98]. This cascade of events trigger the interaction of TRIB3 with the serine-threonine kinase AKT [101] leading to the inhibition of the AKT–mammalian target of rapamycin complex 1 (mTORC1) axis, and the subsequent induction of autophagy [99].

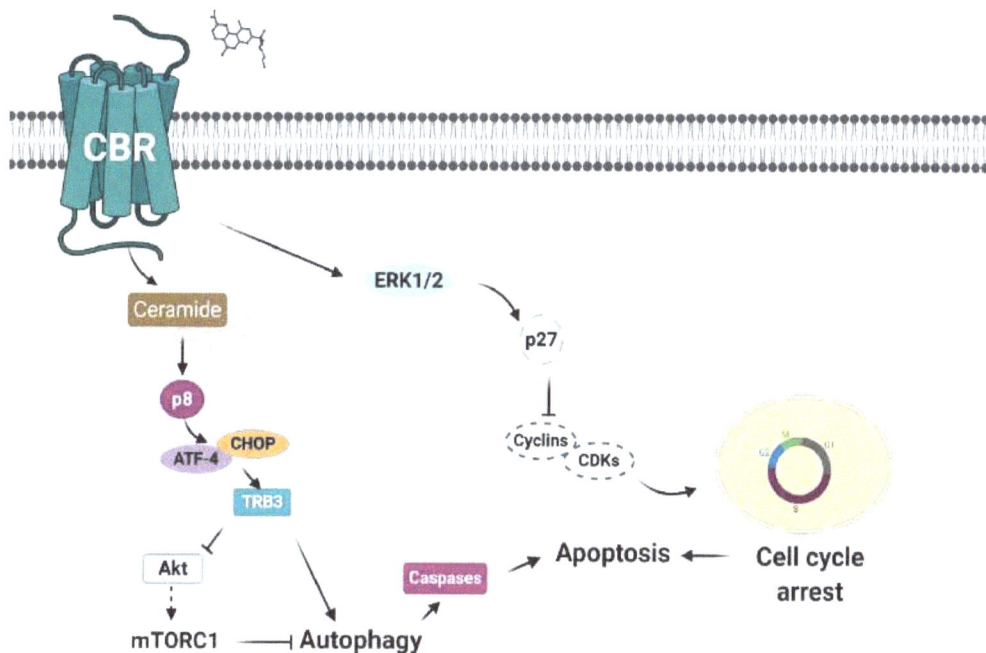

Fig. (1). Schematic representation of the signaling pathways through which cannabinoids impact apoptosis and proliferation. Created with BioRender.com.

Thus, the ceramide accumulation and the activation of the ER-stress related pathway lead to autophagy that has been shown to be upstream of apoptosis in this mechanism of cannabinoid-induced cell death. Additional signalling pathways have been shown to cooperate with the p8/trib3–mediated autophagy pathway. One of them involves ER stress–dependent activation of calcium/calmodulin-dependent protein kinase 2β and AMP-activated protein kinase leads [72]. Activation of CBRs in certain types of cancer cells such as breast cancer and melanoma, inhibits AKT to promote cycle arrest and apoptosis through different pathways that include modulation of cyclins by the cyclin kinase inhibitors (p21 and p27), frequently deregulated in cancers and active in different parts of the cell cycle, or decrease of the phosphorylation of the pro-apoptotic BCL-2 proteins leading to the activation of caspases, which play an essential role in triggering apoptosis [60, 98, 102, 103]. An additional process centered on the activation of an extracellular regulated kinase (ERK) signaling cascade promoting cell cycle arrest and apoptosis have been proposed [54, 55, 59, 104, 105].

There are still many unraveled sides on death pathways activated by cannabinoids as well as on the different contribution of apoptosis and autophagy in cell death depending on the nature of the tumor system.

Effects on Tumor Invasion, Metastasis and Angiogenesis

Angiogenesis has been shown to be inhibited by certain cannabinoids [106]. CBRs activation in cancer cells plays a major role in the vascular endothelial growth factor (VEGF) pathway, known to be inducer of angiogenesis [98]. A down-regulation of the receptors VEGFR1 and VEGFR2 has been observed after cannabinoid pre-clinical treatment in skin carcinomas [107], gliomas [105, 106], and thyroid carcinomas [108]. The cannabinoid-evoked angiogenesis suppression is also associated with a reduced expression of pro-angiogenic cytokine.

Evidence of anti-migrative, anti-adhesive, anti-invasive, and anti-metastatic properties of certain cannabinoids is gathered from a variety of studies [109], including lung [110, 111], glioma [112], cervical [111], and breast [63, 113] cancer cells culture analyses. The potential mechanism of action involves modulation of matrix metalloproteinase 2 (MMP-2), a proteolytic extracellular enzyme that plays a crucial role in tumor invasion allowing tissue breakdown and remodeling during angiogenesis and metastasis. This hypothesis has been confirmed in a cervical cancer cell line [111, 114, 115] and in glioma cells [112] in which the tissue inhibitor of MMPs (TIMP-1) could inhibit the MMPs proteolytic activity suppressing vascular tumor growth and angiogenesis. Ceramide biosynthesis and expression of the stress protein p8 also target these processes [112]. In lung cancer cells, cannabinoids promote the up-regulation of the intercellular adhesion molecule 1 (ICAM-1), a marker for metastatic stage [116].

All these data support the potential of cannabinoids as potent inhibitors of both cancer growth and spreading. However, these effects are generally cell line- or tumor type-dependent. Nonetheless, the potential development of cannabinoids as antitumor drugs has been restricted so far mainly due to their psychoactive properties and the lack of supporting clinical assays.

Towards Clinical Antitumor Application

Cannabis-based medicines have proven benefits in cancer patients as adjunctive treatment to conventional prescriptions for chemotherapy-induced nausea, vomiting, and cancer-related pain. So far, their therapeutic usage in oncology is restricted to treatment-related adverse effects. Despite increasing *in vitro* and *in vivo* preclinical evidence raising their potential in the treatment of tumor progression, only few clinical trials have being reported so far. They engaged a limited number of patients probably due to regulative issues overcoming large randomized clinical trials.

The first pilot clinical trial supporting the antitumor capacity of cannabinoids was performed on 9 patients suffering glioblastoma multiforme refractory to surgical and radiotherapy [117]. The safety profile of intratumoral administration of THC revealed no obvious psychoactive effects. In some of these patients exhibiting clear evidence of tumor progression, a decrease in tumor growth and even induced cell death was observed. Whereas median survival from a surgical operation of tumor relapse was 24 weeks, 2 of the patients survived for approximately 1 year. The very limited number of patients involved in this study does not allow generalizing the outcomes, but it may be considered a first proof-of-concept.

To assess the safety of Sativex® in a combinational therapy with temozolomide (TMZ), a first-line treatment for glioblastoma multiforme, an open-label Phase followed by a randomized Phase have been undertaken in 6-21 recurrent glioblastoma patients (ClinicalTrials.gov Identifier: NCT01812603 and NCT01812616). The outcomes of these studies suggest that a combination of THC/CBD with dose-intensive TMZ led to significant improvements in survival compared with placebo [118]. TMZ monotherapy showed 44% 1-year survival rate in these studies whereas the combinatorial therapy Sativex®/TMZ indicated a 83% 1-year survival rate with a median survival over 662 days compared with 369 days in the control group.

Extensive clinical studies are needed to extract significant conclusions that reinforce the potential utility of cannabinoids as anticancer therapeutics for glioblastoma. In this sense, a clinical Phase Ib, open-label, multicenter, intrapatient dose-escalation clinical trial is recruiting 30 patients to assess the safety profile of a THC/CBD combination at a 1:1 ratio, adding TMZ and radiotherapy in patients with newly-diagnosed glioblastoma (ClinicalTrials.gov Identifier: NCT03529448).

It is worth mentioning here Phase 1 clinical studies realized with dexanabinol (also named HU-211 or ETS2101) in patients with brain (ClinicalTrials.gov Identifier: NCT01654497) and advanced solid tumors (ClinicalTrials.gov Identifier: NCT01489826). These early clinical studies allowed determining the maximum safe dose that can be administered to cancer patients. Even though dexanabinol is the enantiomer of the potent cannabinoid agonist HU-210, it lacks activity at CBRs but has been characterized as a NMDA (N-methyl-D-aspartate) receptor antagonist [119]. It has been suggested to have anti-tumor properties through NFκB, TNFα, COX-2 and additional putative targets suck as HAT, FAT and cyclin dependent kinases [120]. The safety of dexanabinol in monotherapy and in combination with standard chemotherapy (Sorafenib, nab-paclitaxel, or gemcitabine) is assessed in patients with pancreatic cancer or hepatocellular carcinoma (ClinicalTrials.gov Identifier: NCT02423239). Tumor response evaluation outcomes have not been published yet.

Antitumor cannabinoids tested so far in clinical trials are assessed most of the case toxicological profile. Nevertheless, these compounds are not fully appropriate due to elicit CB_1R-mediated psychomimetic activity (THC, Sativex®) and/or high lipophilicity with pharmacokinetic issues (CBD, Sativex®, THC, dexanabinol). Synthetic cannabinoids are still far from clinical assays due to their unknown toxicity for humans.

ANTITUMOR CANNABINOIDS

A range of endogenous, phytogenic and synthetic cannabinoids has shown to impact diverse types of cancer. As discussed above, certain phytocannabinoid-based drugs have already reached the oncological bedside for their palliative effects. However, even though widely proved in preclinical models, their antitumor properties have not been advanced yet into patients. In this section we aim to provide an overview of the compounds that exhibit anticancer therapeutic avenues upon modulation of the ECS.

Endocannabinoids and Endocannabinoid-like Synthetic Derivatives

As aforementioned, abnormal endocannabinoidome regulation in cancer physiopathology is accompanied by dysregulation of the concentration of circulating endocannabinoids and this has been related to cancer progression [3]. In specific tumor types, including hepatocellular carcinoma [121], pituitary adenomas [122], glioma, meningioma [121], or lymphatic metastasis [123] increased AEA levels have been reported in comparison to healthy tissue. Moreover, higher levels of both 2-AG and AEA were detected in colon cancer tissue *versus* its normal counterpart [78]. 2-AG upregulation of was also reported in glioblastomas and meningiomas [121] as well as diffuse in large B-cell lymphoma [124]. Contrariwise, other reports claim minor changes or even lower levels of 2-AG and AEA in cancer samples in comparison to control [122, 123, 125].

Impairment of other endocannabinoids such as oleoylethanolamide (OEA) and palmitoylethanolamide (PEA) have also been detected in human plasma of cancer patients [126]. These monounsaturated (OEA) and fully saturated (PEA) analogues of AEA have shown to target the nuclear the receptor PPARα lacking CB_1R/CB_2R affinity. Interestingly PEA has been reported to synergistically improve AEA's anti proliferative effects in human breast cancer cells [127].

It is also important to note that, as previously mentioned, endocannabinoid degradation enzymes FAAH and MAGL have also shown to be abnormally regulated in cancer tissue correlating with endocannabinoid levels cancer changes [7].

Overall, there is a tendency to observe increased endocannabinoid levels in cancer and correlate with the progression of the disease. However, this might be tumor specific and further investigations remain to be done to obtain consistent data. Therefore, these endogenous molecules cannot be used as reliable general oncology biomarkers.

In addition to expression differences in cancer tissue, numerous studies have evidenced the antitumor potential of endocannabinoids and endocannabinoid-like molecules in diverse cancer models.

Exogenous administration of AEA exhibited antitumorigenic actions in several cancer cell lines and animal models [7]. Its antiproliferative effects are mediated through different mechanisms depending on particular tumor types. For example, AEA has shown to block cancer proliferation *via* CB_1R activation in human breast cancer cells [128, 129], in prostate cancer cell lines activated with epidermal growth factor [130], or in human cutaneous melanoma cells [131], while FAAH-mediated mechanisms have been reported in murine neuroblastoma cells [132]. Moreover, AEA´s apoptotic effect in non-melanoma skin cancer has shown to be mediated through oxidative stress and cannabinoid receptors-independent mechanisms [133]. This endocannabinoid also exhibited ability to inhibit tumor invasion and to provoke antimetastatic effects in a lung cancer *in vivo* model [81]. These properties have been linked to AEA-induced upregulation of TIMP-1.

Stable synthetic derivatives of AEA also demonstrated a promising antiproliferative profile. For instance, (*R*)-(+)-methanandamide (Met-AEA, Fig. **2**) which possesses higher CB_1R potency and metabolic stability than AEA, induces apoptosis in prostate cancer cells [134, 135], in cervical and lung cancer cell lines [136], glioma cells [125, 136] or mantle cell lymphoma [125]. The CB_1R highly selective analog of AEA arachidonyl-2'-chloroethylamide (ACEA, Fig. **2**) was also found to confer inhibition of tumor growth in breast cancer stem cell invasiveness [137] and colorectal carcinoma cells [78] resulting inactive in Kaposi's sarcoma cells [138].

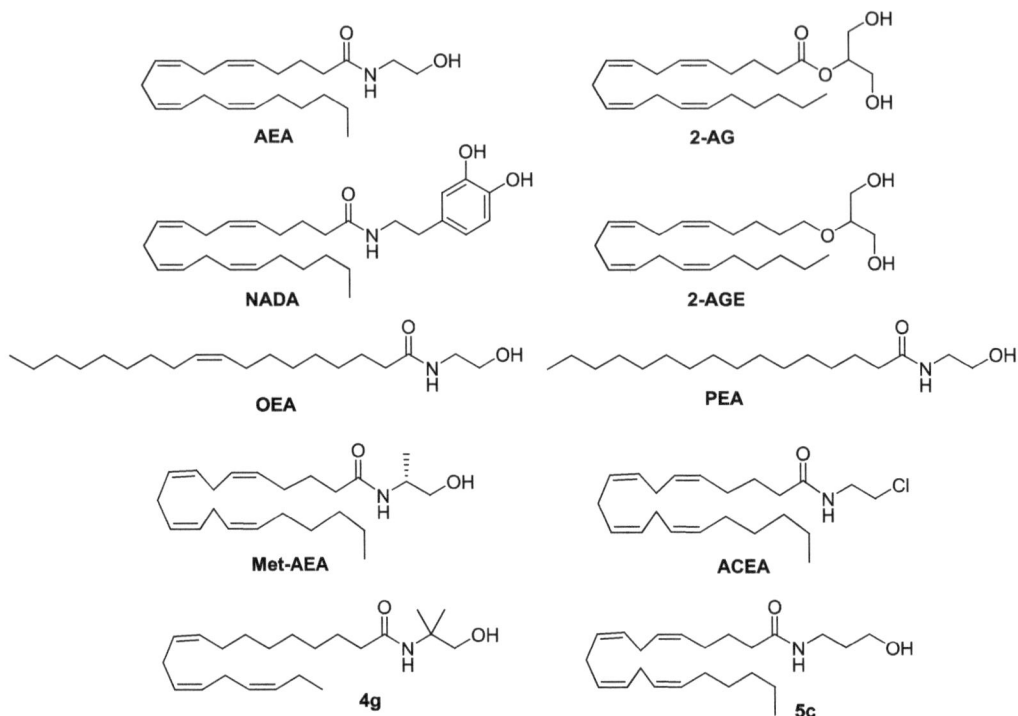

Fig. (2). Chemical structure of endocannabinoids and synthetic derivatives involved in cancer processes.

More recently, biocatalysis was used to obtain N-fatty acylamines from linolenic and arachidonic acids [139]. From this series of compounds, AEA derivatives **4g** and **5c** (Fig. **2**) proved to enhance the antiproliferative properties of AEA in rat glioma C6 cells [139]. The authors suggest that this improved effect is likely due to the FAAH inhibition.

The second major endocannabinoid, 2-AG, has also shown to elicit antitumorigenic actions in a wide range of malignancies. Reduction of tumor growth by 2-AG has been reported in breast cancer cells (CB$_1$R-mediated mechanism) [140], in colorectal carcinoma [78] and in glioma cells [141] among others. Anti-invasive and antimetastatic properties were demonstrated in lung cancer cells in nude mice [81]. Moreover, 2-AG was found to induce anti-invasive effects on androgen-independent prostate cancer cell lines [142] and antiproliferative actions in prostate carcinoma cells [143].

The anticancer properties of the stable 2-AG analog 2-arachidonyl glyceryl ether (2-AGE, noladin ether, Fig. **2**) were demonstrated in prostate cancer cells [142, 143]. 2-AGE inhibits tumor growth *via* nuclear factor (NF)-κB/cyclin D- and cyclin E-dependent pathways [143].

Another endocannabinoid that exerts antitumor actions is *N*-arachidonoyl dopamine (NADA, Fig. **2**). *In vitro* and *in vivo* studies confirmed its ability to reduce proliferation in an array of cancer types including breast adenocarcinoma, neuroblastoma, osteosarcoma, colorectal carcinoma or lymphoma among others [78, 144 - 146].

It is also worth mentioning that exogenous administration of OEA and PEA was reported to counteract tumor progression. Their antiproliferative properties were demonstrated in neuroblastoma [144], while anti-invasive and antimetastatic effects were found in lung cancer models [81].

Besides the growing evidence of the antitumorigenic potential of endocannabinoids in cancer physiopathology, further research is needed to precisely understand their role in the modulation of tumor progression.

Phytocannabinoids and Phytocannabinoid-like Synthetic Derivatives

Phytocannabinoids and their synthetic have not only been approved for palliative cancer care but also are at the forefront of current clinical trials for its antitumor potential. Numerous studies have preclinically confirmed the ability of phytocannabinoids to induce anticancer responses. Although investigations have been mainly focused on the activity of THC and CBD (Fig. **3**), their acidic derivatives Δ^9-tetrahydrocannabinolic acid (THCA, Fig. **3**) and cannabidiolic acid (CBDA, Fig. **3**) have also attracted broad attention because of their antitumor potential [52, 54, 147 - 151]. To a lesser extent, minor phytocannabinoids such as cannabigerol (CBG, Fig. **3**), CBN (Fig. **3**) or cannabichromene (CBC, Fig. **3**) have also shown ability to reduce tumor growth [151].

Antitumorigenic effects of THC have been widely confirmed in different types of cancer including glioblastoma, myeloma, lymphoma, prostate, colon, breast, lung or pancreatic cancers, among others [147, 151, 152]. THC is able to elicit diverse anticancer responses such as inhibition of cell proliferation, induction of apoptosis, impairment of tumor angiogenesis or inhibition of tumor invasion [151]. These effects are largely depending on the cancer type due to molecular changes. Therefore, even though the cannabinoid receptors CB_1R and CB_2R have shown to mediate most of these effects, CBR independent mechanisms have also been observed [153].

As discussed above, the THC synthetic analogs dexanabinol (Fig. **3**) and nabilone (Fig. **3**) have successfully reached the bedside for palliative effects and their antitumor potential is being assessed in ongoing clinical trials.

The non-psychoactive phytocannabinoid CBD was found to inhibit tumor growth, migration, invasion, metastasis or increase autophagy in a variety of malignancies [154]. *In vitro* and *in vivo* studies have demonstrated its antiproliferative potential in glioma, neuroblastoma, myeloma, melanoma, leukemia, cervical, colon, prostate, lung, breast, endometrial and ovarian cancer [148, 151]. The intricate molecular pharmacology of this phytocannabinoid complicates the elucidation of the underlying antitumor mechanisms. Accumulation of reactive oxygen species (ROS) [96], along with its activity at COX-2, 5-LOX, PPARγ, mTOR, p38 MAPK pathway have been suggested to mediate these effects [148]. Clinical trials of CBD alone or in combination with THC and/or other chemotherapeutic agents remain to assess its antitumor actions in cancer patients [154].

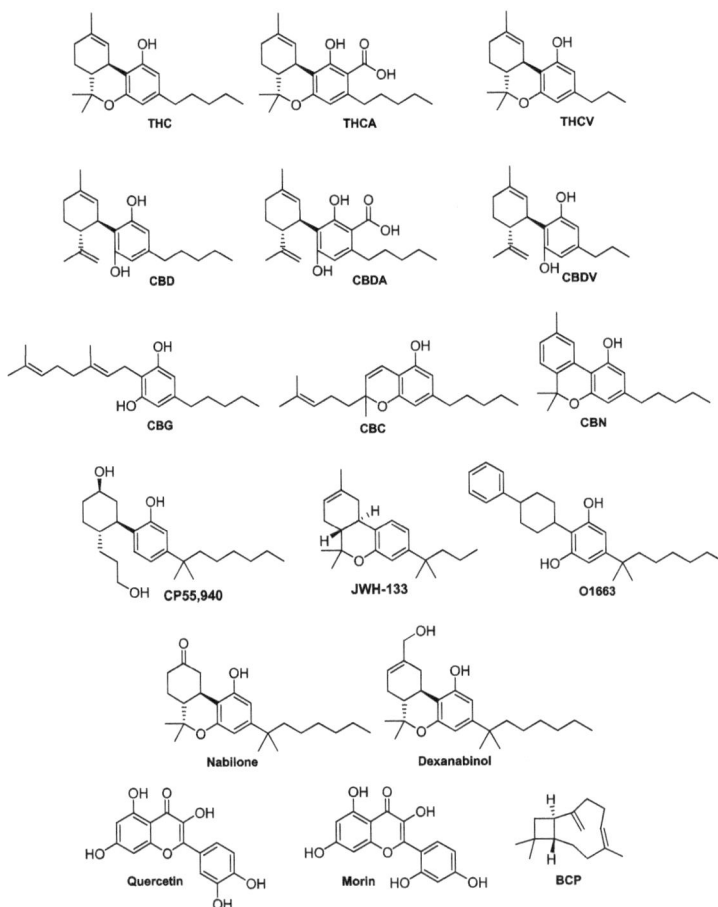

Fig. (3). Chemical structure of phytocannabinoids and synthetic derivatives involved in cancer processes.

The acidic precursors of THC and CBD, THCA and CBDA, have also shown to elicit antiproliferative effects in diverse cancer models. THCA reduces tumor growth in human prostate carcinoma androgen receptor-negative and positive cell lines being slightly less potent than THC [155]. THCA exhibited anticancer effects in other tumor types including glioma, basophilic leukemia, breast, colon, or gastric cancer with comparable *in vitro* activity to its parent compound [96]. CBDA was found to inhibit cell viability and induce apoptosis in breast cancer cells [156].

Even if only a handful of studies claim the potential of minor phytocannabinoids in cancer treatment, promising results have been reported for CBG, CBC and CBN. Emerging data from CBG indicates its antitumorigenic potential in murine models of melanoma and colorectal cancer [157 - 159]. The non-intoxicating phytocannabinoid CBC demonstrated to potently inhibit cell viability in prostate carcinoma [155] and breast cancer cells [96]. In colorectal cancer cells, CBC was only able to reduce proliferation at high doses [158]. CBN, the degraded product of THCA whose psychoactive effects are lower than those of THC, has also been assessed as a cytotoxic agent. Its ability to reduce viability was demonstrated in prostate [155] and aggressive breast cancer cells [160]. Moreover, propyl side chain derivatives of THC and CBD, tetrahydrocannabivarin (THCV, Fig. **3**) and cannabidivarin (CBDV, Fig. **3**), also exhibited potential cytotoxic effects on diverse prostate cancer *in vitro* models [155].

In addition to phytogenic cannabinoids, some synthetic phytocannabinoid-like molecules have shown to counteract tumor progression in a variety of cancer models. For instance, the potent CB_1R/CB_2R agonist CP55,940 (Fig. **3**), displayed apoptotic effects in gastric cancer cells [161]. As aforementioned, CP55,940 has shown to alleviate allodynia in a mouse model of paclitaxel-induced neuropathic pain [162]. Moreover, the potent CB_2R selective agonist JWH-133 was found to inhibit breast cancer growth and metastasis *via* CB_2R [63]. This compound also exerts antinociceptive effects in cisplatin-induced neuropathy [40]. Another synthetic derivative, the resorcinol derivative O-1663 (Fig. **1**), revealed ability to confer inhibition of advanced stages of breast cancer through ROS (reactive oxygen species) stimulation, autophagy upregulation and apoptosis induction [163].

Some flavonoids and terpenes found in diverse plants, including *Cannabis sativa*, can also elicit anticancer effects upon ECS modulation [151]. An example is the flavonoid quercetin (Fig. **1**), a polyphenol present in diverse vegetables and fruits, which reduces cell proliferation in colorectal adenocarcinoma cells *via* CB_1R [66]. Likewise, the structurally related flavonoid morin (Fig. **1**) was shown to induce apoptosis in colorectal carcinoma cells [164]. Although at low levels, over 200 terpenes have been detected in cannabis cultivars [165]. β-caryophyllene (BCP, Fig. **1**) is a relevant anticancer representative of this family [166]. BCP was demonstrated to induce apoptosis and cell cycle arrest in different cancer models including lung and ovarian cancer or glioma [151, 166]. In the latter type, BCP antiproliferative action was proved to be mediated through CB_2R modulation [167]. Furthermore, BCP was found to increase sensitivity to chemotherapeutic agents such as doxorubicin, 5-fluoruracil, oxaliplatin or sorafenib when administered in combination in human cancer cells [168 - 170].

Besides their individual activity, flavonoids and terpenes present in *Cannabis sativa* have been claimed to synergistically improve phytocannabinoids anticancer actions through the so-called "entourage effect" [163]. For instance, a recent study in preclinical breast cancer models compared the effect of pure THC *versus* a botanical extract observing more potent antitumor actions when administering the latter [171]. However, the therapeutic validity of the "entourage effect" has been questioned and needs to be further studied to shed light into its potential [172].

Synthetic Cannabinoids

Synthetic cannabinergic molecules from diverse structural families have been studied in a variety of cancer types. Their antitumor action and/or ability to reduce chemotherapy side effects was demonstrated. Aminoalkyindoles, arylpyrazoles and cannabinoid quinone are among the synthetic chemotypes that have shown most promising results in this pathology.

Aminoalkylindoles

The aminoalkylindole scaffold has been successfully exploited in the cannabinoid field since the early 1990s. The CB_1R/CB_2R potent agonist WIN55,212-2 (Fig. **4**) has been extensively used in research being one of the most relevant synthetic cannabinoids. A number of *in vitro* and *in vivo* studies provide evidence of its anticancer potential. WIN55,212-2 inhibits tumor growth in prostate cancer [173], in hepatocellular carcinoma [174], in triple-negative breast cancer [63], in myeloma [175], in gastric cancer [176], in lung cancer, testicular cancer and neuroblastoma [177], and in renal carcinoma [178]. CB_2R activation seems to primarily mediate WIN55,212-2 antiproliferative effects in renal carcinoma [178], hepatocellular carcinoma [174], or myeloma [175]. Both CBRs are responsible of its antitumor actions in triple-negative breast cancer [63], whereas cyclooxigenase-2 has been implicated on its effects in gastric cancer metastasis [176].

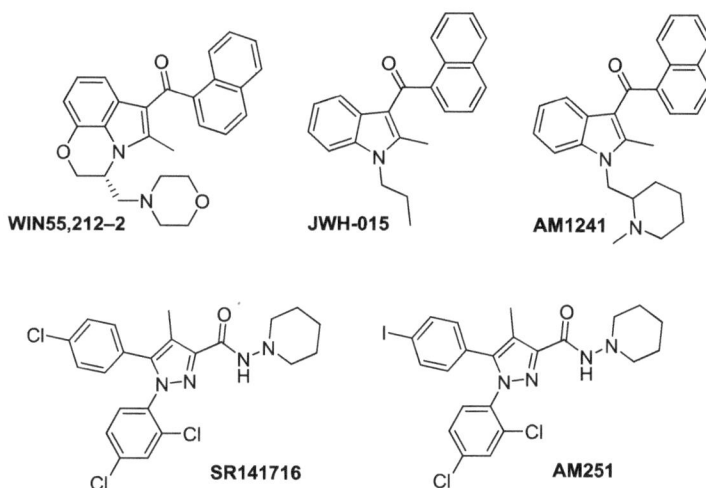

Fig. (4). Chemical structure of aminoalkylindoles and arylpyrazoles involved in cancer processes.

Another synthetic aminoalkylindole with proved antitumorigenic activity is the CB_2R agonist JWH015 (Fig. **4**). This naphtoylindole was found to confer antiproliferative effects in experimental models of breast [179, 180], prostate [181] or lung cancer among others [182]. In most cases, cancer cells viability reduction has seen shown to be mediated through CB_2R. However, in metastatic breast cancer, crosstalk between CB_2R and the chemokine receptor type 4 (CXCR4) seems to be involved in JWH015 cytotoxic properties [179], while no relation with the CBRs has been observed in other mammary carcinomas [180].

Interestingly, a recent study using AM1241 (Fig. **4**), a CB_2R selective aminoalkylindole, highlights the ability of this compound to inhibit morphine tolerance in a rat cancer pain model [183]. This effect was achieved using low doses of AM1241.

Arylpyrazoles

Arylpyrazoles emerged in the cannabinoid field in the late 1990s, providing a robust chemotype for the development of CBR inverse agonists/antagonists for both CB_1R and CB_2R. The CB_1R antagonist SR141716 (Fig. **4**), which reached the clinic for a very short period, as antiobesity drug, was found to exert antitumor actions in specific cell types.

Different studies have confirmed the ability of SR141716 to elicit antiproliferative effects in breast cancer [184], leukemia [185], or colon cancer cells [186 - 188]. While in breast malignacies, the antitumor actions seem to be mediated through CB_1R, preliminary data indicate that in colon cancer and leukimia, this effect is

CB_1R-independent. Synergistic effects with other antineoplastic drugs, such as oxaliplatin have been observed in colon cancer [189]. The closely related analog AM251 (Fig. **4**) was found to confer antitumorigenic activity in Hodgkin lymphoma [190] and rhabdomyosarcoma [191].

Cannabinoid Quinones

Quinoid derivatives of phytocannabinoids were first reported in the early 2000s. Quinones, are well-known for their cytotoxic potential due to inhibition of DNA topoisomerase II enzyme, DNA intercalation, or their ability to form reactive oxygen species [192]. Therefore, cannabinoid quinone derivatives can trigger anticancer effects through diverse mechanisms of action.

Oxidation of phytocannabinoids CBD, Δ^8-THC, and CBN led to the formation of their subsequent paraquinones: HU-331 (Fig. **5**), HU-306, and HU345 [193]. These three cannabinoid quinones were able to reduce tumor growth in glioblastoma, colon cancer, prostate cancer, Burkitt's lymphoma, T-cell lymphoma, lung cancer, and breast cancer cells [193]. *In vivo* studies focused on the antiproliferative profile of HU331 and its mechanism of action [194]. The antitumoral activity of this molecule was found to be mediated through inhibition of topoisomerase II, acting in a CBR independent manner [195].

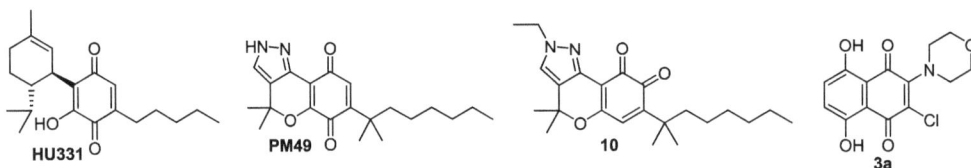

Fig. (5). Chemical structure of cannabinoid quinones involved in cancer processes.

Likewise, the synthetic chromenopyrazole scaffold was oxidized to obtain the corresponding cannabinoid quinone derivatives [196, 197]. *Para*-chromenopyrazolediones yielded remarkable antiproliferative activity *in vitro* and *in vivo* in prostate cancer models. The most promising compound of this series, PM49 (Fig. **5**), a CB_1R/CB_2R agonist, mediates its antitumor actions *via* oxidative stress, PPARγ and partially through CB_1R [196]. On the other hand, *ortho*-chromenopyrazolediones were found to efficiently reduce triple negative breast cancer cell proliferation. Mechanistic studies carried out using the most potent compound, **10** (Fig. **5**), revealed that this effect was mediated by CB_2R activation and ROS production [197].

Moreover, a recent study reported the cytotoxic effects of 1,4-naphthoquinone derivatives in triple-negative breast cancer [198]. The most potent compound in this series, **3a** (Fig. **5**) acts as inverse agonist of GPR55 and since this receptor is highly expressed in this type of cancer [87], its antitumor mechanism could be mediated through this putative cannabinoid receptor. However, further studies are needed to confirm this effect.

Other Antitumor Cannabinergic Ligands

Synthetic cannabinoids from other structural families have also been found to elicit promising therapeutic responses in this pathology. For instance, FAAH inhibitors from diverse chemotypes have confirmed the antitumor potential of endocannabinoid biodegradation [132]. An example is the well-known FAAH inhibitor URB597 (Fig. **6**), which reduces cell viability in lung cancer cells [81]. Another FAAH inhibitor, PF-3845 (Fig. **6**) has shown promising anticancer effects in colon cancer. This compound exhibited better results than the MAGL inhibitor JZL-184 (Fig. **6**) [82]. Nevertheless, other reports demonstrated the antiproliferative activity of JZL-184 in metastatic tumor cell lines [83].

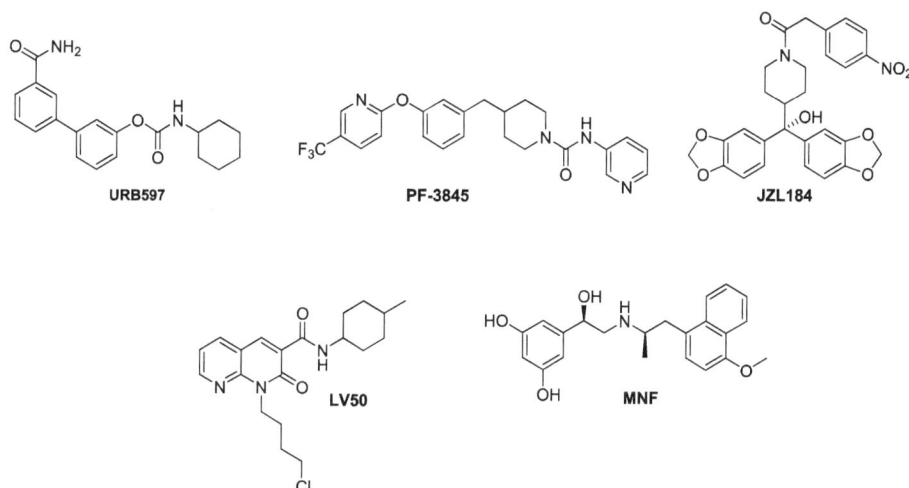

Fig. (6). Chemical structure of synthetic cannabinoids involved in cancer processes.

Naphthyridines and naphtalenes have also emerged as potential cannabinoids antitumor agents. For instance, 1,8-naphthyridin-2-ones, which are potent CB_2R agonists, were able to reduce cell viability in glioblastoma, breast carcinoma, prostate carcinoma and gastric adenocarcinoma cells [199]. The proapoptotic properties of the naphthyridine derivative LV50 (Fig. **6**) were confirmed on Jurkat leukemia cells. This effect was found to be mediated by CB_2R activation [200]. It is also worth mentioning that the naphthylfenoterol MNF (Fig. **6**) reduces tumor growth through a GPR55 mediated mechanism [201].

Besides the activity of a wide variety of cannabinoids in diverse types of cancer models, combinatorial strategies potentiating synergistic effects have also been explored, offering promising results [202].

CONCLUSION AND FUTURE PROSPECTS

The intrinsic complexity of the ECS joined to the multifactorial etiology of cancer intricate the interplay between cannabinoids and oncogenesis. Molecular targets involved in the antitumor effects of cannabinoids include GPCRs, ionic channels, nuclear receptors as well as metabolic enzymes. ECS abnormal regulation in cancer tissue provides a promising targeting strategy for the management of specific types of tumors. Even though a growing body of research has demonstrated the potential of cannabinoids in cancer in the last two decades, ongoing and future clinical trials need to confirm their applicability.

As extensively detailed in this chapter, phytocannabinoids and closely related synthetic analogs are at the forefront of cannabinoid clinical research. They have been successfully prescribed as palliative medicines for the control of chemotherapy side effects in some countries for several years. However, more importantly, their ability to reduce tumor growth is now being assessed in clinical trials. Unfortunately, these clinical trials are still set up to pursue the proof-o--concept issues. Despite extensive preclinical research, no cannabis extracts, cannabis-related, or synthetic cannabinoids are in Phase 3 as anticancer agents. The clinical trials are not large enough to support the cannabinoid anticancer strategies so far. Even though phytocannabinoids are considered medically safe as shown by the regularization of the medical cannabis in diverse countries, their use in cancer therapy is still limited to the palliative care in cancer patients. Drug repurposing for phytocannabinoids could be significantly faster and more economical than synthetic cannabinoids. However, the repurposing is still challenging, probably due to possible legal issues. In this context, synthetic cannabinoids hold many promises, some of them being devoid of psychotropic effects.

The complex physiopathology of cancer underlines the need to contemplate the use of combinatorial approaches. In this context, combination of cannabinoids with other cancer therapies may help overcome oncogenesis from diverse mechanisms of action. Numerous recent reports are focused on the study of the synergistic effects obtained upon co-administration of cannabinoids with standard chemotherapeutic drugs [202]. Specific cannabinoids have been shown to improve sensitivity to conventional cancer treatment in different malignancies. For instance, combinatorial treatment of CBD with bortezomib (currently used myeloma anticancer drug) in myeloma allowed effective cytotoxicity at lower doses [203]. In this sense, clinical trials are currently oriented to combinatorial strategies, such as the study realized on the safety profile of THC/CBD in combination with TMZ and radiotherapy in patients with newly-diagnosed glioblastoma (ClinicalTrials.gov Identifier: NCT03529448).

Most evidence on the use of cannabinoids as anticancer agents are based on preclinical studies. Although phytocannabinoids have a relatively favorable toxicity profile compared to aggressive anticancer drugs used in classical chemotherapies, large clinical trials are needed to support their properties in cancer patients. Synthetic cannabinoids targeting appropriate targets of the ECS can be potential candidates for further exploration, these targets being tumor-specific in most cases, related to the site of origin and to the patient characteristics.

CONSENT FOR PUBLICATION

Not applicable.

CONFLICT OF INTEREST

The author declares no conflict of interest, financial or otherwise.

ACKNOWLEDGEMENTS

This research was funded by the Spanish Ministry of Science and Innovation, grant number MICIU/FEDER: RTI2018-095544-B-I00 and the Spanish National Research Council (CSIC), grant number PIE-201580E033. PM acknowledges the Comunidad de Madrid 'Atracción de Talento' program, fellowship number 2018-T2/BMD-10819.

REFERENCES

[1]   Laezza C, Pagano C, Navarra G, *et al.* The endocannabinoid system: A target for cancer treatment. Int J Mol Sci 2020; 21(3): 747.
[http://dx.doi.org/10.3390/ijms21030747] [PMID: 31979368]

[2]   Moreno E, Cavic M, Krivokuca A, Canela EI. The interplay between cancer biology and the endocannabinoid system—significance for cancer risk, prognosis and response to treatment. Cancers (Basel) 2020; 12(11): 3275.
[http://dx.doi.org/10.3390/cancers12113275] [PMID: 33167409]

[3]   Guindon J, Hohmann AG. The endocannabinoid system and cancer: therapeutic implication. Br J Pharmacol 2011; 163(7): 1447-63.
[http://dx.doi.org/10.1111/j.1476-5381.2011.01327.x] [PMID: 21410463]

[4]   Ramer R, Schwarz R, Hinz B. Modulation of the endocannabinoid system as a potential anticancer strategy. Front Pharmacol 2019; 10: 430.
[http://dx.doi.org/10.3389/fphar.2019.00430] [PMID: 31143113]

[5]   Moreno E, Cavic M, Krivokuca A, Casadó V, Canela E. The endocannabinoid system as a target in

cancer diseases: Are we there yet? Front Pharmacol 2019; 10: 339.
[http://dx.doi.org/10.3389/fphar.2019.00339] [PMID: 31024307]

[6]   Fraguas-Sánchez AI, Martín-Sabroso C, Torres-Suárez AI. Insights into the effects of the
         endocannabinoid system in cancer: a review. Br J Pharmacol 2018; 175(13): 2566-80.
         [http://dx.doi.org/10.1111/bph.14331] [PMID: 29663308]

[7]   Schwarz R, Ramer R, Hinz B. Targeting the endocannabinoid system as a potential anticancer
         approach. Drug Metab Rev 2018; 50(1): 26-53.
         [http://dx.doi.org/10.1080/03602532.2018.1428344] [PMID: 29390896]

[8]   Śledziński P, Zeyland J, Słomski R, Nowak A. The current state and future perspectives of
         cannabinoids in cancer biology. Cancer Med 2018; 7(3): 765-75.
         [http://dx.doi.org/10.1002/cam4.1312] [PMID: 29473338]

[9]   Bogdanović V, Mrdjanović J, Borišev I. A review of the therapeutic antitumor potential of
         cannabinoids. J Altern Complement Med 2017; 23(11): 831-6.
         [http://dx.doi.org/10.1089/acm.2017.0016] [PMID: 28799775]

[10]   Velasco G, Hernández-Tiedra S, Dávila D, Lorente M. The use of cannabinoids as anticancer agents.
         Prog Neuropsychopharmacol Biol Psychiatry 2016; 64: 259-66.
         [http://dx.doi.org/10.1016/j.pnpbp.2015.05.010] [PMID: 26071989]

[11]   Pisanti S, Picardi P, D'Alessandro A, Laezza C, Bifulco M. The endocannabinoid signaling system in
         cancer. Trends Pharmacol Sci 2013; 34(5): 273-82.
         [http://dx.doi.org/10.1016/j.tips.2013.03.003] [PMID: 23602129]

[12]   Pertwee RG. Handbook of Cannabis. New York, NY: Oxford University Press 2014.
         [http://dx.doi.org/10.1093/acprof:oso/9780199662685.001.0001]

[13]   Matsuda LA, Lolait SJ, Brownstein MJ, Young AC, Bonner TI. Structure of a cannabinoid receptor
         and functional expression of the cloned cDNA. Nature 1990; 346(6284): 561-4.
         [http://dx.doi.org/10.1038/346561a0] [PMID: 2165569]

[14]   Munro S, Thomas KL, Abu-Shaar M. Molecular characterization of a peripheral receptor for
         cannabinoids. Nature 1993; 365(6441): 61-5.
         [http://dx.doi.org/10.1038/365061a0] [PMID: 7689702]

[15]   Devane WA, Hanus L, Breuer A, *et al.* Isolation and structure of a brain constituent that binds to the
         cannabinoid receptor. Science 1992; 258(5090): 1946-9.
         [http://dx.doi.org/10.1126/science.1470919] [PMID: 1470919]

[16]   Mechoulam R, Ben-Shabat S, Hanus L, *et al.* Identification of an endogenous 2-monoglyceride,
         present in canine gut, that binds to cannabinoid receptors. Biochem Pharmacol 1995; 50(1): 83-90.
         [http://dx.doi.org/10.1016/0006-2952(95)00109-D] [PMID: 7605349]

[17]   Di Marzo V. New approaches and challenges to targeting the endocannabinoid system. Nat Rev Drug
         Discov 2018; 17(9): 623-39.
         [http://dx.doi.org/10.1038/nrd.2018.115] [PMID: 30116049]

[18]   Laprairie RB, Bagher AM, Kelly MEM, Denovan-Wright EM. Cannabidiol is a negative allosteric
         modulator of the cannabinoid CB1 receptor. Br J Pharmacol 2015; 172(20): 4790-805.
         [http://dx.doi.org/10.1111/bph.13250] [PMID: 26218440]

[19]   Martínez-Pinilla E, Varani K, Reyes-Resina I, *et al.* Binding and signaling studies disclose a potential
         allosteric site for cannabidiol in cannabinoid CB$_2$ receptors. Front Pharmacol 2017; 8: 744.
         [http://dx.doi.org/10.3389/fphar.2017.00744] [PMID: 29109685]

[20]   Tham M, Yilmaz O, Alaverdashvili M, Kelly MEM, Denovan-Wright EM, Laprairie RB. Allosteric
         and orthosteric pharmacology of cannabidiol and cannabidiol-dimethylheptyl at the type 1 and type 2
         cannabinoid receptors. Br J Pharmacol 2019; 176(10): 1455-69.
         [http://dx.doi.org/10.1111/bph.14440] [PMID: 29981240]

[21]   Navarro G, Reyes-Resina I, Rivas-Santisteban R, *et al.* Cannabidiol skews biased agonism at cannabinoid CB_1 and CB_2 receptors with smaller effect in CB_1-CB_2 heteroreceptor complexes. Biochem Pharmacol 2018; 157: 148-58.
[http://dx.doi.org/10.1016/j.bcp.2018.08.046] [PMID: 30194918]

[22]   Morales P, Jagerovic N. Novel approaches and current challenges with targeting the endocannabinoid system. Expert Opin Drug Discov 2020; 15(8): 917-30.
[http://dx.doi.org/10.1080/17460441.2020.1752178] [PMID: 32336154]

[23]   Morales P, Jagerovic N. Antitumor cannabinoid chemotypes: structural insights. Front Pharmacol 2019; 10: 621.
[http://dx.doi.org/10.3389/fphar.2019.00621] [PMID: 31214034]

[24]   Abrams DI, Guzman M. Cannabis in cancer care. Clin Pharmacol Ther 2015; 97(6): 575-86.
[http://dx.doi.org/10.1002/cpt.108] [PMID: 25777363]

[25]   Zalman D, Bar-Sela G. Cannabis and Synthetic Cannabinoids for Cancer Patients : Multiple Palliative.Handbook of Cannabis and Related Pathologies. Elsevier Inc. 2017; pp. 857-68.
[http://dx.doi.org/10.1016/B978-0-12-800756-3.00104-6]

[26]   Chow R, Valdez C, Chow N, *et al.* Oral cannabinoid for the prophylaxis of chemotherapy-induced nausea and vomiting-a systematic review and meta-analysis. Support Care Cancer 2020; 28(5): 2095-103.
[http://dx.doi.org/10.1007/s00520-019-05280-4] [PMID: 31916006]

[27]   Chung M, Kim HK, Abdi S. Update on cannabis and cannabinoids for cancer pain. Curr Opin Anaesthesiol 2020; 33(6): 825-31.
[http://dx.doi.org/10.1097/ACO.0000000000000934] [PMID: 33110020]

[28]   Kleckner AS, Kleckner IR, Kamen CS, *et al.* Opportunities for cannabis in supportive care in cancer. Ther Adv Med Oncol 2019; 11: 1758835919866362.
[http://dx.doi.org/10.1177/1758835919866362] [PMID: 31413731]

[29]   Shin S, Mitchell C, Mannion K, Smolyn J, Meghani SH. An integrated review of cannabis and cannabinoids in adult oncologic pain management. Pain Manag Nurs 2019; 20(3): 185-91.
[http://dx.doi.org/10.1016/j.pmn.2018.09.006] [PMID: 30527857]

[30]   Plasse TF, Gorter RW, Krasnow SH, Lane M, Shepard KV, Wadleigh RG. Recent clinical experience with dronabinol. Pharmacol Biochem Behav 1991; 40(3): 695-700.
[http://dx.doi.org/10.1016/0091-3057(91)90385-F] [PMID: 1666930]

[31]   Einhorn LH, Nagy C, Furnas B, Williams SD. Nabilone: an effective antiemetic in patients receiving cancer chemotherapy. J Clin Pharmacol 1981; 21(S1): 64S-9S.
[http://dx.doi.org/10.1002/j.1552-4604.1981.tb02576.x] [PMID: 6271844]

[32]   Tramèr MR, Carroll D, Campbell FA, Reynolds DJ, Moore RA, McQuay HJ. Cannabinoids for control of chemotherapy induced nausea and vomiting: quantitative systematic review. BMJ 2001; 323(7303): 16-21.
[http://dx.doi.org/10.1136/bmj.323.7303.16] [PMID: 11440936]

[33]   Garcia JM, Shamliyan TA. Cannabinoids in patients with nausea and vomiting associated with malignancy and its treatments. Am J Med 2018; 131(7): 755-9.e2.
[http://dx.doi.org/10.1016/j.amjmed.2017.12.041]

[34]   Sharkey KA, Darmani NA, Parker LA. Regulation of nausea and vomiting by cannabinoids and the endocannabinoid system. Eur J Pharmacol 2014; 722: 134-46.
[http://dx.doi.org/10.1016/j.ejphar.2013.09.068] [PMID: 24184696]

[35]   Mersiades AJ, Tognela A, Haber PS, *et al.* Oral cannabinoid-rich THC/CBD cannabis extract for secondary prevention of chemotherapy-induced nausea and vomiting: a study protocol for a pilot and definitive randomised double-blind placebo-controlled trial (CannabisCINV). BMJ Open 2018; 8(9): e020745.

[http://dx.doi.org/10.1136/bmjopen-2017-020745] [PMID: 30209152]

[36]　Grimison P, Mersiades A, Kirby A, *et al.* Oral THC:CBD cannabis extract for refractory chemotherapy-induced nausea and vomiting: a randomised, placebo-controlled, phase II crossover trial. Ann Oncol 2020; 31(11): 1553-60.
[http://dx.doi.org/10.1016/j.annonc.2020.07.020] [PMID: 32801017]

[37]　Darmani NA, Belkacemi L, Zhong W. Δ^9-THC and related cannabinoids suppress substance P-induced neurokinin NK_1-receptor-mediated vomiting *via* activation of cannabinoid CB_1 receptor. Eur J Pharmacol 2019; 865: 172806.
[http://dx.doi.org/10.1016/j.ejphar.2019.172806] [PMID: 31738934]

[38]　Wang J, Wang Y, Tong M, Pan H, Li D. New prospect for cancer cachexia: Medical cannabinoid. J Cancer 2019; 10(3): 716-20.
[http://dx.doi.org/10.7150/jca.28246] [PMID: 30719170]

[39]　Brown MRD, Farquhar-Smith WP. Cannabinoids and cancer pain: A new hope or a false dawn? Eur J Intern Med 2018; 49: 30-6.
[http://dx.doi.org/10.1016/j.ejim.2018.01.020] [PMID: 29482740]

[40]　Vera G, Cabezos PA, Martín MI, Abalo R. Characterization of cannabinoid-induced relief of neuropathic pain in a rat model of cisplatin-induced neuropathy. Pharmacol Biochem Behav 2013; 105: 205-12.
[http://dx.doi.org/10.1016/j.pbb.2013.02.008] [PMID: 23454533]

[41]　Harris HM, Sufka KJ, Gul W, ElSohly MA. Effects of delta-9-tetrahydrocannabinol and cannabidiol on cisplatin-induced neuropathy in mice. Planta Med 2016; 82(13): 1169-72.
[http://dx.doi.org/10.1055/s-0042-106303] [PMID: 27214593]

[42]　Pascual D, Goicoechea C, Suardíaz M, Martín MI. A cannabinoid agonist, WIN 55,212-2, reduces neuropathic nociception induced by paclitaxel in rats. Pain 2005; 118(1-2): 23-34.
[http://dx.doi.org/10.1016/j.pain.2005.07.008] [PMID: 16213089]

[43]　Rahn EJ, Makriyannis A, Hohmann AG. Activation of cannabinoid CB1 and CB2 receptors suppresses neuropathic nociception evoked by the chemotherapeutic agent vincristine in rats. Br J Pharmacol 2007; 152(5): 765-77.
[http://dx.doi.org/10.1038/sj.bjp.0707333] [PMID: 17572696]

[44]　Mulpuri Y, Marty VN, Munier JJ, *et al.* Synthetic peripherally-restricted cannabinoid suppresses chemotherapy-induced peripheral neuropathy pain symptoms by CB1 receptor activation. Neuropharmacology 2018; 139: 85-97.
[http://dx.doi.org/10.1016/j.neuropharm.2018.07.002] [PMID: 29981335]

[45]　Marino S, Idris AI. Emerging therapeutic targets in cancer induced bone disease: A focus on the peripheral type 2 cannabinoid receptor. Pharmacol Res 2017; 119: 391-403.
[http://dx.doi.org/10.1016/j.phrs.2017.02.023] [PMID: 28274851]

[46]　Khasabova IA, Chandiramani A, Harding-Rose C, Simone DA, Seybold VS. Increasing 2-arachidonoyl glycerol signaling in the periphery attenuates mechanical hyperalgesia in a model of bone cancer pain. Pharmacol Res 2011; 64(1): 60-7.
[http://dx.doi.org/10.1016/j.phrs.2011.03.007] [PMID: 21440630]

[47]　Tateo S. State of the evidence: Cannabinoids and cancer pain-A systematic review. J Am Assoc Nurse Pract 2017; 29(2): 94-103.
[http://dx.doi.org/10.1002/2327-6924.12422] [PMID: 27863159]

[48]　Portenoy RK, Ganae-Motan ED, Allende S, *et al.* Nabiximols for opioid-treated cancer patients with poorly-controlled chronic pain: a randomized, placebo-controlled, graded-dose trial. J Pain 2012; 13(5): 438-49.
[http://dx.doi.org/10.1016/j.jpain.2012.01.003] [PMID: 22483680]

[49]　Hao E, Mukhopadhyay P, Cao Z, *et al.* Cannabidiol protects against doxorubicin-induced

cardiomyopathy by modulating mitochondrial function and biogenesis. Mol Med 2015; 21: 38-45.
[http://dx.doi.org/10.2119/molmed.2014.00261] [PMID: 25569804]

[50]   Pan H, Mukhopadhyay P, Rajesh M, *et al.* Cannabidiol attenuates cisplatin-induced nephrotoxicity by decreasing oxidative/nitrosative stress, inflammation, and cell death. J Pharmacol Exp Ther 2009; 328(3): 708-14.
[http://dx.doi.org/10.1124/jpet.108.147181] [PMID: 19074681]

[51]   Chakravarti B, Ravi J, Ganju RK. Cannabinoids as therapeutic agents in cancer: current status and future implications. Oncotarget 2014; 5(15): 5852-72.
[http://dx.doi.org/10.18632/oncotarget.2233] [PMID: 25115386]

[52]   Guzmán M. Cannabinoids: potential anticancer agents. Nat Rev Cancer 2003; 3(10): 745-55.
[http://dx.doi.org/10.1038/nrc1188] [PMID: 14570037]

[53]   Munson AE, Harris LS, Friedman MA, Dewey WL, Carchman RA. Antineoplastic activity of cannabinoids. J Natl Cancer Inst 1975; 55(3): 597-602.
[http://dx.doi.org/10.1093/jnci/55.3.597] [PMID: 1159836]

[54]   Velasco G, Sánchez C, Guzmán M. Towards the use of cannabinoids as antitumour agents. Nat Rev Cancer 2012; 12(6): 436-44.
[http://dx.doi.org/10.1038/nrc3247] [PMID: 22555283]

[55]   Carracedo A, Gironella M, Lorente M, *et al.* Cannabinoids induce apoptosis of pancreatic tumor cells *via* endoplasmic reticulum stress-related genes. Cancer Res 2006; 66(13): 6748-55.
[http://dx.doi.org/10.1158/0008-5472.CAN-06-0169] [PMID: 16818650]

[56]   Sarfaraz S, Adhami VM, Syed DN, Afaq F, Mukhtar H. Cannabinoids for cancer treatment: progress and promise. Cancer Res 2008; 68(2): 339-42.
[http://dx.doi.org/10.1158/0008-5472.CAN-07-2785] [PMID: 18199524]

[57]   Sarfaraz S, Afaq F, Adhami VM, Malik A, Mukhtar H. Cannabinoid receptor agonist-induced apoptosis of human prostate cancer cells LNCaP proceeds through sustained activation of ERK1/2 leading to G1 cell cycle arrest. J Biol Chem 2006; 281(51): 39480-91.
[http://dx.doi.org/10.1074/jbc.M603495200] [PMID: 17068343]

[58]   Guzmán M, Sánchez C, Galve-Roperh I. Cannabinoids and cell fate. Pharmacol Ther 2002; 95(2): 175-84.
[http://dx.doi.org/10.1016/S0163-7258(02)00256-5] [PMID: 12182964]

[59]   Galve-Roperh I, Sánchez C, Cortés ML, Gómez del Pulgar T, Izquierdo M, Guzmán M. Anti-tumoral action of cannabinoids: involvement of sustained ceramide accumulation and extracellular signal-regulated kinase activation. Nat Med 2000; 6(3): 313-9.
[http://dx.doi.org/10.1038/73171] [PMID: 10700234]

[60]   Caffarel MM, Sarrió D, Palacios J, Guzmán M, Sánchez C. Delta9-tetrahydrocannabinol inhibits cell cycle progression in human breast cancer cells through Cdc2 regulation. Cancer Res 2006; 66(13): 6615-21.
[http://dx.doi.org/10.1158/0008-5472.CAN-05-4566] [PMID: 16818634]

[61]   Malfitano AM, Ciaglia E, Gangemi G, Gazzerro P, Laezza C, Bifulco M. Update on the endocannabinoid system as an anticancer target. Expert Opin Ther Targets 2011; 15(3): 297-308.
[http://dx.doi.org/10.1517/14728222.2011.553606] [PMID: 21244344]

[62]   Schley M, Ständer S, Kerner J, *et al.* Predominant CB2 receptor expression in endothelial cells of glioblastoma in humans. Brain Res Bull 2009; 79(5): 333-7.
[http://dx.doi.org/10.1016/j.brainresbull.2009.01.011] [PMID: 19480992]

[63]   Qamri Z, Preet A, Nasser MW, *et al.* Synthetic cannabinoid receptor agonists inhibit tumor growth and metastasis of breast cancer. Mol Cancer Ther 2009; 8(11): 3117-29.
[http://dx.doi.org/10.1158/1535-7163.MCT-09-0448] [PMID: 19887554]

[64]   Xiang W, Shi R, Kang X, *et al.* Monoacylglycerol lipase regulates cannabinoid receptor 2-dependent

macrophage activation and cancer progression. Nat Commun 2018; 9(1): 2574.
[http://dx.doi.org/10.1038/s41467-018-04999-8] [PMID: 29968710]

[65] Bettiga A, Aureli M, Colciago G, *et al.* Bladder cancer cell growth and motility implicate cannabinoid 2 receptor-mediated modifications of sphingolipids metabolism. Sci Rep 2017; 7: 42157.
[http://dx.doi.org/10.1038/srep42157] [PMID: 28191815]

[66] Refolo MG, D'Alessandro R, Malerba N, *et al.* Anti proliferative and pro apoptotic effects of flavonoid quercetin are mediated by CB1 receptor in human colon cancer cell lines. J Cell Physiol 2015; 230(12): 2973-80.
[http://dx.doi.org/10.1002/jcp.25026] [PMID: 25893829]

[67] Caffarel MM, Andradas C, Mira E, *et al.* Cannabinoids reduce ErbB2-driven breast cancer progression through Akt inhibition. Mol Cancer 2010; 9: 196-206.
[http://dx.doi.org/10.1186/1476-4598-9-196] [PMID: 20649976]

[68] Elbaz M, Ahirwar D, Ravi J, Nasser MW, Ramesh K. Novel role of cannabinoid receptor 2 in inhibiting EGF / EGFR and IGF-I / IGF-IR pathways in breast cancer 2017; 8(18): 29668-78.

[69] Miyato H, Kitayama J, Yamashita H, *et al.* Pharmacological synergism between cannabinoids and paclitaxel in gastric cancer cell lines. J Surg Res 2009; 155(1): 40-7.
[http://dx.doi.org/10.1016/j.jss.2008.06.045] [PMID: 19394652]

[70] Oesch S, Walter D, Wachtel M, *et al.* Cannabinoid receptor 1 is a potential drug target for treatment of translocation-positive rhabdomyosarcoma. Mol Cancer Ther 2009; 8(7): 1838-45.
[http://dx.doi.org/10.1158/1535-7163.MCT-08-1147] [PMID: 19509271]

[71] Carpi S, Fogli S, Polini B, *et al.* Tumor-promoting effects of cannabinoid receptor type 1 in human melanoma cells. Toxicol In vitro 2017; 40: 272-9.
[http://dx.doi.org/10.1016/j.tiv.2017.01.018] [PMID: 28131817]

[72] Vara D, Salazar M, Olea-Herrero N, Guzmán M, Velasco G, Díaz-Laviada I. Anti-tumoral action of cannabinoids on hepatocellular carcinoma: role of AMPK-dependent activation of autophagy. Cell Death Differ 2011; 18(7): 1099-111.
[http://dx.doi.org/10.1038/cdd.2011.32] [PMID: 21475304]

[73] Giuliano M, Pellerito O, Portanova P, *et al.* Apoptosis induced in HepG2 cells by the synthetic cannabinoid WIN: involvement of the transcription factor PPARgamma. Biochimie 2009; 91(4): 457-65.
[http://dx.doi.org/10.1016/j.biochi.2008.11.003] [PMID: 19059457]

[74] Gustafsson K, Wang X, Severa D, *et al.* Expression of cannabinoid receptors type 1 and type 2 in non-Hodgkin lymphoma: growth inhibition by receptor activation. Int J Cancer 2008; 123(5): 1025-33.
[http://dx.doi.org/10.1002/ijc.23584] [PMID: 18546271]

[75] Joseph J, Niggemann B, Zaenker KS, Entschladen F. Anandamide is an endogenous inhibitor for the migration of tumor cells and T lymphocytes. Cancer Immunol Immunother 2004; 53(8): 723-8.
[http://dx.doi.org/10.1007/s00262-004-0509-9] [PMID: 15034673]

[76] Cudaback E, Marrs W, Moeller T, Stella N. The expression level of CB1 and CB2 receptors determines their efficacy at inducing apoptosis in astrocytomas. PLoS One 2010; 5(1): e8702.
[http://dx.doi.org/10.1371/journal.pone.0008702] [PMID: 20090845]

[77] Bifulco M, Laezza C, Pisanti S, Gazzerro P. Cannabinoids and cancer: pros and cons of an antitumour strategy. Br J Pharmacol 2006; 148(2): 123-35.
[http://dx.doi.org/10.1038/sj.bjp.0706632] [PMID: 16501583]

[78] Ligresti A, Bisogno T, Matias I, *et al.* Possible endocannabinoid control of colorectal cancer growth. Gastroenterology 2003; 125(3): 677-87.
[http://dx.doi.org/10.1016/S0016-5085(03)00881-3] [PMID: 12949714]

[79] Thors L, Bergh A, Persson E, *et al.* Fatty acid amide hydrolase in prostate cancer: association with disease severity and outcome, CB1 receptor expression and regulation by IL-4. PLoS One 2010; 5(8):

e12275.
[http://dx.doi.org/10.1371/journal.pone.0012275] [PMID: 20808855]

[80]   Nomura DK, Long JZ, Niessen S, Hoover HS, Ng S-W, Cravatt BF. Monoacylglycerol lipase regulates a fatty acid network that promotes cancer pathogenesis. Cell 2010; 140(1): 49-61.
[http://dx.doi.org/10.1016/j.cell.2009.11.027] [PMID: 20079333]

[81]   Winkler K, Ramer R, Dithmer S, Ivanov I, Merkord J, Hinz B. Fatty acid amide hydrolase inhibitors confer anti-invasive and antimetastatic effects on lung cancer cells. Oncotarget 2016; 7(12): 15047-64.
[http://dx.doi.org/10.18632/oncotarget.7592] [PMID: 26930716]

[82]   Wasilewski A, Krajewska U, Owczarek K, Lewandowska U, Fichna J. Fatty acid amide hydrolase (FAAH) inhibitor PF-3845 reduces viability, migration and invasiveness of human colon adenocarcinoma Colo-205 cell line: an *in vitro* study. Acta Biochim Pol 2017; 64(3): 519-25.
[http://dx.doi.org/10.18388/abp.2017_1520] [PMID: 28850633]

[83]   Ma M, Bai J, Ling Y, *et al.* Monoacylglycerol lipase inhibitor JZL184 regulates apoptosis and migration of colorectal cancer cells. Mol Med Rep 2016; 13(3): 2850-6.
[http://dx.doi.org/10.3892/mmr.2016.4829] [PMID: 26847687]

[84]   Hart S, Fischer OM, Ullrich A. Cannabinoids induce cancer cell proliferation *via* tumor necrosis factor alpha-converting enzyme (TACE/ADAM17)-mediated transactivation of the epidermal growth factor receptor. Cancer Res 2004; 64(6): 1943-50.
[http://dx.doi.org/10.1158/0008-5472.CAN-03-3720] [PMID: 15026328]

[85]   Oka S, Kimura S, Toshida T, Ota R, Yamashita A, Sugiura T. Lysophosphatidylinositol induces rapid phosphorylation of p38 mitogen-activated protein kinase and activating transcription factor 2 in HEK293 cells expressing GPR55 and IM-9 lymphoblastoid cells. J Biochem 2010; 147(5): 671-8.
[http://dx.doi.org/10.1093/jb/mvp208] [PMID: 20051382]

[86]   Pérez-Gómez E, Andradas C, Flores JM, *et al.* The orphan receptor GPR55 drives skin carcinogenesis and is upregulated in human squamous cell carcinomas. Oncogene 2013; 32(20): 2534-42.
[http://dx.doi.org/10.1038/onc.2012.278] [PMID: 22751111]

[87]   Andradas C, Caffarel MM, Pérez-Gómez E, *et al.* The orphan G protein-coupled receptor GPR55 promotes cancer cell proliferation *via* ERK. Oncogene 2011; 30(2): 245-52.
[http://dx.doi.org/10.1038/onc.2010.402] [PMID: 20818416]

[88]   Leyva-Illades D, Demorrow S. Orphan G protein receptor GPR55 as an emerging target in cancer therapy and management. Cancer Manag Res 2013; 5: 147-55.
[PMID: 23869178]

[89]   Hasenoehrl C, Feuersinger D, Sturm EM, *et al.* G protein-coupled receptor GPR55 promotes colorectal cancer and has opposing effects to cannabinoid receptor 1. Int J Cancer 2018; 142(1): 121-32.
[http://dx.doi.org/10.1002/ijc.31030] [PMID: 28875496]

[90]   Henstridge CM, Balenga NA, Kargl J, *et al.* Minireview: recent developments in the physiology and pathology of the lysophosphatidylinositol-sensitive receptor GPR55. Mol Endocrinol 2011; 25(11): 1835-48.
[http://dx.doi.org/10.1210/me.2011-1197] [PMID: 21964594]

[91]   Balenga NA, Martínez-Pinilla E, Kargl J, *et al.* Heteromerization of GPR55 and cannabinoid CB2 receptors modulates signalling. Br J Pharmacol 2014; 171(23): 5387-406.
[http://dx.doi.org/10.1111/bph.12850] [PMID: 25048571]

[92]   Moreno E, Andradas C, Medrano M, *et al.* Targeting CB2-GPR55 receptor heteromers modulates cancer cell signaling. J Biol Chem 2014; 289(32): 21960-72.
[http://dx.doi.org/10.1074/jbc.M114.561761] [PMID: 24942731]

[93]   Di Marzo V, De Petrocellis L, Fezza F, Ligresti A, Bisogno T. Anandamide receptors. Prostaglandins Leukot Essent Fatty Acids 2002; 66(2-3): 377-91.

[http://dx.doi.org/10.1054/plef.2001.0349] [PMID: 12052051]

[94]   Badolato M, Carullo G, Caroleo MC, Cione E, Aiello F, Manetti F. Discovery of 1,4-Naphthoquinones as a New Class of Antiproliferative Agents Targeting GPR55. ACS Med Chem Lett 2019; 10(4): 402-6.
[http://dx.doi.org/10.1021/acsmedchemlett.8b00333] [PMID: 30996770]

[95]   Fonseca BM, Correia-da-Silva G, Teixeira NA. Cannabinoid-induced cell death in endometrial cancer cells: involvement of TRPV1 receptors in apoptosis. J Physiol Biochem 2018; 74(2): 261-72.
[http://dx.doi.org/10.1007/s13105-018-0611-7] [PMID: 29441458]

[96]   Ligresti A, Moriello AS, Starowicz K, *et al.* Antitumor activity of plant cannabinoids with emphasis on the effect of cannabidiol on human breast carcinoma. J Pharmacol Exp Ther 2006; 318(3): 1375-87.
[http://dx.doi.org/10.1124/jpet.106.105247] [PMID: 16728591]

[97]   Lago-Fernandez A, Zarzo-Arias S, Jagerovic N, Morales P. Relevance of Peroxisome Proliferator Activated Receptors in Multitarget Paradigm Associated with the Endocannabinoid System. Int J Mol Sci 2021; 22(3): 1001.
[http://dx.doi.org/10.3390/ijms22031001] [PMID: 33498245]

[98]   Velasco G, Sánchez C, Guzmán M. Anticancer mechanisms of cannabinoids. Curr Oncol 2016; 23(2): S23-32.
[http://dx.doi.org/10.3747/co.23.3080] [PMID: 27022311]

[99]   Salazar M, Carracedo A, Salanueva IJ, *et al.* Cannabinoid action induces autophagy-mediated cell death through stimulation of ER stress in human glioma cells. J Clin Invest 2009; 119(5): 1359-72.
[http://dx.doi.org/10.1172/JCI37948] [PMID: 19425170]

[100]   Armstrong JL, Hill DS, McKee CS, *et al.* Exploiting cannabinoid-induced cytotoxic autophagy to drive melanoma cell death. J Invest Dermatol 2015; 135(6): 1629-37.
[http://dx.doi.org/10.1038/jid.2015.45] [PMID: 25674907]

[101]   Du K, Herzig S, Kulkarni RN, Montminy M. TRB3: a tribbles homolog that inhibits Akt/PKB activation by insulin in liver. Science 2003; 300(5625): 1574-7.
[http://dx.doi.org/10.1126/science.1079817] [PMID: 12791994]

[102]   Blázquez C, Carracedo A, Barrado L, *et al.* Cannabinoid receptors as novel targets for the treatment of melanoma. FASEB J 2006; 20(14): 2633-5.
[http://dx.doi.org/10.1096/fj.06-6638fje] [PMID: 17065222]

[103]   Caffarel MM, Moreno-Bueno G, Cerutti C, *et al.* JunD is involved in the antiproliferative effect of Delta9-tetrahydrocannabinol on human breast cancer cells. Oncogene 2008; 27(37): 5033-44.
[http://dx.doi.org/10.1038/onc.2008.145] [PMID: 18454173]

[104]   Sánchez C, Rueda D, Ségui B, Galve-Roperh I, Levade T, Guzmán M. The CB(1) cannabinoid receptor of astrocytes is coupled to sphingomyelin hydrolysis through the adaptor protein fan. Mol Pharmacol 2001; 59(5): 955-9.
[http://dx.doi.org/10.1124/mol.59.5.955] [PMID: 11306675]

[105]   Blázquez C, González-Feria L, Alvarez L, Haro A, Casanova ML, Guzmán M. Cannabinoids inhibit the vascular endothelial growth factor pathway in gliomas. Cancer Res 2004; 64(16): 5617-23.
[http://dx.doi.org/10.1158/0008-5472.CAN-03-3927] [PMID: 15313899]

[106]   Blázquez C, Casanova ML, Planas A, *et al.* Inhibition of tumor angiogenesis by cannabinoids. FASEB J 2003; 17(3): 529-31.
[http://dx.doi.org/10.1096/fj.02-0795fje] [PMID: 12514108]

[107]   Casanova ML, Blázquez C, Martínez-Palacio J, *et al.* Inhibition of skin tumor growth and angiogenesis *in vivo* by activation of cannabinoid receptors. J Clin Invest 2003; 111(1): 43-50.
[http://dx.doi.org/10.1172/JCI200316116] [PMID: 12511587]

[108]   Portella G, Laezza C, Laccetti P, De Petrocellis L, Di Marzo V, Bifulco M. Inhibitory effects of cannabinoid CB1 receptor stimulation on tumor growth and metastatic spreading: actions on signals

involved in angiogenesis and metastasis. FASEB J 2003; 17(12): 1771-3.
[http://dx.doi.org/10.1096/fj.02-1129fje] [PMID: 12958205]

[109]   Freimuth N, Ramer R, Hinz B. Antitumorigenic effects of cannabinoids beyond apoptosis. J Pharmacol Exp Ther 2010; 332(2): 336-44.
[http://dx.doi.org/10.1124/jpet.109.157735] [PMID: 19889794]

[110]   Preet A, Ganju RK, Groopman JE. Delta9-Tetrahydrocannabinol inhibits epithelial growth factor-induced lung cancer cell migration *in vitro* as well as its growth and metastasis *in vivo*. Oncogene 2008; 27(3): 339-46.
[http://dx.doi.org/10.1038/sj.onc.1210641] [PMID: 17621270]

[111]   Ramer R, Hinz B. Inhibition of cancer cell invasion by cannabinoids *via* increased expression of tissue inhibitor of matrix metalloproteinases-1. J Natl Cancer Inst 2008; 100(1): 59-69.
[http://dx.doi.org/10.1093/jnci/djm268] [PMID: 18159069]

[112]   Blázquez C, Salazar M, Carracedo A, *et al.* Cannabinoids inhibit glioma cell invasion by down-regulating matrix metalloproteinase-2 expression. Cancer Res 2008; 68(6): 1945-52.
[http://dx.doi.org/10.1158/0008-5472.CAN-07-5176] [PMID: 18339876]

[113]   Grimaldi C, Pisanti S, Laezza C, *et al.* Anandamide inhibits adhesion and migration of breast cancer cells. Exp Cell Res 2006; 312(4): 363-73.
[http://dx.doi.org/10.1016/j.yexcr.2005.10.024] [PMID: 16343481]

[114]   Ramer R, Merkord J, Rohde H, Hinz B. Cannabidiol inhibits cancer cell invasion *via* upregulation of tissue inhibitor of matrix metalloproteinases-1. Biochem Pharmacol 2010; 79(7): 955-66.
[http://dx.doi.org/10.1016/j.bcp.2009.11.007] [PMID: 19914218]

[115]   Ramer R, Fischer S, Haustein M, Manda K, Hinz B. Cannabinoids inhibit angiogenic capacities of endothelial cells *via* release of tissue inhibitor of matrix metalloproteinases-1 from lung cancer cells. Biochem Pharmacol 2014; 91(2): 202-16.
[http://dx.doi.org/10.1016/j.bcp.2014.06.017] [PMID: 24976505]

[116]   Haustein M, Ramer R, Linnebacher M, Manda K, Hinz B. Cannabinoids increase lung cancer cell lysis by lymphokine-activated killer cells *via* upregulation of ICAM-1. Biochem Pharmacol 2014; 92(2): 312-25.
[http://dx.doi.org/10.1016/j.bcp.2014.07.014] [PMID: 25069049]

[117]   Guzmán M, Duarte MJ, Blázquez C, *et al.* A pilot clinical study of Delta9-tetrahydrocannabinol in patients with recurrent glioblastoma multiforme. Br J Cancer 2006; 95(2): 197-203.
[http://dx.doi.org/10.1038/sj.bjc.6603236] [PMID: 16804518]

[118]   GW pharmaceuticals achieves positive results in phase 2 proof of concept study in glioma [Internet] [cited 2020 Oct 11]. Available from: http://ir.gwpharm.com/static-files/ cde942fe-555c-4b2f-9-c9-f34d24c7ad27.

[119]   Striem S, Bar-Joseph A, Berkovitch Y, Biegon A. Interaction of dexanabinol (HU-211), a novel NMDA receptor antagonist, with the dopaminergic system. Eur J Pharmacol 1997; 338(3): 205-13.
[http://dx.doi.org/10.1016/S0014-2999(97)81923-1] [PMID: 9424014]

[120]   Dexanabinol in Patients With Brain Cancer [Internet]. ClinicalTrials.gov. [cited 2019 Feb 27]. Available from: https://clinicaltrials.gov/ct2/ show/NCT01654497.

[121]   Petersen G, Moesgaard B, Schmid PC, *et al.* Endocannabinoid metabolism in human glioblastomas and meningiomas compared to human non-tumour brain tissue. J Neurochem 2005; 93(2): 299-309.
[http://dx.doi.org/10.1111/j.1471-4159.2005.03013.x] [PMID: 15816853]

[122]   Wu X, Han L, Zhang X, *et al.* Alteration of endocannabinoid system in human gliomas. J Neurochem 2012; 120(5): 842-9.
[http://dx.doi.org/10.1111/j.1471-4159.2011.07625.x] [PMID: 22176552]

[123]   Maccarrone M, Attinà M, Cartoni A, Bari M, Finazzi-Agrò A. Gas chromatography-mass spectrometry analysis of endogenous cannabinoids in healthy and tumoral human brain and human

cells in culture. J Neurochem 2001; 76(2): 594-601.
[http://dx.doi.org/10.1046/j.1471-4159.2001.00092.x] [PMID: 11208922]

[124] Zhang J, Medina-Cleghorn D, Bernal-Mizrachi L, *et al.* The potential relevance of the endocannabinoid, 2-arachidonoylglycerol, in diffuse large B-cell lymphoma. Oncoscience 2016; 3(1): 31-41.
[http://dx.doi.org/10.18632/oncoscience.289] [PMID: 26973858]

[125] Hinz B, Ramer R, Eichele K, Weinzierl U, Brune K. Up-regulation of cyclooxygenase-2 expression is involved in R(+)-methanandamide-induced apoptotic death of human neuroglioma cells. Mol Pharmacol 2004; 66(6): 1643-51.
[http://dx.doi.org/10.1124/mol.104.002618] [PMID: 15361550]

[126] Sailler S, Schmitz K, Jäger E, *et al.* Regulation of circulating endocannabinoids associated with cancer and metastases in mice and humans. Oncoscience 2014; 1(4): 272-82.
[http://dx.doi.org/10.18632/oncoscience.33] [PMID: 25594019]

[127] Di Marzo V, Melck D, Orlando P, *et al.* Palmitoylethanolamide inhibits the expression of fatty acid amide hydrolase and enhances the anti-proliferative effect of anandamide in human breast cancer cells. Biochem J 2001; 358(Pt 1): 249-55.
[http://dx.doi.org/10.1042/bj3580249] [PMID: 11485574]

[128] De Petrocellis L, Melck D, Palmisano A, *et al.* The endogenous cannabinoid anandamide inhibits human breast cancer cell proliferation. Proc Natl Acad Sci USA 1998; 95(14): 8375-80.
[http://dx.doi.org/10.1073/pnas.95.14.8375] [PMID: 9653194]

[129] Laezza C, Pisanti S, Crescenzi E, Bifulco M. Anandamide inhibits Cdk2 and activates Chk1 leading to cell cycle arrest in human breast cancer cells. FEBS Lett 2006; 580(26): 6076-82.
[http://dx.doi.org/10.1016/j.febslet.2006.09.074] [PMID: 17055492]

[130] Mimeault M, Pommery N, Wattez N, Bailly C, Hénichart JP. Anti-proliferative and apoptotic effects of anandamide in human prostatic cancer cell lines: implication of epidermal growth factor receptor down-regulation and ceramide production. Prostate 2003; 56(1): 1-12.
[http://dx.doi.org/10.1002/pros.10190] [PMID: 12746841]

[131] Adinolfi B, Romanini A, Vanni A, *et al.* Anticancer activity of anandamide in human cutaneous melanoma cells. Eur J Pharmacol 2013; 718(1-3): 154-9.
[http://dx.doi.org/10.1016/j.ejphar.2013.08.039] [PMID: 24041928]

[132] Matas D, Juknat A, Pietr M, Klin Y, Vogel Z. Anandamide protects from low serum-induced apoptosis *via* its degradation to ethanolamine. J Biol Chem 2007; 282(11): 7885-92.
[http://dx.doi.org/10.1074/jbc.M608646200] [PMID: 17227767]

[133] Soliman E, Van Dross R. Anandamide-induced endoplasmic reticulum stress and apoptosis are mediated by oxidative stress in non-melanoma skin cancer: Receptor-independent endocannabinoid signaling. Mol Carcinog 2016; 55(11): 1807-21.
[http://dx.doi.org/10.1002/mc.22429] [PMID: 26513129]

[134] Sánchez MG, Sánchez AM, Ruiz-Llorente L, Díaz-Laviada I. Enhancement of androgen receptor expression induced by (R)-methanandamide in prostate LNCaP cells. FEBS Lett 2003; 555(3): 561-6.
[http://dx.doi.org/10.1016/S0014-5793(03)01349-8] [PMID: 14675774]

[135] Orellana-Serradell O, Poblete CE, Sanchez C, *et al.* Proapoptotic effect of endocannabinoids in prostate cancer cells. Oncol Rep 2015; 33(4): 1599-608.
[http://dx.doi.org/10.3892/or.2015.3746] [PMID: 25606819]

[136] Eichele K, Ramer R, Hinz B. R(+)-methanandamide-induced apoptosis of human cervical carcinoma cells involves a cyclooxygenase-2-dependent pathway. Pharm Res 2009; 26(2): 346-55.
[http://dx.doi.org/10.1007/s11095-008-9748-3] [PMID: 19015962]

[137] Mohammadpour F, Ostad SN, Aliebrahimi S, Daman Z. Anti-invasion effects of cannabinoids agonist and antagonist on human breast cancer stem cells. Iran J Pharm Res 2017; 16(4): 1479-86.

[PMID: 29552056]

[138] Luca T, Di Benedetto G, Scuderi MR, *et al.* The CB1/CB2 receptor agonist WIN-55,212-2 reduces viability of human Kaposi's sarcoma cells *in vitro.* Eur J Pharmacol 2009; 616(1-3): 16-21.
[http://dx.doi.org/10.1016/j.ejphar.2009.06.004] [PMID: 19539619]

[139] Quintana PG, García Liñares G, Chanquia SN, Gorojod RM, Kotler ML, Baldessari A. Improved enzymatic procedure for the synthesis of anandamide and N-fatty acylalkanolamine analogues: A combination strategy to antitumor activity. Eur J Org Chem 2016; 2016(3): 518-28.
[http://dx.doi.org/10.1002/ejoc.201501263]

[140] Melck D, De Petrocellis L, Orlando P, *et al.* Suppression of nerve growth factor Trk receptors and prolactin receptors by endocannabinoids leads to inhibition of human breast and prostate cancer cell proliferation. Endocrinology 2000; 141(1): 118-26.
[http://dx.doi.org/10.1210/endo.141.1.7239] [PMID: 10614630]

[141] Jacobsson SOP, Wallin T, Fowler CJ. Inhibition of rat C6 glioma cell proliferation by endogenous and synthetic cannabinoids. Relative involvement of cannabinoid and vanilloid receptors. J Pharmacol Exp Ther 2001; 299(3): 951-9.
[PMID: 11714882]

[142] Nithipatikom K, Endsley MP, Isbell MA, *et al.* 2-arachidonoylglycerol: a novel inhibitor of androgen-independent prostate cancer cell invasion. Cancer Res 2004; 64(24): 8826-30.
[http://dx.doi.org/10.1158/0008-5472.CAN-04-3136] [PMID: 15604240]

[143] Nithipatikom K, Isbell MA, Endsley MP, Woodliff JE, Campbell WB. Anti-proliferative effect of a putative endocannabinoid, 2-arachidonylglyceryl ether in prostate carcinoma cells. Prostaglandins Other Lipid Mediat 2011; 94(1-2): 34-43.
[http://dx.doi.org/10.1016/j.prostaglandins.2010.12.002] [PMID: 21167293]

[144] Wu M, Huang J, Zhang J, Benes C, Jiao B, Ren R. N-Arachidonoyl Dopamine Inhibits NRAS Neoplastic Transformation by Suppressing Its Plasma Membrane Translocation. Mol Cancer Ther 2017; 16(1): 57-67.
[http://dx.doi.org/10.1158/1535-7163.MCT-16-0419] [PMID: 27760835]

[145] Davies JW, Hainsworth AH, Guerin CJ, Lambert DG. Pharmacology of capsaicin-, anandamide-, and N-arachidonoyl-dopamine-evoked cell death in a homogeneous transient receptor potential vanilloid subtype 1 receptor population. Br J Anaesth 2010; 104(5): 596-602.
[http://dx.doi.org/10.1093/bja/aeq067] [PMID: 20354008]

[146] Akimov MG, Gretskaya NM, Zinchenko GN, Bezuglov VV. Cytotoxicity of endogenous lipids n-acyl dopamines and their possible metabolic derivatives for human cancer cell lines of different histological origin. Anticancer Res 2015; 35(5): 2657-61.
[PMID: 25964542]

[147] Fowler CJ. Delta(9) -tetrahydrocannabinol and cannabidiol as potential curative agents for cancer: A critical examination of the preclinical literature. Clin Pharmacol Ther 2015; 97(6): 587-96.
[http://dx.doi.org/10.1002/cpt.84] [PMID: 25669486]

[148] Hinz B, Ramer R. Anti-tumour actions of cannabinoids. Br J Pharmacol 2019; 176(10): 1384-94.
[http://dx.doi.org/10.1111/bph.14426] [PMID: 30019449]

[149] Pellati F, Borgonetti V, Brighenti V, Biagi M, Benvenuti S, Corsi L. *Cannabis sativa* L. and nonpsychoactive cannabinoids: their chemistry and role against oxidative stress, inflammation, and cancer. BioMed Res Int 2018; 2018: 1691428.
[http://dx.doi.org/10.1155/2018/1691428] [PMID: 30627539]

[150] Lal S, Shekher A, Puneet , Narula AS, Abrahamse H, Gupta SC. Cannabis and its constituents for cancer: History, biogenesis, chemistry and pharmacological activities. Pharmacol Res 2021; 163: 105302.
[http://dx.doi.org/10.1016/j.phrs.2020.105302] [PMID: 33246167]

[151]   Tomko AM, Whynot EG, Ellis LD, Dupré DJ. Anti-cancer potential of cannabinoids, terpenes, and flavonoids present in cannabis. Cancers (Basel) 2020; 12(7): 1-81.
[http://dx.doi.org/10.3390/cancers12071985] [PMID: 32708138]

[152]   Fraguas-Sánchez AI, Fernández-Carballido A, Torres-Suárez AI. Phyto-, endo- and synthetic cannabinoids: promising chemotherapeutic agents in the treatment of breast and prostate carcinomas. Expert Opin Investig Drugs 2016; 25(11): 1311-23.
[http://dx.doi.org/10.1080/13543784.2016.1236913] [PMID: 27633508]

[153]   Powles T, te Poele R, Shamash J, *et al.* Cannabis-induced cytotoxicity in leukemic cell lines: the role of the cannabinoid receptors and the MAPK pathway. Blood 2005; 105(3): 1214-21.
[http://dx.doi.org/10.1182/blood-2004-03-1182] [PMID: 15454482]

[154]   Seltzer ES, Watters AK, MacKenzie D Jr, Granat LM, Zhang D. Cannabidiol (CBD) as a promising anti-cancer drug. Cancers (Basel) 2020; 12(11): 1-26.
[http://dx.doi.org/10.3390/cancers12113203] [PMID: 33143283]

[155]   De Petrocellis L, Ligresti A, Schiano Moriello A, *et al.* Non-THC cannabinoids inhibit prostate carcinoma growth *in vitro* and *in vivo*: pro-apoptotic effects and underlying mechanisms. Br J Pharmacol 2013; 168(1): 79-102.
[http://dx.doi.org/10.1111/j.1476-5381.2012.02027.x] [PMID: 22594963]

[156]   Takeda S, Himeno T, Kakizoe K, *et al.* Cannabidiolic acid-mediated selective down-regulation of c-fos in highly aggressive breast cancer MDA-MB-231 cells: possible involvement of its down-regulation in the abrogation of aggressiveness. J Nat Med 2017; 71(1): 286-91.
[http://dx.doi.org/10.1007/s11418-016-1030-0] [PMID: 27530354]

[157]   Baek SH, Kim YO, Kwag JS, Choi KE, Jung WY, Han DS. Boron trifluoride etherate on silica-A modified Lewis acid reagent (VII). Antitumor activity of cannabigerol against human oral epitheloid carcinoma cells. Arch Pharm Res 1998; 21(3): 353-6.
[http://dx.doi.org/10.1007/BF02975301] [PMID: 9875457]

[158]   Borrelli F, Pagano E, Romano B, *et al.* Colon carcinogenesis is inhibited by the TRPM8 antagonist cannabigerol, a Cannabis-derived non-psychotropic cannabinoid. Carcinogenesis 2014; 35(12): 2787-97.
[http://dx.doi.org/10.1093/carcin/bgu205] [PMID: 25269802]

[159]   Baek S-H, Du Han S, Yook CN, Kim YC, Kwak JS. Synthesis and antitumor activity of cannabigerol. Arch Pharm Res 1996; 19(3): 228-30.
[http://dx.doi.org/10.1007/BF02976895]

[160]   McAllister SD, Christian RT, Horowitz MP, Garcia A, Desprez PY. Cannabidiol as a novel inhibitor of Id-1 gene expression in aggressive breast cancer cells. Mol Cancer Ther 2007; 6(11): 2921-7.
[http://dx.doi.org/10.1158/1535-7163.MCT-07-0371] [PMID: 18025276]

[161]   Ortega A, García-Hernández VM, Ruiz-García E, *et al.* Comparing the effects of endogenous and synthetic cannabinoid receptor agonists on survival of gastric cancer cells. Life Sci 2016; 165: 56-62.
[http://dx.doi.org/10.1016/j.lfs.2016.09.010] [PMID: 27640887]

[162]   Deng L, Cornett BL, Mackie K, Hohmann AG. CB1 knockout mice unveil sustained CB2-mediated antiallodynic effects of the mixed CB1/CB2 agonist CP55,940 in a mouse model of paclitaxel-induced neuropathic pain. Mol Pharmacol 2015; 88(1): 64-74.
[http://dx.doi.org/10.1124/mol.115.098483] [PMID: 25904556]

[163]   Murase R, Kawamura R, Singer E, *et al.* Targeting multiple cannabinoid anti-tumour pathways with a resorcinol derivative leads to inhibition of advanced stages of breast cancer. Br J Pharmacol 2014; 171(19): 4464-77.
[http://dx.doi.org/10.1111/bph.12803] [PMID: 24910342]

[164]   Hyun HB, Lee WS, Go SI, *et al.* The flavonoid morin from Moraceae induces apoptosis by modulation of Bcl-2 family members and Fas receptor in HCT 116 cells. Int J Oncol 2015; 46(6): 2670-8.

[http://dx.doi.org/10.3892/ijo.2015.2967] [PMID: 25892545]

[165]   Booth JK, Bohlmann J. Terpenes in Cannabis sativa - From plant genome to humans. Plant Sci 2019; 284: 67-72.
[http://dx.doi.org/10.1016/j.plantsci.2019.03.022] [PMID: 31084880]

[166]   Fidyt K, Fiedorowicz A, Strządała L, Szumny A. β-caryophyllene and β-caryophyllene oxide-natural compounds of anticancer and analgesic properties. Cancer Med 2016; 5(10): 3007-17.
[http://dx.doi.org/10.1002/cam4.816] [PMID: 27696789]

[167]   Irrera N, D'Ascola A, Pallio G, *et al.* β-caryophyllene inhibits cell proliferation through a direct modulation of CB2 receptors in glioblastoma cells. Cancers (Basel) 2020; 12(4): 1038.
[http://dx.doi.org/10.3390/cancers12041038] [PMID: 32340197]

[168]   Ambrož M, Šmatová M, Šadibolová M, *et al.* Sesquiterpenes α-humulene and β-caryophyllene oxide enhance the efficacy of 5-fluorouracil and oxaliplatin in colon cancer cells. Acta Pharm 2019; 69(1): 121-8.
[http://dx.doi.org/10.2478/acph-2019-0003] [PMID: 31259712]

[169]   Di Giacomo S, Briz O, Monte MJ, *et al.* Chemosensitization of hepatocellular carcinoma cells to sorafenib by β-caryophyllene oxide-induced inhibition of ABC export pumps. Arch Toxicol 2019; 93(3): 623-34.
[http://dx.doi.org/10.1007/s00204-019-02395-9] [PMID: 30659321]

[170]   DI Giacomo S, DI Sotto A, Mazzanti G, Wink M. Chemosensitizing properties of β-caryophyllene and β-caryophyllene oxide in combination with doxorubicin in human cancer cells. Anticancer Res 2017; 37(3): 1191-6.
[http://dx.doi.org/10.21873/anticanres.11433] [PMID: 28314281]

[171]   Blasco-Benito S, Seijo-Vila M, Caro-Villalobos M, *et al.* Appraising the "entourage effect": Antitumor action of a pure cannabinoid *versus* a botanical drug preparation in preclinical models of breast cancer. Biochem Pharmacol 2018; 157: 285-93.
[http://dx.doi.org/10.1016/j.bcp.2018.06.025] [PMID: 29940172]

[172]   Cogan PS. The 'entourage effect' or 'hodge-podge hashish': the questionable rebranding, marketing, and expectations of cannabis polypharmacy. Expert Rev Clin Pharmacol 2020; 13(8): 835-45.
[http://dx.doi.org/10.1080/17512433.2020.1721281] [PMID: 32116073]

[173]   Morell C, Bort A, Vara D, Ramos-Torres A, Rodríguez-Henche N, Díaz-Laviada I. The cannabinoid WIN 55,212-2 prevents neuroendocrine differentiation of LNCaP prostate cancer cells. Prostate Cancer Prostatic Dis 2016; 19(3): 248-57.
[http://dx.doi.org/10.1038/pcan.2016.19] [PMID: 27324222]

[174]   Xu D, Wang J, Zhou Z, He Z, Zhao Q. Cannabinoid WIN55, 212-2 induces cell cycle arrest and inhibits the proliferation and migration of human BEL7402 hepatocellular carcinoma cells. Mol Med Rep 2015; 12(6): 7963-70.
[http://dx.doi.org/10.3892/mmr.2015.4477] [PMID: 26500101]

[175]   Barbado MV, Medrano M, Caballero-Velázquez T, *et al.* Cannabinoid derivatives exert a potent anti-myeloma activity both *in vitro* and *in vivo*. Int J Cancer 2017; 140(3): 674-85.
[http://dx.doi.org/10.1002/ijc.30483] [PMID: 27778331]

[176]   Xian X, Huang L, Zhang B, Wu C, Cui J, Wang Z. WIN 55,212-2 Inhibits the Epithelial Mesenchymal Transition of Gastric Cancer Cells *via* COX-2 Signals. Cell Physiol Biochem 2016; 39(6): 2149-57.
[http://dx.doi.org/10.1159/000447910] [PMID: 27802436]

[177]   Müller L, Radtke A, Decker J, Koch M, Belge G. The Synthetic Cannabinoid WIN 55,212-2 Elicits Death in Human Cancer Cell Lines. Anticancer Res 2017; 37(11): 6341-5.
[PMID: 29061818]

[178]   Khan MI, Sobocińska AA, Brodaczewska KK, *et al.* Involvement of the CB_2 cannabinoid receptor in cell growth inhibition and G0/G1 cell cycle arrest *via* the cannabinoid agonist WIN 55,212-2 in renal

cell carcinoma. BMC Cancer 2018; 18(1): 583.
[http://dx.doi.org/10.1186/s12885-018-4496-1] [PMID: 29792186]

[179]   Nasser MW, Qamri Z, Deol YS, *et al.* Crosstalk between chemokine receptor CXCR4 and cannabinoid receptor CB2 in modulating breast cancer growth and invasion. PLoS One 2011; 6(9): e23901.
[http://dx.doi.org/10.1371/journal.pone.0023901] [PMID: 21915267]

[180]   Hanlon KE, Lozano-Ondoua AN, Umaretiya PJ, Symons-Liguori AM, Chandramouli A, Moy JK, *et al.* Modulation of breast cancer cell viability by a cannabinoid receptor 2 agonist, JWH-015, is calcium dependent. Breast cancer Targets Ther 2016; 8: 59-71.

[181]   Olea-Herrero N, Vara D, Malagarie-Cazenave S, Díaz-Laviada I. Inhibition of human tumour prostate PC-3 cell growth by cannabinoids R(+)-Methanandamide and JWH-015: involvement of CB2. Br J Cancer 2009; 101(6): 940-50.
[http://dx.doi.org/10.1038/sj.bjc.6605248] [PMID: 19690545]

[182]   Preet A, Qamri Z, Nasser MW, *et al.* Cannabinoid receptors, CB1 and CB2, as novel targets for inhibition of non-small cell lung cancer growth and metastasis. Cancer Prev Res (Phila) 2011; 4(1): 65-75.
[http://dx.doi.org/10.1158/1940-6207.CAPR-10-0181] [PMID: 21097714]

[183]   Ma C, Zhang M, Liu L, *et al.* Low-dose cannabinoid receptor 2 agonist induces microglial activation in a cancer pain-morphine tolerance rat model. Life Sci 2021; 264: 118635.

[184]   Sarnataro D, Pisanti S, Santoro A, *et al.* The cannabinoid CB1 receptor antagonist rimonabant (SR141716) inhibits human breast cancer cell proliferation through a lipid raft-mediated mechanism. Mol Pharmacol 2006; 70(4): 1298-306.
[http://dx.doi.org/10.1124/mol.106.025601] [PMID: 16822929]

[185]   Gallotta D, Nigro P, Cotugno R, Gazzerro P, Bifulco M, Belisario MA. Rimonabant-induced apoptosis in leukemia cell lines: activation of caspase-dependent and -independent pathways. Biochem Pharmacol 2010; 80(3): 370-80.
[http://dx.doi.org/10.1016/j.bcp.2010.04.023] [PMID: 20417624]

[186]   Santoro A, Pisanti S, Grimaldi C, *et al.* Rimonabant inhibits human colon cancer cell growth and reduces the formation of precancerous lesions in the mouse colon. Int J Cancer 2009; 125(5): 996-1003.
[http://dx.doi.org/10.1002/ijc.24483] [PMID: 19479993]

[187]   Proto MC, Fiore D, Piscopo C, *et al.* Inhibition of Wnt/β-Catenin pathway and Histone acetyltransferase activity by Rimonabant: a therapeutic target for colon cancer. Sci Rep 2017; 7(1): 11678.
[http://dx.doi.org/10.1038/s41598-017-11688-x] [PMID: 28916833]

[188]   Fiore D, Ramesh P, Proto MC, *et al.* Rimonabant kills colon cancer stem cells without inducing toxicity in normal colon organoids. Front Pharmacol 2018; 8: 949.
[http://dx.doi.org/10.3389/fphar.2017.00949] [PMID: 29354056]

[189]   Gazzerro P, Malfitano AM, Proto MC, *et al.* Synergistic inhibition of human colon cancer cell growth by the cannabinoid CB1 receptor antagonist rimonabant and oxaliplatin. Oncol Rep 2010; 23(1): 171-5.
[PMID: 19956878]

[190]   Benz AH, Renné C, Maronde E, *et al.* Expression and functional relevance of cannabinoid receptor 1 in Hodgkin lymphoma. PLoS One 2013; 8(12): e81675.
[http://dx.doi.org/10.1371/journal.pone.0081675] [PMID: 24349109]

[191]   Marshall AD, Lagutina I, Grosveld GC. PAX3-FOXO1 induces cannabinoid receptor 1 to enhance cell invasion and metastasis. Cancer Res 2011; 71(24): 7471-80.
[http://dx.doi.org/10.1158/0008-5472.CAN-11-0924] [PMID: 22037868]

[192]   Asche C. Antitumour quinones. Mini-Reviews Med Chem 2005; 5: 449-67.

[http://dx.doi.org/10.2174/1389557053765556]

[193] Kogan NM, Rabinowitz R, Levi P, *et al.* Synthesis and antitumor activity of quinonoid derivatives of cannabinoids. J Med Chem 2004; 47(15): 3800-6.
[http://dx.doi.org/10.1021/jm040042o] [PMID: 15239658]

[194] Kogan NM, Blázquez C, Alvarez L, *et al.* A cannabinoid quinone inhibits angiogenesis by targeting vascular endothelial cells. Mol Pharmacol 2006; 70(1): 51-9.
[http://dx.doi.org/10.1124/mol.105.021089] [PMID: 16571653]

[195] Kogan NM, Schlesinger M, Priel E, *et al.* HU-331, a novel cannabinoid-based anticancer topoisomerase II inhibitor. Mol Cancer Ther 2007; 6(1): 173-83.
[http://dx.doi.org/10.1158/1535-7163.MCT-06-0039] [PMID: 17237277]

[196] Morales P, Vara D, Goméz-Cañas M, *et al.* Synthetic cannabinoid quinones: preparation, *in vitro* antiproliferative effects and *in vivo* prostate antitumor activity. Eur J Med Chem 2013; 70: 111-9.
[http://dx.doi.org/10.1016/j.ejmech.2013.09.043] [PMID: 24141201]

[197] Morales P, Blasco-Benito S, Andradas C, *et al.* Selective, nontoxic CB(2) cannabinoid o-quinone with *in vivo* activity against triple-negative breast cancer. J Med Chem 2015; 58(5): 2256-64.
[http://dx.doi.org/10.1021/acs.jmedchem.5b00078] [PMID: 25671648]

[198] Badolato M, Carullo G, Caroleo MC, Cione E, Aiello F, Manetti F. Discovery of 1,4-naphthoquinones as a new class of antiproliferative agents targeting GPR55. ACS Med Chem Lett. 2019.

[199] Manera C, Saccomanni G, Malfitano AM, *et al.* Rational design, synthesis and anti-proliferative properties of new CB2 selective cannabinoid receptor ligands: an investigation of the 1,8-naphthyridin-2(1H)-one scaffold. Eur J Med Chem 2012; 52: 284-94.
[http://dx.doi.org/10.1016/j.ejmech.2012.03.031] [PMID: 22483967]

[200] Capozzi A, Mattei V, Martellucci S, *et al.* Anti-proliferative properties and proapoptotic function of new CB2 selective cannabinoid receptor agonist in jurkat leukemia cells. Int J Mol Sci 2018; 19(7): 1958.
[http://dx.doi.org/10.3390/ijms19071958] [PMID: 29973514]

[201] Paul RK, Wnorowski A, Gonzalez-Mariscal I, *et al.* (R,R′)-4′-methoxy-1-naphthylfenoterol targets GPR55-mediated ligand internalization and impairs cancer cell motility. Biochem Pharmacol 2014; 87(4): 547-61.
[http://dx.doi.org/10.1016/j.bcp.2013.11.020] [PMID: 24355564]

[202] Malhotra P, Casari I, Falasca M. Therapeutic potential of cannabinoids in combination cancer therapy. Adv Biol Regul 2021; 79: 100774.

[203] Morelli MB, Offidani M, Alesiani F, *et al.* The effects of cannabidiol and its synergism with bortezomib in multiple myeloma cell lines. A role for transient receptor potential vanilloid type-2. Int J Cancer 2014; 134(11): 2534-46.
[http://dx.doi.org/10.1002/ijc.28591] [PMID: 24293211]

The Beneficial Effects of Turmeric and its Active Constituent in Cancer Treatment: Current and Future Trends

Giftson J. Senapathy[1], Blassan P. George[1] and **Heidi Abrahamse[1,*]**

[1] *Laser Research Centre, Faculty of Health Sciences, University of Johannesburg, P.O. Box 17011, Doornfontein 2028, South Africa*

Abstract: 'Turmeric' (*Curcuma longa* L.) is an important spice found almost in every culinary preparation of Asian cooking, especially in India. This yellow rhizome is known for its medicinal and nutritional properties for many centuries and hence in Chinese and Indian traditional medicine it has been used for treating internal diseases and common ailments. It has various pharmacological properties including anticancer activity, which is mainly centered on its orange colored curcuminoid polyphenol called "curcumin". Cancer is a deadly multifactorial disease originating from cells affecting many parts of the body in later stages. New cancer drugs and treatment methods become an everyday search due to the genetic complexity of the disease. Nowadays, natural products like turmeric are gaining importance as cancer therapeutics since their dietary intake reduces the cancer risk. In this chapter, the background, importance and pharmacological activities of turmeric and its chemical constituent curcumin were discussed with reference to the recent anticancer studies. Numerous reports are available on the anticancer potential of turmeric and curcumin. As reflected from these study results, curcumin was observed to inhibit the proliferation of cells, invasion, angiogenesis and metastasis in tumor cells. It increases the accumulation of free radicals through the reactive oxygen species resulting in apoptosis. It also sensitizes cancer cells for other cancer therapies. Due to its antioxidant and pharmacological activities, it can even reverse the cancer progression in the early stages. In contrast, the poor absorption limits its clinical use but the conversion into nanoforms improves its solubility. Curcumin is nongenotoxic and nonmutagenic and hence it is approved as a safe substance in various clinical trials.

Keywords: Anticancer, Antioxidant, Apoptosis, Cancer, Chemotherapy, Curcumin, Nutraceutical, Pharmacology, Phytotherapy, Signaling pathways, Turmeric.

* **Corresponding author Heidi Abrahamse:** Laser Research Centre, Faculty of Health Sciences, University of Johannesburg, P.O. Box 17011, Doornfontein 2028, South Africa; Tel: +27 115596448; Fax: +27115596550; E-mail: habrahamse@uj.ac.za

Atta-ur-Rahman & M. Iqbal Choudhary (Eds.)
All rights reserved-© 2021 Bentham Science Publishers

INTRODUCTION

Curcuma longa (Zingiberaceae) or Turmeric is a known spice and condiment used in food preparations throughout the world (Fig. **1**). Due to its catchy natural yellow color and flavor, it became a common food additive and dietary coloring agent. The powdered or finely minced form of its rhizome (turmeric powder) is a common dietary spice in the cuisines of India, Iran, Thailand, Malaysia and China. Because of its rich pharmacological activities, turmeric powder is used for treating common ailments like flu, body pain, skin burns, dermatologic diseases, bacterial and fungal infections, external wounds and for treating stress, depression and internal diseases in traditional Chinese and Indian Ayurvedic medicine [1].

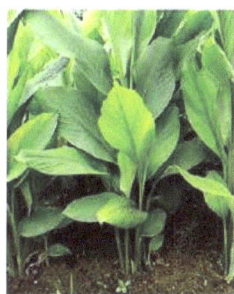

Turmeric Plant   Fresh rhizome

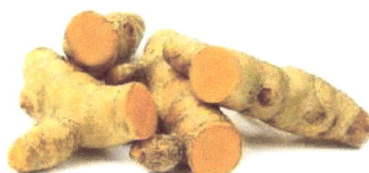

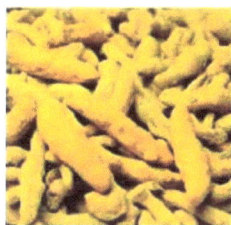

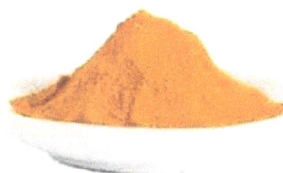

Dry rhizome   Powdered rhizome or
                         Turmeric powder

Fig. (1). Different parts of turmeric plant used for its medicinal and beneficial properties.

The name 'nutraceutical' was first given by Stephen De Felice in the year 1989 to a group of compounds which has both nutritional effect and pharmaceutical use. Nutraceutical refers to a food substance (whole or a portion of it) that has the capacity to increase nutrition and reduce occurrence of a disease, which in turn can be used to treat certain diseases or health conditions [2]. Several reports have proven that the intake of nutraceuticals from the categories of natural food substances including probiotics, antioxidants, polyunsaturated fatty acids, dietary fibers, spices and vitamins and parts of a plants such as leaves, flowers has beneficial effects on health and also reduces the risk of diseases. Turmeric is one such nutraceutical since it is a food substance with important medicinal properties. Besides being an ingredient of food, it also possesses antimicrobial, antitumor, analgesic, lipid modifier, anti-hyperlipidemic and anti-inflammatory properties [3].

Cancer still considered to be a deadly disease, is the second most leading factor for disease associated deaths in the whole world. Several treatment strategies were employed in recent decades to fight cancer evasion, including chemotherapy, surgery, radiation and immuno therapies. Chemotherapy involves cytotoxic anti-neoplastic drugs such as antimetabolites and alkylating agents for the treatment of cancers. Though it is effective in many cases, it is always accompanied with side-effects resulting in cancer cell chemoresistance. Drug resistance may be due to the acquired mutations in the cellular therapeutic targets or due to the molecular heterogeneity of cancer cells [4]. The normal cells have controlled growth, whereas cancer cells exhibit an anomalous growth with increased life span resulting in chronic proliferation [5]. This uncontrolled exponential cell growth as a result of evading programmed cell death by the circumvention of signaling pathways, epigenetic and genetic alterations, is observed in all the stages of cancer progression. Bypassing apoptosis is an important contributing factor for the resistance of cancer cells to cancer therapies, including chemo and radiotherapy [6].

Phytotherapy is a method of treating chronic illnesses including cancer using plants or plant derived drugs. Phytotherapy in the recent decades is attracting the interest of oncologists and cancer researchers as it is relatively harmless than chemical drugs [7]. This led to the copious explorations on pharmacologically active chemicals of plant origin called as phytochemicals which has an array of biomedical applications. Due to this, the phytochemicals were also called phytopharmaceuticals, which include their entire sub classes namely flavonoids, phytoalexins and phenolic compounds. They possess anticancer properties and were employed in adjuvant therapy because of their low range of toxicities and side effects. They were known to potentially modulate a variety of metabolic processes concerned to carcinogenesis [8, 9]. Plants rich in phytochemicals especially polyphenols were found to have antimicrobial, anticancer, antioxidant and antimutagenic properties. The phenolics were derived mainly from the amino acid phenylalanine and less frequently from tyrosine from the plants. Phyto phenols were known for its inhibitory effect on cancer cells and control metastasis [10].

Curcumin, a diarylheptanoid and polyphone, is an essential curcuminoid found in turmeric. It has its own pride for being the most-studied compound among natural medicines, for its various pharmacological properties. Among few other polyphenols, it is also identified as a chemotherapeutic and preventive agent. Extensive research evidence in the past six decades have explored significant functions of curcumin in cancer therapy [11]. Many reports were published on the impact of curcumin on multiple cellular targets and molecules like cytokines, transcription factors, enzymes, kinases, growth factors and other cancer receptors. In addition to this, curcumin is recognized as a safe substance at relatively high drug concentrations in various *in vivo* models and clinical trials. Even when administered at 500 mg (two times per day for 30 days), it was proven to be safe for humans [12]. In contrast to its pharmacological activities as reported by several studies, turmeric and curcumin are not accepted for clinical applications to masses due to its low absorption by gastrointestinal tract, low bioavailability, poor stability and solubility [13, 14]. Research findings have suggested that the use of nano formulations, nanoparticle drug delivery system, curcumin analogs, co-administration with other phytochemicals like piperine and ginger can overcome the limitations of curcumin in clinical applications [15].

This chapter is prepared to give the reader a clear overview about the phytochemistry and pharmacological effects of turmeric and its bioactive compound curcumin, their structure activity relationship, antioxidant, prooxidant and anticancer activity of curcumin, multiple targets in cancer treatments, recent studies on curcumin combinations, challenges and future prospects in cancer treatment using curcumin and turmeric.

PHYTOCHEMISTRY OF CURCUMIN

Curcumin or diferuloylmethane (Fig. **2a**), a yellow-orange crystal, has a molar mass of 368.38 g/mole. The IUPAC designation of curcumin is 1, 7-bis (4-hyd roxy-3-methoxyphenyl)-1,6-heptadiene-3,5- dione and its molecular formula is $C_{21}H_{20}O_6$ [16]. Its chemical structure reveals three distinct structures comprising of two aromatic ring structures with 4-hydroxy-3-methoxy-phenyl groups linked to a 7C linker molecule, which has ß-unsaturated ß-diketone carbon bridge. This seven-carbon linker molecule behaves as a Michael acceptor. Curcumin exists in its tautomeric forms (keto and enol forms) with a higher concentration of the enol form in solution. The keto–enol tautomerism of curcumin is pH dependent and has a direct influence on its photochemical properties in the solution form (Fig. **2b**). It is also sensitive to alkaline solutions resulting in quick degradation [17]. Apart from curcumin, other non-curcumin entities were also present in turmeric. Turmerin, furanodiene, turmerone, curdione, calebin A bisacurone, germacrone, elemene and cyclocurcumin were some of them. All these non-curcuminoids also exert anti-inflammatory activities [18].

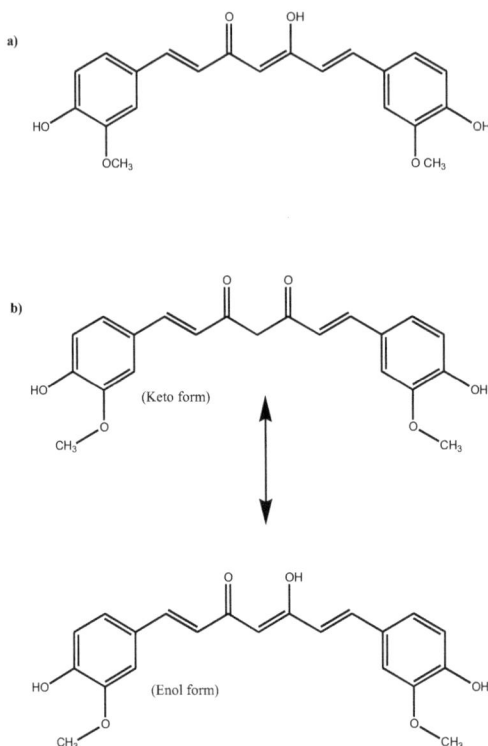

Fig. (2). a) Symmetrical chemical arrangement of curcumin; **b)** Keto-enol tautomerism of curcumin molecule.

STRUCTURE ACTIVITY RELATIONSHIP

The chemical arrangement of curcumin reveals 2 symmetrical aromatic rings as shown in Fig. (**2a**). The tautomeric forms (keto and enol forms) and aromatic rings might be responsible for the hydrophobicity of curcumin making it poorly soluble. Chemical interactions with other molecules and drugs brands curcumin a chemically active molecule. Hydrophobic nature of curcumin, ability of hydrogen bond formation, tautomeric conversions, symmetrical aromatic rings and availability of pairing groups on the linking molecules might together facilitate the non-covalent interactions of curcumin. Also diketo groups in the enol form and the unsaturated bonds promote the covalent interactions with -SH groups of the proteins. Metal ions are essential for many important biochemical processes in the body and hence they should be present in the cells and plasma to carry out these functions but at their physiological levels. An increase or decrease in the levels of metals ions beyond their physiological limits necessitates an external mechanism such as chelation therapy to bring the levels in control. The diketo groups (enol form) can form complexes with transition metals thereby reducing its toxicity. Due to this property of curcumin could be employed as a chelator in chelation therapy to bind to toxic metals and scavenge or neutralize them [19]. It also facilitates the selective transport of metal ions to the intracellular components of the cells, especially the nucleus enabling them to interact with DNA and inhibiting cancer cell proliferation [20]. However, during chemical modifications of curcumin, done in order to enhance their pharmacological activities, this property might be decreased due to the *O*-methoxy groups, which may affect the metal chelating ability of diketo groups of curcumin by changing its electron density [21].

PHARMACOLOGICAL PROPERTIES OF CURCUMIN

Reports from traditional medicines revealed that curcumin was employed in treating inflammatory diseases for more than 5000 years in the form of an oral supplement. Well known for its healing properties, the earliest mention of curcumin was reported by Albert Oppenheimer in 1937 for the treatment of cholecystitis [22]. Later, it is used in the treatment of other illnesses such as liver diseases, urinary diseases, inflammation of joints and skin problems occurred by parasitic infections [23]. Subsequently, curcumin has been found to be effective in most of the known diseases like cancer, arthritis, depression, liver disease, dyslipidemia, chronic obstructive pulmonary disease and gastrointestinal disorders [22, 24, 25, 26 - 30]. These abilities were mainly because of its antioxidant and anti-inflammatory properties. Many research reports carried out in diseases such as autoimmune neuritis, atherosclerosis, encephalomyelitis and arthritis suggest that curcumin reduces inflammation in these conditions [31]. The neuroprotective action of turmeric was reported in multiple studies on nerve cells like microglia, neurons and astrocytes [32 - 34]. In the recent decades, extensive researches conducted on various *in vivo* and *in vitro* models sufficiently proved the antitumor, anticarcinogenic, antineoplastic, antiangiogenic, chemopreventive, chemotherapeutic and antioxidant activities of curcumin [25, 35].

In clinical trials, when curcumin is administered to individuals affected by cardiovascular illnesses such as acute myocardial infarction, dyslipidemia and acute coronary heart disease, the treatment was proven to be beneficial. Even at high concentrations, curcumin acted as a cardioprotective, antidiabetic and neuroprotective agent. Curcumin was also found to diminish the levels of fats such as cholesterol, triglycerides (TGs) and low-density lipoprotein (LDL). At the same time it increases the levels of high-density lipoprotein which could be a positive effect in the lipoprotein metabolism [36]. In line with its proven anti-inflammatory effect, curcumin showed therapeutic effects over the chronic rare auto immune disease systemic lupus erythematosus (SLE) occurring mostly in aged women characterized by infilteration of auto-antibodies in important organs such as liver, kidney, heart and in plasma [37, 38]. The antiviral and immunomodulatory activities of curcumin suggest that it can be employed in handling HIV (Human Immunodeficiency Virus) infections and Acquired Immunodeficiency Syndrome (AIDS) at later stages [39].

Antioxidant and Prooxidant Nature of Curcumin

Curcumin is a potential antioxidant due to its structural arrangement of atoms. The conjugated-double bonds in the arrangement of curcumin make it to serve as an effective electron donor. It readily donates its electron during redox reactions and helps in scavenging the reactive oxygen species (ROS) thus, exhibiting its antioxidant activity [4]. Similar to many polyphenols, curcumin exerts both antioxidant and prooxidant activities. The prooxidant mechanism of curcumin remains unclear. However, factors such as, low pH, high doses, increased concentration of transition metal ions facilitate the prooxidant nature of curcumin [40]. It was found that it scavenges ROS in low doses and stimulates ROS generation at high doses [41].

ANTICANCER ACTIVITY OF CURCUMIN

The anti-proliferative property of whole turmeric and curcumin has been extensively reported in genito-urinary, lung, breast, melanoma, ovarian, cervical, brain, head and neck, prostate and gastrointestinal cancers (Fig. **3**) [42 - 47]. It was reported to be inhibitory and efficient against melanoma [48], pancreatic cancer [49], colon cancer [50] and glioblastoma [51] either alone or with other chemotherapeutic drugs. Some of the recent results of curcumin on above mentioned cancers were summarized below (Table **1**).

Table 1. Anticancer activity of curcumin expressed in different cancers.

S.No.	Curcumin/Curcumin Derivatives	Cancer Type	Mechanism of Action	References
1	Curcumin	Bladder cancer	Sonic Hedgehog pathway	[52]
2	Curcumin	Bladder cancer	β-catenin pathway	[53]
3	Curcumin	Bladder cancer	Tumor-associated calcium signal transducer gene family	[54]
4	Curcumin	Lung cancer	Sonic Hedgehog pathway and Wnt/β-catenin pathway Lung CSC markers such as (Oct4, CD133, ALDHA1, CD44 and Nanog)	[55]
5	Curcumin	Lung cancer	ERK/MEK pathways and AKT/S6K pathways Autophagic cell death	[57]

(Table 1) cont.....

S.No.	Curcumin/Curcumin Derivatives	Cancer Type	Mechanism of Action	References
6	Curcumin	Breast cancer	Downregulated expression of β-catenin, Fibro nectin and Vimentin, upregulated E-Cadherin expression	[58]
7	Curcumin and paclitaxel combination	Breast cancer	Caspase mediated apoptosis, necrosis PARP and NF- κB activation	[59]
8	Curcumin analog -WZ35	Breast cancer	ROS generation and YAP (Yes Associated Protein)-JNK activation	[60]
9	Curcumin	Melanoma	Cytochrome c release and ROS mediated apoptosis	[62]
10	Curcumin	Melanoma	ROS mediated DNA damage and apoptosis accompanied by loss of mitochondrial membrane potential	[63]
11	Curcumin analog – Compound A combined with tamoxifen	Melanoma	Oxidative stress mediated apoptosis	[64]
12	Curcumin	Ovarian cancer	AKT/mTOR/p70S6K signaling pathways Protective autophagy	[65]
13	Curcumin derivatives ST03 and ST08	Ovarian cancer	MMP1 inhibition	[66]
14	Curcumin and paclitaxel combination	Ovarian cancer	CD44 targeted drug delivery	[67]
15	Curcumin	Cervical cancer	Reduction in epithelial-mesenchymal transition (EMT) and Vimentin, Slug and N-Cadherin protein levels Reduction in Pirin-dependent epithelial mesenchymal transition	[68]
16	Curcumin	Cervical cancer	Regulation of NF-kB and Wnt pathways	[69]
17	Curcumin	Glioblastoma multiforme	Multitargeted cancer control	[70]
18	Curcumin	Prostate cancer	Reduction in the steroidogenic acute regulatory proteins CYP11A1 and HSD3B2 Decreased androgen production	[71]
19	Curcumin	Prostate cancer	Inhibition of JNK signaling pathway	[72]
20	Curcumin and metformin combination	Head and neck squamous cell carcinoma	Multi targeted signaling mechanism	[74]

(Table 1) cont.....

S.No.	Curcumin/Curcumin Derivatives	Cancer Type	Mechanism of Action	References
21	Novel curcumin gum formulation	Head and neck squamous cell carcinoma	Increased curcumin release and transmucosal absorption Reduction of serum Reduction of serum CXL1 (GRO –α) and TNF – α levels	[75]
22	Curcumin nanomicelle	Head and neck cancer	Reduction in radiotherapy induced oral mucositis	[76]
23	Curcumin	Pancreatic cancer	Inhibition of Enhancer of Zeste Homolog-2 (EZH2) subunit of Polycomb Repressive Complex 2 (PRC2)	[77]
24	Curcumin	Esophageal cancer	Inhibition of ROS inhibitors and JAK/STAT3 signaling pathways	[78]
25	Curcumin	Gastric cancer	Suppression of miRNA-21 Inhibition of PTEN/PI3K/AKT pathway	[79]
26	Curcumin	Colon cancer	Suppression of Yes- Associated Proteins (YAP) Promotion of cancer cell autophagy	[80]

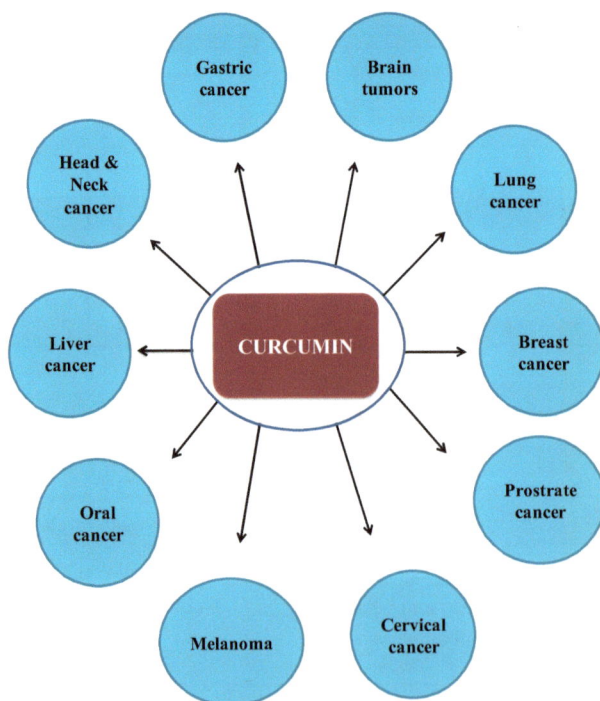

Fig. (3). Anticancer potential of curcumin against variety of cancers.

Genitourinary Cancer

In a study by Wang *et al.* curcumin was found to inhibit bladder cancer stem cells by inhibiting the formation of cell spheres, cell proliferation and reduced the expression of cancer stem cell (CSC) markers. It was also found that the overall inhibition of bladder cancer cells by curcumin is coupled with the suppression of Sonic Hedgehog pathway [52]. Another study by Shi *et al.* on the effects of curcumin on bladder cancer revealed that the flavonoid reduced the cancer progression by inhibiting cancer cell proliferation, reducing the capacity of cell migration and invasiveness by regulating the expression of β-catenin [53]. Similarly, curcumin was reported to inhibit the cell proliferation of bladder cancer cells through the suppression of tumor-associated calcium signal transducer gene family by inhibiting the expression of human trophoblast cell surface antigen 2 (Trop 2) [54].

Lung Cancer

Jian-Yun Zhu and his collaborators showed that curcumin inhibits lung CSC through the suppression of Sonic Hedgehog pathway and Wnt/β-catenin pathway. A significant reduction in the levels of lung CSC markers such as (Oct4, CD133, ALDHA1, CD44 and Nanog) was observed in curcumin treatments evidencing the inhibitory effect of curcumin over lung CSC [55]. In a study on non-small-cell lung cancer cells, administration of curcumin reduced the cell proliferation and ROS levels and also observed the inhibition in the expression of p-GSK3β (Ser9), β-catenin, c-Myc and cyclin D1 proteins [56]. Recently, curcumin was found to overcome the resistance of lung cancer cells H157 and H1299 for the chemotherapeutic drug gefitinib by inducing autophagy related cell death. The results showed that curcumin downregulated the EGFR (Epidermal Growth Factor Receptor) activity, ERK/MEK pathways and AKT/S6K pathways resulting in autophagic cell death [57].

Breast Cancer

Recently, curcumin was reported to express anti-metastatic activity and stem cell like expression in breast cancer cells. Curcumin treatment suppressed the proliferation of MCF7 and MDA-MB-231 breast cancer cells and downregulated the expression of β-catenin, Fibro nectin and Vimentin, upregulated E-Cadherin expression and most importantly reduced the stem cell genes (Sox2 and Nanog) expression [58]. The combination with the chemotherapeutic drug paclitaxel, curcumin significantly induced caspase 3/7 mediated apoptosis, necrosis, PARP and NF- κB activation in breast cancer cells revealing the chemosensitizing effect of curcumin in combination with paclitaxel [59]. Coker-Gurkan and colleagues reported a curcumin analog (WZ35) to have breast cancer cell growth inhibiting effect through increased ROS generation and YAP (Yes Associated Protein)-JNK activation. The curcumin analog also induced mitochondrial dysfunction of breast cancer cells [60]. In a study on breast cancer, it was found to increase the down regulation of oncogenic stem cell markers namely Oct4, ALDH1A1 and CD44 [61].

Melanoma

Liao *et al.* reported that the curcumin treatment resulted in the elevation of ROS levels, cytochrome c release, and increased apoptosis through ROS dependent HIF-1α proteins in A375 melanoma cells [62]. Similarly, in another study on B16-F10 mouse melanoma cells, curcumin augmented ROS mediated DNA damage and apoptosis through reduction in the mitochondrial membrane potential. The authors suggested that the increased cytotoxicity and apoptosis of melanoma cells by curcumin may be due to the expression of prooxidant nature of curcumin [63]. A recent study by Parashar *et al.* (2019) showed that curcumin analog compound A induced oxidative stress mediated apoptosis in human melanoma cells in combination with tamoxifen [64].

Ovarian Cancer

Curcumin induced apoptosis in human ovarian cancer cells SK-OV-3 and A2780. Apart from the reduction in cell viability and colony forming ability, it was reported that curcumin treatment could induce protective autophagy by inducing AKT/mTOR/p70S6K signaling pathways [65]. The curcumin derivatives ST03 and ST08, showed a hundred-fold increase than curcumin on apoptosis induction and inhibition of MMP1 (matrix metalloproteinase 1) in metastatic ovarian cancer cell line PA-1 [66]. The co-delivery of curcumin and paclitaxel though a nano formulation for CD44 targeted drug delivery for ovarian cancer cells, showed synergistic anticancer effects of these drug combinations on ovarian cancer *in vitro* and *in vivo*. A drug resistance effected by the SKOV-TR30 ovarian cancer cells was significantly reversed by this curcumin-drug combination [67].

Cervical Cancer

Aedo-Aguilera *et al.* reported that, administration of curcumin to SiHa cervical cancer cells, reduced the epithelial-mesenchymal transition (EMT) and Vimentin, Slug and N-Cadherin protein levels. Also, a further reduction in PIR expression and Pirin protein levels, which is an oxidative stress sensor protein, were observed in curcumin treatments. The results collected revealed that curcumin could reduce the Pirin-dependent epithelial mesenchymal transition in cervical cancer cells [68]. Curcumin also inhibited the cell growth of cervical cancer cells through the regulation of NF-kB and Wnt pathways [69].

Brain Tumor

Although data related to the inhibitory effects of curcumin on brain tumors are limited, earlier preclinical data (*in vitro* and *in vivo*) have shown that curcumin could offer effective treatment for brain tumors including glioblastoma multiforme [70].

Prostate Cancer

Ide *et al.* reported that curcumin administration in human prostrate cancer cells LNCaP and 22Rv1 resulted in a dose dependent inhibition of cell proliferation and apoptosis. Also, the treatment reduced the levels of CYP11A1 and HSD3B2 which belongs to the category of steroidogenic acute regulatory proteins expressed in prostate cancers. Overall, the anticancer activity of curcumin contributed to the reduction in androgen production thereby inhibiting prostate cancer cell proliferation [71]. Similarly, curcumin suppressed the growth of prostate cancer cells by inhibiting JNK signaling pathway and induced apoptosis in LNCaP cells [72]. In prostate cancer cells (Du145 and 22RV1), curcumin showed strong antitumor effect (cell lines and animal models) by inhibiting cell cycle and multiplication [73].

Head and Neck Cancer

Cancers that are formed on oral cavity, salivary glands, thoracic cavity and other areas around head and neck are collectively termed as head and neck cancers. Recently, Lindsay *et al.* explored the anticancer activity of curcumin in combination with the standard drug metformin in HPV+ and HPV- head and neck squamous cell carcinoma cell lines (HNSCC). It was observed that curcumin inhibited cancer cell viability and proliferation effected through a multi targeted signaling mechanism as evidenced from the protein and RNA expression data. However, there were no synergistic anticancer effects observed in these drug combinations [74]. Recently, a novel gum formulation using curcumin was developed to treat head and neck squamous cell carcinoma and tested in a clinical trial comprising of 30 volunteers. The results revealed a high release and transmucosal absorption of curcumin was observed in this formulation with a significant reduction in the chemoprevention biomarkers CXL1 (GRO –α) and TNF – α in serum [75]. Similarly, in a randomized controlled trial performed on 32 head and neck cancer patients, a nanomicelle formulation of curcumin was administered orally to study its effect on oral mucositis observed during the radiotherapy of head and neck cancers. The results showed that only 32% of oral mucositis cases were observed among the patients administered with curcumin in nanomicelle form revealing the possibility of nanocurcumin administration for head and neck cancer patients undergoing radiotherapy [76].

Gastro Intestinal Cancer

Cancers affecting the associating organs of Gastro intestinal (GI) tract are termed as GI cancers. Various reports show the therapeutic effects of curcumin against GI cancers. Yoshida *et al.* reported that curcumin treatment resensitizes gemcitabine resistant pancreatic ductal adenocarcinoma cells (PDAC) through the inhibition of Enhancer of Zeste Homolog-2 (EZH2) subunit of Polycomb Repressive Complex 2 (PRC2), a key regulator of chemoresistance [77]. Zhen *et al.* studied the effect of curcumin in human esophageal cancer cells Eca-109. The polyphenol increased the cell adhesion of cancer cells by inhibiting ROS inhibitors and JAK/STAT3 signaling pathway [78]. Also in a study on gastric cancer, curcumin suppressed the metabolism and expression of gastric cancer by regulating miRNA-21 and inhibiting the proteins of PTEN/PI3K/AKT pathway [79]. Administration of curcumin in gastric cancer cells reduced VEGFR-3 and LYVE-1 expression, which belong to the important category of metastatic proteins [80]. To treat colon cancer, curcumin is employed for many years as it significantly controls the propagation of cancer cells in all the stages of tumor progression starting from pre-initiation, initiation, post-initiation and metastasis of colon cancer [81]. Curcumin treatment in human colon cancer cells, suppressed the expression of Yes- Associated Proteins (YAP) leading to the inhibition of cell proliferation and promotion of cancer cell autophagy [82].

Mode of Action of Curcumin

Curcumin was reported to modulate various patho-physio processes of cancer, such as cell survival, modulation of immune system, signal transduction, cell proliferation, cell death, mitochondrial and death receptor pathways, tumor suppressor pathways and protein kinase pathways [83 - 85]. It reacts with numerous intra and extra cellular molecules involved in cancer initiation and progression. It is reported to be an anti-angiogenic agent resulting in cancer suppression. An anti-telomerase effect of curcumin was recorded against some cancers [86].

Effect of Curcumin on Cancer Signaling Pathways

Extensive research evidence indicates that curcumin could act in a multi-targeted fashion (Fig. **4**) by interfering with various cell signaling pathways by targeting bioactive proteins or epigenetically regulating gene expression, in key cancer signalling pathways [85, 87, 88]. Curcumin suppressed cancer cell invasion, proliferation, angiogenesis and metastasis [89 - 91]. Apart from targeting the key signaling pathways leading to apoptosis curcumin exerts its anticancer potential by enhancing the activity of immune system through its immunomodulating efficacy. This contributes for the eradication of cancers at early and later stages

[8]. It was found to inhibit the inflammatory pathways of STAT3 (Signal Transducer and Activator of Transcription 3) and NF-κB (Nuclear Factor kappa-B) which is important for the progression of cancer. In a study on gastric cancer, curcumin application lowered gastrin secretion to increase the pH of gastric fluid which further represses the multiplication of cancer cells [92].

Literature shows (Fig. **5**) that curcumin influences a various cell adhesion molecules (CAMs), downstream proteins like COX-2 (Cyclooxygenase 2), NOS (Nitric Oxide Synthase), Cyclin D1, TNF-α (Tumor Necrosis Factor α), Bcl-2 (B-cell lymphoma 2), interleukins, P-gp (P glycoprotein), MMP9 Matrix Metallo peptidase 9), MDR (Multi Drug Resistance) and growth factor receptors involved in tumor growth [85, 93, 94, 13, 14]. The PD-L1 (Programmed Death Ligand) blockade is currently considered to be a promising immune intervention for the therapy of malignant diseases. Studies have revealed that curcumin has the potential to augment antitumor activity of PD-1/PD-L1 blockage by significantly reducing the expression of PD-L1 in treated cells [95]. Tregs (Regulatory T cells) is an immune-suppressive group of T cells subgroup observed in surroundings of cancer tissues were often increased in cancers [96]. Furthermore, curcumin treatment were found augment the immune response to cancers by increasing CD8+ (Cluster of Differentiation 8) T cells and diminishing Tregs and Myeloid-derived suppressor cells (MDSCs). Thus, curcumin could be useful as an adjuvant for immunotherapy for patients with malignant diseases [1].

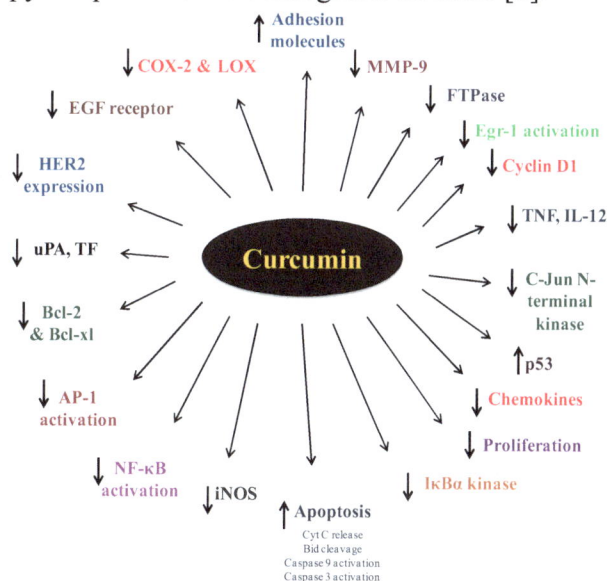

Fig. (4). Multitargeted anticancer activity of curcumin [adopted from 12]. Curcumin was found to show its anticancer activity by targeting multiple cancer target proteins as evidenced from the results of both the preclinical and clinical studies.

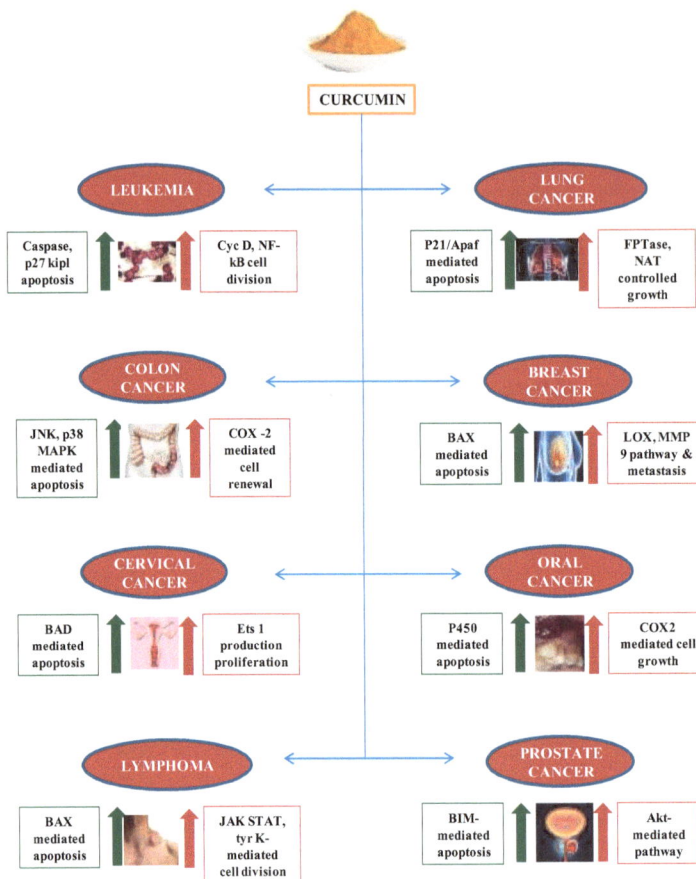

Fig. (5). Targeted signaling pathways by curcumin in anticancer therapy (adopted from reference [87]). Curcumin upregulates/downregulates different signaling pathways in cervical, colorectal, oral, leukemia, lymphoma, prostrate and breast cancers.

Shah *et al.* reported that curcumin could synergistically combine with chemo-therapeutic drug cytarabine or ara-C to impede the multiplication of tumor cells by MDR genes down regulation in primary leukemia [97]. The inhibition of cancer by curcumin is operated in a multi targeted fashion targeting growth factor, transcription factors, kinases and cell proliferation proteins. In cancer cells, the anticancer and anti-metastatic activities of this yellow flavonoid were expressed by inhibiting growth factors (EGF, FGF, VEGF, TGF-b1, HGF, PDGF); transcription factors (PPAR-gamma, EpRE, p53, STATs, HIF-1, b-catenin, NFkb, ERE, AP-1), protein kinases (MAPK, JNK, AMPK, Akt) and cell proliferation proteins (c-myc, cyclin D1). Reduction of tumor metastasis by curcumin has a remarkable significance on cancer therapy [98].

Next to the anti-metastatic activity, anti-angiogenic property of an antitumor drug is an important feature of its antitumor potential. VEGF and MMPs contribute to the tumor angiogenesis and tumor invasion. VEGF pathways promote angiogenesis and MMPs facilitate tumor invasion to ECM (extra cellular matrix). Studies revealed that curcumin administration suppressed VEGFs and MMPs indicating the suppression of cancer angiogenesis and progression [99].

Combination Therapies of Curcumin with other Drugs

Many recent researches have reported synergistic actions of curcumin and anticancer drugs, pharmacological agents and phytochemicals.

Many reports suggest that curcumin could augment the effect of chemotherapeutic chemicals in multidrug resistant tumors. Curcumin administration increased the sensitivity of various cancer cells for radio and chemotherapies [100]. Zhou *et al.* stated the sensitivity of breast and lung malignant cells for paclitaxel, cisplatin and doxorubicin treatments was improved by curcumin administration [94].

Co-administration of *Curcuma longa* extracts with chemotherapeutic drugs cisplatin, 5-fluorouracil and docetaxel demonstrated synergistic effects between these drug combinations with a significant improvement in the survival rate than the placebo. Similarly, in a study, on oxaliplatin-resistant tumor mice, combination of curcumin and oxaliplatin showed significant tumor inhibiting effects [101]. In another study, combination of curcumin with a similar anticancer flavonoid quercetin increased the cancer inhibiting effect than the single treatments by inhibiting the anti-apoptotic pathways and phosphorylation of ERK and Akt [102]. Nanoparticles of curcumin have shown to improve the anticancer properties of curcumin. In a research report by Chaurasia *et al.* [103], the polymeric curcumin nanoparticles exhibited a significant improvement in the bioavailability in animal models further increasing the antitumor activity by reducing tumor growth and increasing the survival rate of animals. A novel structural analogue of curcumin, Dehydrozingerone showed accumulation of intracellular ROS, inhibition of cell cycle at G2/M phase and upregulation of p21 genes in HT-29 cells, suggesting the anticancer potential of curcumin analogues in large bowel cancer [104].

In photodynamic therapy of cancer, the internal molecular resonance stability of curcumin helped to give better results suggesting the photosensitizing activity of curcumin [105, 106]. In a study by Yue *et al*, the turmerones present in turmeric extract facilitated the colonic infiltration of curcumin which in turn contributed the increased antitumor effects on colon cancer induced animals [107].

Curcumin Analogs and Cancer Stem Cells

Curcumin and its analogs were reported to express its cytotoxic action against various cancer stem cells such as colon, breast, pancreas, brain, bladder, and lung cancer stem cells. Few notable works of curcumin on cancer stem cells were briefly summarized in Table **2**.

Table 2. Effect of curcumin and curcumin analogs on cancer stem cells.

S.No.	Curcumin/ Curcumin Analogs	Cancer Type	References
1	Difluorinated- curcumin	Colon CSC	[108]
2	Curcumin and FOLFOX combination	Colon CSC	[109]
3	Curcumin polymeric nanoparticles formulation	Malignant brain tumor	[110]
4	Micelle formulation of curcumin	Colon CSC	[111]
5	Curcumin combination with gemicitabine	Pancreatic cancer patients (Phase 1/II trials)	[112]
6	Docetaxel and curcumin combination	Metastatic breast cancer patients (Phase I trial)	[113]
7	Oral curcumin	High risk patients with pre-malignant lesions (Phase I trial)	[114]
8	GO-Y030 – curcumin analog	Colon CSC	[115]
9	Curcumin	Colon CSC	[116]
10	Curcumin	Bladder CSC	[52]
11	Curcumin	Lung CSC	[55]
12	Curcumin in combination with irinotecan	Colon CSC	[117]

CHALLENGES IN TURMERIC AND CURCUMIN TREATMENTS

Although curcumin's potential in cancer chemoprevention and chemotherapy was affirmed by plenty of preclinical and clinical studies, there are some concerns regarding the bioavailability and poor water solubility (about 11 ng/mL) of curcumin following the oral ingestion. Studies revealed that oral administration of curcumin resulted in poor retention and intestinal absorption with a large excretion of unabsorbed curcumin in the feces. The very low amounts of ingested curcumin in turn is metabolized rapidly resulting in the non- availability of curcumin for action limiting its application as cancer drug [25, 118]. However, curcumin is hydrophobic and hence it can be easily transported through the cell membranes. The minimal amounts of free curcumin absorbed in turn will be easily degraded in the alkaline pH reducing its bioavailability further. Hence, an increased dose is always required for exhibiting a possible therapeutic action

[119 - 122]. Intraperitoneal (i.p.) or intravenous (i.v.) injections of curcumin also result in the excretion of it through bile as tetrahydrocurcumin glucuronide and hexahydrocurcumin derivatives [123, 124]. To manage these practical limitations for the bioavailability, numerous approaches have been adopted to enhance its systemic absorption [125]. Various formulations of curcumin such as curcumin nanoparticles, curcumin phosphor lipid complexes, liposomes and curcumin anolgues were developed in the recent decades to enhance its systemic bioavailability [25].

Curcumin also has certain other limitations in clinical trials. Several phase I clinical studies have clearly showed the safety efficacy of its oral form. However, there are a couple of studies that have indicated potential caution with curcumin's use in the clinical trials. It was found that high concentrations of curcumin could potentially induce the depletion of glutathione, liver toxicity and activation of caspases [126]. Another research reported that curcumin can interfere with systemic iron metabolism by repressing hepcidin synthesis, indicating limited application of curcumin in cancer patients who are affected with chronic anemia or with marginal iron stores [127]. Administration of curcumin with other chemotherapeutic drugs is an alternative approach for effective utilization [81, 128, 129]. Nanoparticles of curcumin, synthesis of curcumin analogues and adjuvant therapy also would help to balance the challenges of curcumin and turmeric anticancer treatments. Piperine, a phytochemical was used as an adjuvant with curcumin which resulted in an increased bioavailability of curcumin by 20 times with an elevated anticancer effect of curcumin [130, 131]. The effects of curcumin and its formulations in clinical trials of various cancers were summarized in Table **3**. Besides these limitations, literature shows the safety of curcumin in clinical studies, as novel preparations of curcumin allow superior absorption and consequently improved the efficacy in cancer treatments.

Table 3. A review on various clinical trials on curcumin in various cancers [132].

S.No.	Curcumin/Curcumin Formulations Used	Administration Route	Cancer Type Investigated	Duration	Overall Effect	Adverse Side Effects
1	Curcumin capsules (500mg) combined with Docetaxal	-	Breast cancer	1.5 months	Positive	Nil
2	Curcumin capsule (18 mg) and curcumin derivative (Desmetoxy curcumin-2mg) suspended in curcumin oil	Oral	Colon cancer	1 month	Positive	Nil
3	Capsules of curcumin c3 complex (0.4g/day)	Oral	Colon cancer	1 week followed by surgery	Positive	Nil

(Table 3) cont.....

S.No.	Curcumin/Curcumin Formulations Used	Administration Route	Cancer Type Investigated	Duration	Overall Effect	Adverse Side Effects
4	Curcumin capsules (2-4g/day)	Oral	Colon cancer	1 month	Positive	Nil
5	Capsules of curcumin c3 complex	Oral	Colon cancer	4 months	Positive	Nil
6	Oxy curcumin (480 mg) with quercetin (20 mg) in tablets form	Oral	Colon cancer	9 months maximum	Positive	Nil
7	Curcumin capsule (360 mg)	Oral	Colon cancer	1 month	Positive	Nil
8	Curcumin (100mg) with Soy isoflavones (40mg) as food supplements	Oral	Prostate cancer	6 months	Positive	Nil
9	Curcumin (750 mg) in tablet form	Oral	Lung cancer	1 month	Positive	Nil
10	Curcumin (900 mg) with bidesmethoxycurcumin and desmethoxy curcumin combinations. Altogether not exceeding 8g/day. Capsule form		Pancreatic cancer	2 months	Positive	Nil
11	Curcumin (900 mg) with bidesmethoxycurcumin and desmethoxy curcumin combinations. Altogether not exceeding 8g/day. Treated in combination with germicitabine	Oral	Pancreatic cancer	1 year	Positive	Nil
12	Curcumin with bidesmethoxycurcumin and desmethoxy curcumin (450 mg, 20mg and 40 mg respectively). Combined with germicitabine. Capsule form	Oral	Pancreatic cancer	1.5 months	No positive effect	Abdominal discomfort and pain felt in few patients
13	Theocurcumin (400 mg/ day maximum). Combined with germicitabine	Oral	Pancreatic cancer	Not applicable	Positive effect	Abdominal discomfort and pain felt in few patients
14	Curcumin chewable tablets (1g)	Oral	Head and neck cancer	1 day	Positive	Nil

(Table 3) cont.....

S.No.	Curcumin/Curcumin Formulations Used	Administration Route	Cancer Type Investigated	Duration	Overall Effect	Adverse Side Effects
15	Curcumin c3 complex tablets with bidesmethoxycurcumin and desmethoxy curcumin (900mg, 20mg, 80 mg respectively)	Oral	Multiple myeloma	1 year	Positive	Not investigated
16	Ointment containing curcumin	Topical application	Skin lesions	Not applicable	Positive	99% Nil except 1 patient
17	Curcumin tablets (8g maximum)	Oral	Skin lesions	3 months	Positive	Nil
18	Turmeric oil, resin and extract (600mg, 600mg and 3g respectively) in capsule form	Oral	Skin lesions	3 months	Positive	Not investigated
19	Curcumin with desmethoxycurcumin and bidesmethoxycurcumin (900mg, 80mg and 20 mg respectively)	Oral	Skin lesions	1 week	Positive	Not investigated

FUTURE PROSPECTS

Due to its many promising therapeutic potentials, various pharmaceutical and cosmetic firms make multiple products like tablets, coloring agents, ointments, tablets, energy beverages, extracts, gels, soap, cosmetics, nasal sprays and creams using curcumin and other turmeric compounds [23]. Curcumin treatment was found to be beneficial in many cancers including colon, lung, breast, cervical, pancreatic, colon and gastric cancers and with less or no side effects. Inhalable curcumin combinations were successfully synthesized and tested for positive therapeutic results in lung cancer. Clinical trials done earlier using curcumin on breast, pancreatic, colorectal cancers and myeloma showed promising results both on sides of treatment and patient survival. Various formulations of curcumin like ointment, capsules, tablets, oral supplements were used in the clinical trials [103]. This suggests the possible use of curcumin in clinics for various cancer treatments. Hence, the practice of curcumin as a potential agent for anticancer therapy will be a promising strategy. The research findings from various reports as mentioned above, have kindled the possibility of using curcumin in single and combination treatments along with drugs and other treatment strategies like radiotherapy or immunotherapy.

CONCLUDING REMARKS

Turmeric is an important and remarkable nutraceutical in view of its safety and health beneficial actions on health. In this chapter, the phytochemistry of turmeric and curcumin, its pharmacological effects, phytochemistry, structure activity relationship, antioxidant and pro-oxidant activities, potential anticancer activities, signaling mechanism and anticancer cellular targets, its effect in combination therapies, challenges and future prospects of curcumin treatments in cancer were briefly presented. The studies displayed here demonstrated the potential efficacy of turmeric, as a whole drug or its active constituent curcumin for cancer treatments. As reported in this review, several reports confirmed the effects of curcumin, on various diseases and different types of cancers. Based on these evidence, it can be concluded that treatment using curcumin can have a positive influence on various anticancer agents, chemotherapeutic drug combinations, radiotherapy, and photodynamic therapy of cancer(s). In a few clinical trials, it was often observed that the negative results were always associated with the poor bioavailability of curcumin [133]. Also, recently many efforts have been attempted to enhance the oral delivery and bioavailability of curcumin. The main limitations of curcumin delivery were its low bioavailability, solubility and metabolic stability. Many alternative suggestions were carried out to overcome these drawbacks. The usage of different carrier systems, adjuvants, enhanced specific formulations, curcumin nanoparticles, phospholipid complexes of curcumin, association with metabolic inhibitors, co-administration with similar natural products and chemotherapeutic drugs could offer promising results facilitating its application further towards treating chronic diseases like cancer. On a big picture, the highly promiscuous nature of curcumin increases its probability of a potent novel anticancer medicine of the future.

CONSENT FOR PUBLICATION

Not Applicable.

CONFLICT OF INTEREST

The author declares that there is no conflict of interest in this chapter.

ACKNOWLEDGEMENTS

This work is based on the research supported by the South African Research Chairs Initiative of the Department of Science and Technology and National Research Foundation of South Africa (Grant No. 98337). The authors sincerely thank the University of Johannesburg, South Africa for their support.

REFERENCES

[1]   Weng W, Goel A. Curcumin and colorectal cancer: An update and current perspective on this natural medicine. Semin Cancer Biol 2020; S1044-579X(20): 30044-4.
[http://dx.doi.org/10.1016/j.semcancer.2020.02.011]

[2]   Kalra EK. Nutraceutical--definition and introduction. AAPS PharmSci 2003; 5(3): E25.
[http://dx.doi.org/10.1208/ps050325] [PMID: 14621960]

[3]   Pandey M, Verma RK, Saraf SA. Nutraceuticals: new era of medicine and health. Asian J Pharm Clin Res 2010; 3(1): 11-5.

[4]   Hanahan D, Weinberg RA. Hallmarks of cancer: the next generation. Cell 2011; 144(5): 646-74.
[http://dx.doi.org/10.1016/j.cell.2011.02.013] [PMID: 21376230]

[5]   Sa G, Das T. Anti cancer effects of curcumin: cycle of life and death. Cell Div 2008; 3(1): 14.
[http://dx.doi.org/10.1186/1747-1028-3-14] [PMID: 18834508]

[6]   Bidram E, Esmaeili Y, Ranji-Burachaloo H, *et al.* A concise review on cancer treatment methods and delivery systems. J Drug Deliv Sci Technol 2019; 54: 101350.
[http://dx.doi.org/10.1016/j.jddst.2019.101350]

[7]   Das T, Sa G, Saha B, Das K. Multifocal signal modulation therapy of cancer: ancient weapon, modern targets. Mol Cell Biochem 2010; 336(1-2): 85-95.
[http://dx.doi.org/10.1007/s11010-009-0269-0] [PMID: 19826768]

[8]   Bose S, Panda AK, Mukherjee S, Sa G. Curcumin and tumor immune-editing: resurrecting the immune system. Cell Div 2015; 10(1): 6.
[http://dx.doi.org/10.1186/s13008-015-0012-z] [PMID: 26464579]

[9]   Iranshahi M, Sahebkar A, Takasaki M, Konoshima T, Tokuda H. Cancer chemopreventive activity of the prenylated coumarin, umbelliprenin, *in vivo*. Eur J Cancer Prev 2009; 18(5): 412-5.
[http://dx.doi.org/10.1097/CEJ.0b013e32832c389e] [PMID: 19531956]

[10]   Zhang CY, Zhang L, Yu HX, Bao JD, Lu RR. Curcumin inhibits the metastasis of K1 papillary thyroid cancer cells *via* modulating E-cadherin and matrix metalloproteinase-9 expression. Biotechnol Lett 2013; 35(7): 995-1000.
[http://dx.doi.org/10.1007/s10529-013-1173-y] [PMID: 23474829]

[11]   Lai CS, Ho CT, Pan MH. The cancer chemopreventive and therapeutic potential of tetrahydrocurcumin. Biomolecules 2020; 10(6): 831.
[http://dx.doi.org/10.3390/biom10060831] [PMID: 32486019]

[12]   Aggarwal BB, Kumar A, Bharti AC. Anticancer potential of curcumin: preclinical and clinical studies. 2003; 1;23(1/A): 363-98.

[13]   Peng S, Li Z, Zou L, Liu W, Liu C, McClements DJ. Enhancement of curcumin bioavailability by encapsulation in sophorolipid-coated nanoparticles: an *in vitro* and *in vivo* study. J Agric Food Chem 2018; 66(6): 1488-97.
[http://dx.doi.org/10.1021/acs.jafc.7b05478] [PMID: 29378117]

[14]   Nelson KM, Dahlin JL, Bisson J, Graham J, Pauli GF, Walters MA. The essential medicinal chemistry of curcumin: miniperspective. J Med Chem 2017; 60(5): 1620-37.
[http://dx.doi.org/10.1021/acs.jmedchem.6b00975] [PMID: 28074653]

[15]   Mahran RI, Hagras MM, Sun D, Brenner DE. Bringing curcumin to the clinic in cancer prevention: a review of strategies to enhance bioavailability and efficacy. AAPS J 2017; 19(1): 54-81.
[http://dx.doi.org/10.1208/s12248-016-0003-2] [PMID: 27783266]

[16]   Shehzad A, Qureshi M, Anwar MN, Lee YS. Multifunctional curcumin mediate multitherapeutic effects. J Food Sci 2017; 82(9): 2006-15.
[http://dx.doi.org/10.1111/1750-3841.13793] [PMID: 28771714]

[17]   Shishodia S, Misra K, Aggarwal BB. Turmeric as cure-cumin: promises, problems, and solutions. In: Dong Z, Surh YJ. Dietary modulation of cell signaling pathways. Boca Raton: CRC Press 2008; pp. 91-136.
[http://dx.doi.org/10.1201/9780849381492.ch4]

[18]   Nair A, Amalraj A, Jacob J, Kunnumakkara AB, Gopi S. Non-curcuminoids from turmeric and their potential in cancer therapy and anticancer drug delivery formulations. Biomolecules 2019; 9(1): 13.
[http://dx.doi.org/10.3390/biom9010013] [PMID: 30609771]

[19]   Kunnumakkara AB, Bordoloi D, Padmavathi G, *et al.* Curcumin, the golden nutraceutical: multitargeting for multiple chronic diseases. Br J Pharmacol 2017; 174(11): 1325-48.
[http://dx.doi.org/10.1111/bph.13621] [PMID: 27638428]

[20]   Teymouri M, Pirro M, Johnston TP, Sahebkar A. Curcumin as a multifaceted compound against human papilloma virus infection and cervical cancers: A review of chemistry, cellular, molecular, and preclinical features. Biofactors 2017; 43(3): 331-46.
[http://dx.doi.org/10.1002/biof.1344] [PMID: 27896883]

[21]   Golonko A, Lewandowska H, Świsłocka R, Jasińska UT, Priebe W, Lewandowski W. Curcumin as tyrosine kinase inhibitor in cancer treatment. Eur J Med Chem 2019; 181: 111512.
[http://dx.doi.org/10.1016/j.ejmech.2019.07.015] [PMID: 31404861]

[22]   Hewlings SJ, Douglas S. Kalman. curcumin: a review of its' effects on human health. Foods 2017; 6: 10-92.
[http://dx.doi.org/10.3390/foods6100092]

[23]   Gupta SC, Patchva S, Aggarwal BB. Therapeutic roles of curcumin: lessons learned from clinical trials. AAPS J 2013; 15(1): 195-218.
[http://dx.doi.org/10.1208/s12248-012-9432-8] [PMID: 23143785]

[24]   Gupta SC, Kismali G, Aggarwal BB. Curcumin, a component of turmeric: from farm to pharmacy. Biofactors 2013; 39(1): 2-13.
[http://dx.doi.org/10.1002/biof.1079] [PMID: 23339055]

[25]   Anand P, Kunnumakkara AB, Newman RA, Aggarwal BB. Bioavailability of curcumin: problems and promises. Mol Pharm 2007; 4(6): 807-18.
[http://dx.doi.org/10.1021/mp700113r] [PMID: 17999464]

[26]   Kim JH, Gupta SC, Park B, Yadav VR, Aggarwal BB. Turmeric (*Curcuma longa*) inhibits inflammatory nuclear factor (NF)-κB and NF-κB-regulated gene products and induces death receptors leading to suppressed proliferation, induced chemosensitization, and suppressed osteoclastogenesis. Mol Nutr Food Res 2012; 56(3): 454-65.
[http://dx.doi.org/10.1002/mnfr.201100270] [PMID: 22147524]

[27]   Yue GG, Kwok HF, Lee JK, *et al.* Combined therapy using bevacizumab and turmeric ethanolic extract (with absorbable curcumin) exhibited beneficial efficacy in colon cancer mice. Pharmacol Res 2016; 111: 43-57.
[http://dx.doi.org/10.1016/j.phrs.2016.05.025] [PMID: 27241019]

[28]   Johnson JJ, Mukhtar H. Curcumin for chemoprevention of colon cancer. Cancer Lett 2007; 255(2): 170-81.
[http://dx.doi.org/10.1016/j.canlet.2007.03.005] [PMID: 17448598]

[29]   Park SY, Jin ML, Kim YH, Kim Y, Lee SJ. Anti-inflammatory effects of aromatic-turmerone through blocking of NF-κB, JNK, and p38 MAPK signaling pathways in amyloid β-stimulated microglia. Int Immunopharmacol 2012; 14(1): 13-20.
[http://dx.doi.org/10.1016/j.intimp.2012.06.003] [PMID: 22728094]

[30]   Parian AM, Limketkai BN, Shah ND, Mullin GE. Nutraceutical supplements for inflammatory bowel disease. Nutr Clin Pract 2015; 30(4): 551-8.
[http://dx.doi.org/10.1177/0884533615586598] [PMID: 26024677]

[31]   Zhu J, Sanidad KZ, Sukamtoh E, Zhang G. Potential roles of chemical degradation in the biological activities of curcumin. Food Funct 2017; 8(3): 907-14.
[http://dx.doi.org/10.1039/C6FO01770C] [PMID: 28138677]

[32]   Aggarwal BB, Yuan W, Li S, Gupta SC. Curcumin-free turmeric exhibits anti-inflammatory and anticancer activities: Identification of novel components of turmeric. Mol Nutr Food Res 2013; 57(9): 1529-42.
[http://dx.doi.org/10.1002/mnfr.201200838] [PMID: 23847105]

[33]   Priyadarsini KI. Chemical and structural features influencing the biological activity of curcumin. Curr Pharm Des 2013; 19(11): 2093-100.
[PMID: 23116315]

[34]   Srichairatanakool S, Thephinlap C, Phisalaphong C, Porter JB, Fucharoen S. Curcumin contributes to *in vitro* removal of non-transferrin bound iron by deferiprone and desferrioxamine in thalassemic plasma. Med Chem 2007; 3(5): 469-74.
[http://dx.doi.org/10.2174/157340607781745447] [PMID: 17897073]

[35]   Teiten MH, Dicato M, Diederich M. Hybrid curcumin compounds: a new strategy for cancer treatment. Molecules 2014; 19(12): 20839-63.
[http://dx.doi.org/10.3390/molecules191220839] [PMID: 25514225]

[36]   Hu RW, Carey EJ, Lindor KD, Tabibian JH. Curcumin in hepatobiliary disease: pharmacotherapeutic properties and emerging potential clinical applications. Ann Hepatol 2017; 16(6): 835-41.
[http://dx.doi.org/10.5604/01.3001.0010.5273] [PMID: 29055920]

[37]   Revathy S, Elumalai S, Antony MB. Isolation, purification and identification of curcuminoids from turmeric (*Curcuma longa* L.) by column chromatography. J Exp Sci 2011; 2.

[38]   Manente L, Lucariello A, Costanzo C, *et al.* Suppression of pre adipocyte differentiation and promotion of adipocyte death by anti-HIV drugs. In Vivo 2012; 26(2): 287-91.
[PMID: 22351671]

[39]   Willenbacher E, Khan SZ, Mujica SCA, *et al.* Curcumin: new insights into an ancient ingredient against cancer. Int J Mol Sci 2019; 20(8): 1808.
[http://dx.doi.org/10.3390/ijms20081808] [PMID: 31013694]

[40]   Gonçalves PB, Romeiro NC. Multi-target natural products as alternatives against oxidative stress in Chronic Obstructive Pulmonary Disease (COPD). Eur J Med Chem 2019; 163: 911-31.
[http://dx.doi.org/10.1016/j.ejmech.2018.12.020] [PMID: 30612088]

[41]   Khan H, Ullah H, Nabavi SM. Mechanistic insights of hepatoprotective effects of curcumin: Therapeutic updates and future prospects. Food Chem Toxicol 2019; 124: 182-91.
[http://dx.doi.org/10.1016/j.fct.2018.12.002] [PMID: 30529260]

[42]   Chen CY, Kao CL, Liu CM. The cancer prevention, anti-inflammatory and anti-oxidation of bioactive phytochemicals targeting the TLR4 signaling pathway. Int J Mol Sci 2018; 19(9): 2729.
[http://dx.doi.org/10.3390/ijms19092729] [PMID: 30213077]

[43]   Chandran B, Goel A. A randomized, pilot study to assess the efficacy and safety of curcumin in patients with active rheumatoid arthritis. Phytother Res 2012; 26(11): 1719-25.
[http://dx.doi.org/10.1002/ptr.4639] [PMID: 22407780]

[44]   Sanmukhani J, Satodia V, Trivedi J, *et al.* Efficacy and safety of curcumin in major depressive disorder: a randomized controlled trial. Phytother Res 2014; 28(4): 579-85.
[http://dx.doi.org/10.1002/ptr.5025] [PMID: 23832433]

[45]   Shehzad A, Rehman G, Lee YS. Curcumin in inflammatory diseases. Biofactors 2013; 39(1): 69-77.
[http://dx.doi.org/10.1002/biof.1066] [PMID: 23281076]

[46]   Karlstetter M, Lippe E, Walczak Y, *et al.* Curcumin is a potent modulator of microglial gene expression and migration. J Neuroinflammation 2011; 8(1): 125.

[http://dx.doi.org/10.1186/1742-2094-8-125] [PMID: 21958395]

[47]   Lavoie S, Chen Y, Dalton TP, *et al.* Curcumin, quercetin, and tBHQ modulate glutathione levels in astrocytes and neurons: importance of the glutamate cysteine ligase modifier subunit. J Neurochem 2009; 108(6): 1410-22.
[http://dx.doi.org/10.1111/j.1471-4159.2009.05908.x] [PMID: 19183254]

[48]   Mirzaei H, Naseri G, Rezaee R, *et al.* Curcumin: A new candidate for melanoma therapy? Int J Cancer 2016; 139(8): 1683-95.
[http://dx.doi.org/10.1002/ijc.30224] [PMID: 27280688]

[49]   Bimonte S, Barbieri A, Leongito M, *et al.* Curcumin anticancer studies in pancreatic cancer. Nutrients 2016; 8(7): 433.
[http://dx.doi.org/10.3390/nu8070433] [PMID: 27438851]

[50]   Chauhan DP. Chemotherapeutic potential of curcumin for colorectal cancer. Curr Pharm Des 2002; 8(19): 1695-706.
[http://dx.doi.org/10.2174/1381612023394016] [PMID: 12171541]

[51]   Sordillo LA, Sordillo PP, Helson L. Curcumin for the treatment of glioblastoma. Anticancer Res 2015; 35(12): 6373-8.
[PMID: 26637846]

[52]   Wang D, Kong X, Li Y, *et al.* Curcumin inhibits bladder cancer stem cells by suppressing Sonic Hedgehog pathway. Biochem Biophys Res Commun 2017; 493(1): 521-7.
[http://dx.doi.org/10.1016/j.bbrc.2017.08.158] [PMID: 28870814]

[53]   Shi J, Wang Y, Jia Z, Gao Y, Zhao C, Yao Y. Curcumin inhibits bladder cancer progression *via* regulation of β-catenin expression. Tumour Biol 2017; 39(7): 1010428317702548.
[http://dx.doi.org/10.1177/1010428317702548] [PMID: 28705118]

[54]   Zhang L, Yang G, Zhang R, *et al.* Curcumin inhibits cell proliferation and motility *via* suppression of TROP2 in bladder cancer cells. Int J Oncol 2018; 53(2): 515-26.
[http://dx.doi.org/10.3892/ijo.2018.4423] [PMID: 29901071]

[55]   Zhu JY, Yang X, Chen Y, *et al.* Curcumin suppresses lung cancer stem cells *via* inhibiting Wnt/β catenin and sonic hedgehog pathways. Phytother Res 2017; 31(4): 680-8.
[http://dx.doi.org/10.1002/ptr.5791] [PMID: 28198062]

[56]   Wang JY, Wang X, Wang XJ, *et al.* Curcumin inhibits the growth via Wnt/β-catenin pathway in non-small-cell lung cancer cells. Eur Rev Med Pharmacol Sci 2018; 22(21): 7492-9.
[PMID: 30468498]

[57]   Chen P, Huang HP, Wang Y, *et al.* Curcumin overcome primary gefitinib resistance in non-small-cell lung cancer cells through inducing autophagy-related cell death. J Exp Clin Cancer Res 2019; 38(1): 254.
[http://dx.doi.org/10.1186/s13046-019-1234-8] [PMID: 31196210]

[58]   Hu C, Li M, Guo T, *et al.* Anti-metastasis activity of curcumin against breast cancer *via* the inhibition of stem cell-like properties and EMT. Phytomedicine 2019; 58: 152740.
[http://dx.doi.org/10.1016/j.phymed.2018.11.001] [PMID: 31005718]

[59]   Calaf GM, Ponce-Cusi R, Carrión F. Curcumin and paclitaxel induce cell death in breast cancer cell lines. Oncol Rep 2018; 40(4): 2381-8.
[http://dx.doi.org/10.3892/or.2018.6603] [PMID: 30066930]

[60]   Coker-Gurkan A, Celik M, Ugur M, *et al.* Curcumin inhibits autocrine growth hormone-mediated invasion and metastasis by targeting NF-κB signaling and polyamine metabolism in breast cancer cells. Amino Acids 2018; 50(8): 1045-69.
[http://dx.doi.org/10.1007/s00726-018-2581-z] [PMID: 29770869]

[61]   Li M, Yue GG, Tsui SK, Fung KP, Lau CB. Turmeric extract, with absorbable curcumin, has potent anti-metastatic effect *in vitro* and *in vivo*. Phytomedicine 2018; 46: 131-41.

[http://dx.doi.org/10.1016/j.phymed.2018.03.065] [PMID: 30097113]

[62]   Liao W, Xiang W, Wang FF, Wang R, Ding Y. Curcumin inhibited growth of human melanoma A375 cells *via* inciting oxidative stress. Biomed Pharmacother 2017; 95: 1177-86.
[http://dx.doi.org/10.1016/j.biopha.2017.09.026] [PMID: 28926928]

[63]   Kocyigit A, Guler EM. Curcumin induce DNA damage and apoptosis through generation of reactive oxygen species and reducing mitochondrial membrane potential in melanoma cancer cells. Cell Mol Biol 2017; 63(11): 97-105.
[http://dx.doi.org/10.14715/cmb/2017.63.11.17] [PMID: 29208180]

[64]   Parashar K, Sood S, Mehaidli A, *et al.* Evaluating the anti-cancer efficacy of a synthetic curcumin analog on human melanoma cells and its interaction with standard chemotherapeutics. Molecules 2019; 24(13): 2483.
[http://dx.doi.org/10.3390/molecules24132483] [PMID: 31284561]

[65]   Liu LD, Pang YX, Zhao XR, *et al.* Curcumin induces apoptotic cell death and protective autophagy by inhibiting AKT/mTOR/p70S6K pathway in human ovarian cancer cells. Arch Gynecol Obstet 2019; 299(6): 1627-39.
[http://dx.doi.org/10.1007/s00404-019-05058-3] [PMID: 31006841]

[66]   Koroth J, Nirgude S, Tiwari S, *et al.* Investigation of anti-cancer and migrastatic properties of novel curcumin derivatives on breast and ovarian cancer cell lines. BMC Complement Altern Med 2019; 19(1): 273.
[http://dx.doi.org/10.1186/s12906-019-2685-3] [PMID: 31638975]

[67]   Zhao MD, Li JQ, Chen FY, *et al.* Co-Delivery of curcumin and paclitaxel by "core-shell" targeting amphiphilic copolymer to reverse resistance in the treatment of ovarian cancer. Int J Nanomedicine 2019; 14: 9453-67.
[http://dx.doi.org/10.2147/IJN.S224579] [PMID: 31819443]

[68]   Aedo-Aguilera V, Carrillo-Beltrán D, Calaf GM, *et al.* Curcumin decreases epithelial-mesenchymal transition by a Pirin-dependent mechanism in cervical cancer cells. Oncol Rep 2019; 42(5): 2139-48.
[http://dx.doi.org/10.3892/or.2019.7288] [PMID: 31436299]

[69]   Ghasemi F, Shafiee M, Banikazemi Z, *et al.* Curcumin inhibits NF-kB and Wnt/β-catenin pathways in cervical cancer cells. Pathol Res Pract 2019; 215(10): 152556.
[http://dx.doi.org/10.1016/j.prp.2019.152556] [PMID: 31358480]

[70]   Klinger NV, Mittal S. Therapeutic potential of curcumin for the treatment of brain tumors. Oxid Med Cell Longev 2016; 2016: 9324085.
[http://dx.doi.org/10.1155/2016/9324085] [PMID: 27807473]

[71]   Ide H, Lu Y, Noguchi T, *et al.* Modulation of AKR1C2 by curcumin decreases testosterone production in prostate cancer. Cancer Sci 2018; 109(4): 1230-8.
[http://dx.doi.org/10.1111/cas.13517] [PMID: 29369461]

[72]   Zhao W, Zhou X, Qi G, Guo Y. Curcumin suppressed the prostate cancer by inhibiting JNK pathways *via* epigenetic regulation. J Biochem Mol Toxicol 2018; 32(5): e22049.
[http://dx.doi.org/10.1002/jbt.22049] [PMID: 29485738]

[73]   Liu T, Chi H, Chen J, *et al.* Curcumin suppresses proliferation and *in vitro* invasion of human prostate cancer stem cells by ceRNA effect of miR-145 and lncRNA-ROR. Gene 2017; 631: 29-38.
[http://dx.doi.org/10.1016/j.gene.2017.08.008] [PMID: 28843521]

[74]   Lindsay C, Kostiuk M, Conrad D, *et al.* Antitumour effects of metformin and curcumin in human papillomavirus positive and negative head and neck cancer cells. Mol Carcinog 2019; 58(11): 1946-59.
[http://dx.doi.org/10.1002/mc.23087] [PMID: 31338907]

[75]   Boven L, Holmes SP, Latimer B, *et al.* Curcumin gum formulation for prevention of oral cavity head and neck squamous cell carcinoma. Laryngoscope 2019; 129(7): 1597-603.

[http://dx.doi.org/10.1002/lary.27542] [PMID: 30421467]

[76] Delavarian Z, Pakfetrat A, Ghazi A, *et al.* Oral administration of nanomicelle curcumin in the prevention of radiotherapy-induced mucositis in head and neck cancers. Spec Care Dentist 2019; 39(2): 166-72.
      [http://dx.doi.org/10.1111/scd.12358] [PMID: 30761565]

[77] Yoshida K, Toden S, Ravindranathan P, Han H, Goel A. Curcumin sensitizes pancreatic cancer cells to gemcitabine by attenuating PRC2 subunit EZH2, and the lncRNA PVT1 expression. Carcinogenesis 2017; 38(10): 1036-46.
      [http://dx.doi.org/10.1093/carcin/bgx065] [PMID: 29048549]

[78] Zheng BZ, Liu TD, Chen G, Zhang JX, Kang X. The effect of curcumin on cell adhesion of human esophageal cancer cell. Eur Rev Med Pharmacol Sci 2018; 22(2): 551-60.
      [PMID: 29424917]

[79] Liu W, Huang M, Zou Q, Lin W. Curcumin suppresses gastric cancer biological activity by regulation of miRNA-21: an *in vitro* study. Int J Clin Exp Pathol 2018; 11(12): 5820-9.
      [PMID: 31949668]

[80] Wang XM, Zhang QZ, Yang J, *et al.* Validated HPLC–MS/MS method for simultaneous determination of curcumin and piperine in human plasma. Trop J Pharm Res 2012; 11(4): 621-9.
      [http://dx.doi.org/10.4314/tjpr.v11i4.13]

[81] Sankpal UT, Nagaraju GP, Gottipolu SR, *et al.* Combination of tolfenamic acid and curcumin induces colon cancer cell growth inhibition through modulating specific transcription factors and reactive oxygen species. Oncotarget 2016; 7(3): 3186-200.
      [http://dx.doi.org/10.18632/oncotarget.6553] [PMID: 26672603]

[82] Zhu J, Zhao B, Xiong P, *et al.* Curcumin induces autophagy *via* inhibition of yes-associated protein (YAP) in human colon cancer cells. Med Sci Monit 2018; 24: 7035-42.
      [http://dx.doi.org/10.12659/MSM.910650] [PMID: 30281585]

[83] Hossain DM, Bhattacharyya S, Das T, Sa G. Curcumin: the multi-targeted therapy for cancer regression. Front Biosci (Schol Ed) 2012; 4: 335-55.
      [http://dx.doi.org/10.2741/s272] [PMID: 22202064]

[84] Wilken R, Veena MS, Wang MB, Srivatsan ES. Curcumin: A review of anti-cancer properties and therapeutic activity in head and neck squamous cell carcinoma. Mol Cancer 2011; 10(1): 12.
      [http://dx.doi.org/10.1186/1476-4598-10-12] [PMID: 21299897]

[85] Mirzaei H, Masoudifar A, Sahebkar A, *et al.* MicroRNA: A novel target of curcumin in cancer therapy. J Cell Physiol 2018; 233(4): 3004-15.
      [http://dx.doi.org/10.1002/jcp.26055] [PMID: 28617957]

[86] Vallianou NG, Evangelopoulos A, Schizas N, Kazazis C. Potential anticancer properties and mechanisms of action of curcumin. Anticancer Res 2015; 35(2): 645-51.
      [PMID: 25667441]

[87] Carlos-Reyes Á, López-González JS, Meneses-Flores M, *et al.* Dietary compounds as epigenetic modulating agents in cancer. Front Genet 2019; 10: 79.
      [http://dx.doi.org/10.3389/fgene.2019.00079] [PMID: 30881375]

[88] Bahrami A, Amerizadeh F, ShahidSales S, *et al.* Therapeutic potential of targeting Wnt/β-catenin pathway in treatment of colorectal cancer: rational and progress. J Cell Biochem 2017; 118(8): 1979-83.
      [http://dx.doi.org/10.1002/jcb.25903] [PMID: 28109136]

[89] Moradi-Marjaneh R, Hassanian SM, Rahmani F, Aghaee-Bakhtiari SH, Avan A, Khazaei M. Phytosomal curcumin elicits antitumor properties through suppression of angiogenesis, cell proliferation and induction of oxidative stress in colorectal cancer. Curr Pharm Des 2018; 24(39): 4626-38.

[http://dx.doi.org/10.2174/1381612825666190110145151] [PMID: 30636578]

[90] Hosseini S, Chamani J, Hadipanah MR, *et al.* Nano-curcumin's suppression of breast cancer cells (MCF7) through the inhibition of cyclinD1 expression. Breast cancer: targets and therapy 2019; 11: 137.

[91] Hashemzehi M, Behnam-Rassouli R, Hassanian SM, *et al.* Phytosomal-curcumin antagonizes cell growth and migration, induced by thrombin through AMP-Kinase in breast cancer. J Cell Biochem 2018; 119(7): 5996-6007.
[http://dx.doi.org/10.1002/jcb.26796] [PMID: 29600521]

[92] Banala RR, Vemuri SK, Gurava Reddy AV, Subbaiah GP. Aqueous extract of Acalypha indica leaves for the treatment of psoriasis: in-vitro studies. Int J Bioassays 2017; 6(04): 5360-4.
[http://dx.doi.org/10.21746/ijbio.2017.04.007]

[93] Martinez-Cifuentes M, Weiss-Lopez B, Santos LS, Araya-Maturana R. Heterocyclic curcumin derivatives of pharmacological interest: Recent progress. Curr Top Med Chem 2015; 15(17): 1663-72.
[http://dx.doi.org/10.2174/1568026615666150427111837] [PMID: 25915614]

[94] Zhou GZ, Li AF, Sun YH, Sun GC. A novel synthetic curcumin derivative MHMM-41 induces ROS-mediated apoptosis and migration blocking of human lung cancer cells A549. Biomed Pharmacother 2018; 103: 391-8.
[http://dx.doi.org/10.1016/j.biopha.2018.04.086] [PMID: 29674274]

[95] Liao F, Liu L, Luo E, Hu J. Curcumin enhances anti-tumor immune response in tongue squamous cell carcinoma. Arch Oral Biol 2018; 92: 32-7.
[http://dx.doi.org/10.1016/j.archoralbio.2018.04.015] [PMID: 29751146]

[96] Link A, Balaguer F, Shen Y, *et al.* Curcumin modulates DNA methylation in colorectal cancer cells. PLoS One 2013; 8(2): e57709.
[http://dx.doi.org/10.1371/journal.pone.0057709] [PMID: 23460897]

[97] Shah K, Mirza S, Desai U, Jain N, Rawal R. Synergism of curcumin and cytarabine in the down regulation of multi-drug resistance genes in acute myeloid leukemia. Anticancer Agents Med Chem 2016; 16(1): 128-35.
[http://dx.doi.org/10.2174/1871520615666150817115718] [PMID: 26278546]

[98] Giordano A, Tommonaro G. Curcumin and Cancer. Nutrients 2019; 11(10): 2376.
[http://dx.doi.org/10.3390/nu11102376] [PMID: 31590362]

[99] Quintero-Fabián S, Arreola R, Becerril-Villanueva E, *et al.* Role of matrix metalloproteinases in angiogenesis and cancer. Front Oncol 2019; 9: 1370.
[http://dx.doi.org/10.3389/fonc.2019.01370] [PMID: 31921634]

[100] Prasad S, Tyagi AK, Aggarwal BB. Recent developments in delivery, bioavailability, absorption and metabolism of curcumin: the golden pigment from golden spice. Cancer Research and Treatment: Official J Korean Cancer Association 2014; 46(1): 2.
[http://dx.doi.org/10.4143/crt.2014.46.1.2]

[101] Howells LM, Sale S, Sriramareddy SN, *et al.* Curcumin ameliorates oxaliplatin-induced chemoresistance in HCT116 colorectal cancer cells *in vitro* and *in vivo*. Int J Cancer 2011; 129(2): 476-86.
[http://dx.doi.org/10.1002/ijc.25670] [PMID: 20839263]

[102] Mutlu Altundağ E, Yılmaz AM, Koçtürk S, Taga Y, Yalçın AS. Synergistic induction of apoptosis by quercetin and curcumin in chronic myeloid leukemia (K562) cells. Nutr Cancer 2018; 70(1): 97-108.
[http://dx.doi.org/10.1080/01635581.2018.1380208] [PMID: 29161179]

[103] Chaurasia S, Chaubey P, Patel RR, Kumar N, Mishra B. Curcumin-polymeric nanoparticles against colon-26 tumor-bearing mice: cytotoxicity, pharmacokinetic and anticancer efficacy studies. Drug Dev Ind Pharm 2016; 42(5): 694-700.
[http://dx.doi.org/10.3109/03639045.2015.1064941] [PMID: 26165247]

[104] Yogosawa S, Yamada Y, Yasuda S, Sun Q, Takizawa K, Sakai T. Dehydrozingerone, a structural analogue of curcumin, induces cell-cycle arrest at the G2/M phase and accumulates intracellular ROS in HT-29 human colon cancer cells. J Nat Prod 2012; 75(12): 2088-93.
[http://dx.doi.org/10.1021/np300465f] [PMID: 23245566]

[105] Shanmugam MK, Rane G, Kanchi MM, *et al.* The multifaceted role of curcumin in cancer prevention and treatment. Molecules 2015; 20(2): 2728-69.
[http://dx.doi.org/10.3390/molecules20022728] [PMID: 25665066]

[106] Ravindran J, Prasad S, Aggarwal BB. Curcumin and cancer cells: how many ways can curry kill tumor cells selectively? AAPS J 2009; 11(3): 495-510.
[http://dx.doi.org/10.1208/s12248-009-9128-x] [PMID: 19590964]

[107] Yue GG, Cheng SW, Yu H, *et al.* The role of turmerones on curcumin transportation and P-glycoprotein activities in intestinal Caco-2 cells. J Med Food 2012; 15(3): 242-52.
[http://dx.doi.org/10.1089/jmf.2011.1845] [PMID: 22181075]

[108] Kanwar SS, Yu Y, Nautiyal J, *et al.* Difluorinated-curcumin (CDF): a novel curcumin analog is a potent inhibitor of colon cancer stem-like cells. Pharm Res 2011; 28(4): 827-38.
[http://dx.doi.org/10.1007/s11095-010-0336-y] [PMID: 21161336]

[109] Yu Y, Kanwar SS, Patel BB, Nautiyal J, Sarkar FH, Majumdar AP. Elimination of colon cancer stem-like cells by the combination of curcumin and FOLFOX. Transl Oncol 2009; 2(4): 321-8.
[http://dx.doi.org/10.1593/tlo.09193] [PMID: 19956394]

[110] Lim KJ, Bisht S, Bar EE, Maitra A, Eberhart CG. A polymeric nanoparticle formulation of curcumin inhibits growth, clonogenicity and stem-like fraction in malignant brain tumors. Cancer Biol Ther 2011; 11(5): 464-73.
[http://dx.doi.org/10.4161/cbt.11.5.14410] [PMID: 21193839]

[111] Wang K, Zhang T, Liu L, *et al.* Novel micelle formulation of curcumin for enhancing antitumor activity and inhibiting colorectal cancer stem cells. Int J Nanomedicine 2012; 7: 4487-97.
[PMID: 22927762]

[112] Kanai M, Yoshimura K, Asada M, *et al.* A phase I/II study of gemcitabine-based chemotherapy plus curcumin for patients with gemcitabine-resistant pancreatic cancer. Cancer Chemother Pharmacol 2011; 68(1): 157-64.
[http://dx.doi.org/10.1007/s00280-010-1470-2] [PMID: 20859741]

[113] Bayet-Robert M, Kwiatkowski F, Leheurteur M, *et al.* Phase I dose escalation trial of docetaxel plus curcumin in patients with advanced and metastatic breast cancer. Cancer Biol Ther 2010; 9(1): 8-14.
[http://dx.doi.org/10.4161/cbt.9.1.10392] [PMID: 19901561]

[114] Cheng AL, Hsu CH, Lin JK, *et al.* Phase I clinical trial of curcumin, a chemopreventive agent, in patients with high-risk or pre-malignant lesions. Anticancer Res 2001; 21(4B): 2895-900.
[PMID: 11712783]

[115] Lin L, Liu Y, Li H, *et al.* Targeting colon cancer stem cells using a new curcumin analogue, GO-Y030. Br J Cancer 2011; 105(2): 212-20.
[http://dx.doi.org/10.1038/bjc.2011.200] [PMID: 21694723]

[116] Buhrmann C, Kraehe P, Lueders C, Shayan P, Goel A, Shakibaei M. Curcumin suppresses crosstalk between colon cancer stem cells and stromal fibroblasts in the tumor microenvironment: potential role of EMT. PLoS One 2014; 9(9): e107514.
[http://dx.doi.org/10.1371/journal.pone.0107514] [PMID: 25238234]

[117] Su P, Yang Y, Wang G, Chen X, Ju Y. Curcumin attenuates resistance to irinotecan *via* induction of apoptosis of cancer stem cells in chemoresistant colon cancer cells. Int J Oncol 2018; 53(3): 1343-53.
[http://dx.doi.org/10.3892/ijo.2018.4461] [PMID: 29956726]

[118] Liu W, Zhai Y, Heng X, *et al.* Oral bioavailability of curcumin: problems and advancements. J Drug Target 2016; 24(8): 694-702.

[http://dx.doi.org/10.3109/1061186X.2016.1157883] [PMID: 26942997]

[119] Anand P, Thomas SG, Kunnumakkara AB, *et al.* Biological activities of curcumin and its analogues (Congeners) made by man and Mother Nature. Biochem Pharmacol 2008; 76(11): 1590-611.
[http://dx.doi.org/10.1016/j.bcp.2008.08.008] [PMID: 18775680]

[120] Wang Y, Ying X, Xu H, Yan H, Li X, Tang H. The functional curcumin liposomes induce apoptosis in C6 glioblastoma cells and C6 glioblastoma stem cells *in vitro* and in animals. Int J Nanomedicine 2017; 12: 1369-84.
[http://dx.doi.org/10.2147/IJN.S124276] [PMID: 28260885]

[121] Maeda H. The enhanced permeability and retention (EPR) effect in tumor vasculature: the key role of tumor-selective macromolecular drug targeting. Adv Enzyme Regul 2001; 41: 189-207.
[http://dx.doi.org/10.1016/S0065-2571(00)00013-3] [PMID: 11384745]

[122] Zheng B, McClements DJ. Formulation of more efficacious curcumin delivery systems using colloid science: enhanced solubility, stability, and bioavailability. Molecules 2020; 25(12): 2791.
[http://dx.doi.org/10.3390/molecules25122791] [PMID: 32560351]

[123] Ireson C, Orr S, Jones DJ, *et al.* Characterization of metabolites of the chemopreventive agent curcumin in human and rat hepatocytes and in the rat *in vivo*, and evaluation of their ability to inhibit phorbol ester-induced prostaglandin E2 production. Cancer Res 2001; 61(3): 1058-64.
[PMID: 11221833]

[124] Anand P, Sundaram C, Jhurani S, Kunnumakkara AB, Aggarwal BB. Curcumin and cancer: an "old-age" disease with an "age-old" solution. Cancer Lett 2008; 267(1): 133-64.
[http://dx.doi.org/10.1016/j.canlet.2008.03.025] [PMID: 18462866]

[125] Toden S, Goel A. The holy grail of curcumin and its efficacy in various diseases: is bioavailability truly a big concern? J Restor Med 2017; 6(1): 27-36.
[http://dx.doi.org/10.14200/jrm.2017.6.0101] [PMID: 30899605]

[126] Ghoneim AI. Effects of curcumin on ethanol-induced hepatocyte necrosis and apoptosis: implication of lipid peroxidation and cytochrome c. Naunyn Schmiedebergs Arch Pharmacol 2009; 379(1): 47-60.
[http://dx.doi.org/10.1007/s00210-008-0335-2] [PMID: 18716759]

[127] Jiao Y, Wilkinson J IV, Di X, *et al.* Curcumin, a cancer chemopreventive and chemotherapeutic agent, is a biologically active iron chelator. Blood 2009; 113(2): 462-9.
[http://dx.doi.org/10.1182/blood-2008-05-155952] [PMID: 18815282]

[128] Toden S, Okugawa Y, Jascur T, *et al.* Curcumin mediates chemosensitization to 5-fluorouracil through miRNA-induced suppression of epithelial-to-mesenchymal transition in chemoresistant colorectal cancer. Carcinogenesis 2015; 36(3): 355-67.
[http://dx.doi.org/10.1093/carcin/bgv006] [PMID: 25653233]

[129] Shen F, Cai WS, Li JL, *et al.* Synergism from the combination of ulinastatin and curcumin offers greater inhibition against colorectal cancer liver metastases *via* modulating matrix metalloproteinase-9 and E-cadherin expression. OncoTargets Ther 2014; 7: 305-14.
[PMID: 24570592]

[130] Bolat ZB, Islek Z, Demir BN, Yilmaz EN, Sahin F, Ucisik MH. Curcumin-and Piperine-loaded emulsomes as combinational treatment approach enhance the anticancer activity of Curcumin on HCT116 colorectal cancer model. Front Bioeng Biotechnol 2020; 8: 50.
[http://dx.doi.org/10.3389/fbioe.2020.00050] [PMID: 32117930]

[131] Hay E, Lucariello A, Contieri M, *et al.* Therapeutic effects of turmeric in several diseases: An overview. Chem Biol Interact 2019; 310: 108729.
[http://dx.doi.org/10.1016/j.cbi.2019.108729] [PMID: 31255636]

[132] Salehi B, Stojanović-Radić Z, Matejić J, *et al.* The therapeutic potential of curcumin: A review of clinical trials. Eur J Med Chem 2019; 163: 527-45.
[http://dx.doi.org/10.1016/j.ejmech.2018.12.016] [PMID: 30553144]

[133] Pagano E, Romano B, Izzo AA, Borrelli F. The clinical efficacy of curcumin-containing nutraceuticals: An overview of systematic reviews. Pharmacol Res 2018; 134: 79-91.
[http://dx.doi.org/10.1016/j.phrs.2018.06.007] [PMID: 29890252]

CHAPTER 3

Immunotherapy Approaches Focusing on Cancer Stem Cells

Marcela Rodrigues de Camargo[1,*], **Rafael Carneiro Ortiz**[2], **Carolina Mendonça Gorgulho**[3], **Vanessa Soares Lara**[1] and **Camila Oliveira Rodini**[2]

[1] *Department of Surgery, Stomatology, Pathology and Radiology, Bauru School of Dentistry, University of São Paulo, Bauru, São Paulo, Brazil*

[2] *Department of Biological Sciences, Bauru School of Dentistry, University of São Paulo, Bauru, São Paulo, Brazil*

[3] *ImmunoSurgery/Immunotherapy Unit, Champalimaud Foundation - Champalimaud Centre for the Unknown, Brasilia Avenue, 1400-038 Lisbon, Portugal*

Abstract: Metastasis and relapses are still one of the main causes of death in many cancer patients, and they probably occur since cytotoxic chemotherapy as well as the the stress from surgery itself can impair the steady immunological state, the ability to develop an antitumor immune response and also because of poor cancer stem cells (CSC) elimination. CSC appear to use features of both cancer cells and stem cells, including self-renewal and resistance to apoptosis for survival and proliferation, making cancer elimination even more difficult, which then becomes a potential therapeutic target. In this scenario, the successful generation of immunity is the key that can help fight against cancer. Techniques such as monoclonal antibodies, dendritic cell vaccine, and adoptive T cell therapies have been developed, targeting CSC to eliminate tumor mass. In this chapter, some features and aspects of CSC, as well as their relation with patients' prognosis and therapeutic values, will be listed.

Keywords: Anti-tumor response, Cancer stem cells, Immunotherapy, Inflammation, Vaccines.

INTRODUCTION

"The global cancer burden is estimated to have risen to 18.1 million new cases and 9.6 million deaths in 2018; it means that one in 5 men and one in 6 women worldwide develop cancer during their lifetime, and one in 8 men and one in 11 women die from the disease" [1]. These data highlight cancer as one of the main public health problems in the world.

---

[*] **Corresponding author Marcela Rodrigues de Camargo:** Department of Surgery, Stomatology, Pathology and Radiology, Bauru School of Dentistry, University of São Paulo, Bauru, São Paulo, Brazil; Tel: +55 14 32358000; E-mail: marcelarcv@gmail.com

Atta-ur-Rahman & M. Iqbal Choudhary (Eds.)
All rights reserved-© 2021 Bentham Science Publishers

Millions of researches have been conducted all over the world in order to decrease these numbers and increase patients' quality of life. Different techniques have been developed, aiming at this goal. Among them, the most common technique to reduce the tumor mass and facilitate surgical intervention is perioperative chemotherapy, also called neoadjuvant therapy administered before surgery [2, 3]. But even though chemotherapy can be effective against tumor cells and contribute to the reduction of tumor burden, the conventional regimen based on the administration of maximum tolerated dose (MTD) is also toxic to normal cells and the immune system.

MTD frequently promotes deep myelosuppression, followed by a depressive effect on immune system functions, leading to the selection of drug-resistant cells, and increasing the possibility of relapse [4]. Metastasis and relapse are still the main causes of death in many patients, and they probably occur since cytotoxic chemotherapy, as well as the surgery stress itself, can impair the steady immunological state, the ability to develop an antitumor immune response and effectively eliminate cancer stem cells (CSC).

CSCs are a rare subpopulation within the whole tumor cells that are able to extensively proliferate and initiate tumor growth [5]. CSCs are also the most migratory and highly metastatic cellular subpopulation within the tumor. CSCs appear to use features of both cancer cells and stem cells, including self-renewal and resistance to apoptosis, favoring survival and proliferation [6].

Furthermore, changes in metabolic conditions during normal physiologic conditions and disease can modify the inflammatory response, requiring cells to integrate signals, such as interleukins, cytokines, and chemokines, with resources such as the local oxygen concentrations and other metabolites, promoting damages that can lead to tumor development [7]. Inflammation can be driven according to the regulation of its components and in the tumor microenvironment (TME). There are several types of components, such as malignant cells, non-cancerous and non-cellular ones [8 - 10], making it difficult to assign a single role to inflammation. The orchestration of all these components with tumorigenesis and the immune system is not so clear and is very important for a successful response against cancer [11 - 13]. Inflammatory cells can hold tumor-suppressing properties but are frequently polarized into invasion and metastasis, promoting tumor progression [14 - 16].

In this scenario, the successful generation of an immune response is the key to many steps that can help fight against cancer, such as tumor uptake and presentation by antigen-presenting cells (APCs). After APCs migration to lymph nodes, several immune phenomena occur sequentially, including the promotion of naïve T cells to effector (tumor-specific) T cells and their migration to blood and tumor tissues, T cells recognition to tumor lysis, and the generation of tumor-specific memory T cells, which will help in the maintenance and prevention of cancer recurrences and metastasis. However, as a survival strategy, cancer cells develop many pathways to bypass antitumor immunity. These strategies, named "immune evasion mechanisms", generally collapse the already developed specific antitumor immunity, leading to successful tumor growth. These mechanisms are always in development during cancer progression and can be even more complex in late-stage cancers [17].

Based on the understanding of the cancer microenvironment and immune system mechanisms, various types of immunotherapies can be developed to improve the quality of immune activation, and to modulate mechanisms that can activate and increase the immune response. This chapter highlights immunotherapeutic approaches towards CSC, then a brief section of stem cells (SC) concepts is presented, followed by a section describing the relevance of CSC theory to tumorigenesis and metastasis, as well as Cancer Immunotherapy principles preceding and supporting the main idea.

STEM CELLS

Multicellular organisms are complex and made up of different types of specialized cells that carry out different functions, comprising the tissues that compose an organism as a whole [18]. Most somatic cells have a limited life span and are susceptible to different kinds of damage [19]. Hence, a reservoir of progenitor cells called Stem Cells (SC) is necessary for embryogenesis, damage repair, and to prevent tissue aging.

SCs are classified as undifferentiated cells capable of self-renewal during mitosis (cell proliferation), basically in two different ways. First, SCs can self-renew to replicate themselves for maintenance of an SC pool. Second, SCs can also give rise to specialized cells under appropriate conditions [20]. Specific cell signaling pathways determine the course of an SC towards stemness maintenance or differentiation. There are different types of SCs that can be classified according to distinct mechanisms that lead to self-renewal and pluripotency. These cells can be programmed to determine functions as they are at a stage where they are not yet fully specialized [21].

Postnatal organisms have a small population of adult SCs spread throughout the body that can be either multipotent or unipotent [22]. Multipotent SCs have a lower capacity to self-renewal by division as compared to pluripotent SC, but can develop into multiple somatic cell types present in a specific tissue or organ [23]. A great example of a SC niche is the bone marrow, which has multipotent SCs capable of regenerating the entire hematopoietic system. However, multipotent SCs remain quiescent (without dividing or differentiating) for a long period of time with the purpose of maintaining SC pool within the tissue, until a stimulus occurs; even the most stable organs, such as the heart and brain, present adult SCs to maintain tissue homeostasis and carry out repair [24]. SC self-renewal can be symmetric and/or asymmetric, where symmetric division produces two daughter SC, exactly like the progenitor, contributing to a reservoir of SC. On the other hand, the asymmetric division also provides two daughter cells, where one of them remains as their progenitor (self-renewal), while the other enters a specialized program, being a differentiated cell [25]. Since adult SCs are referred to their tissue of origin, it is possible to further classify them as their source. Fig. (**1**) demonstrates adult SC niches and their respectively differentiated cell lines [26 - 28].

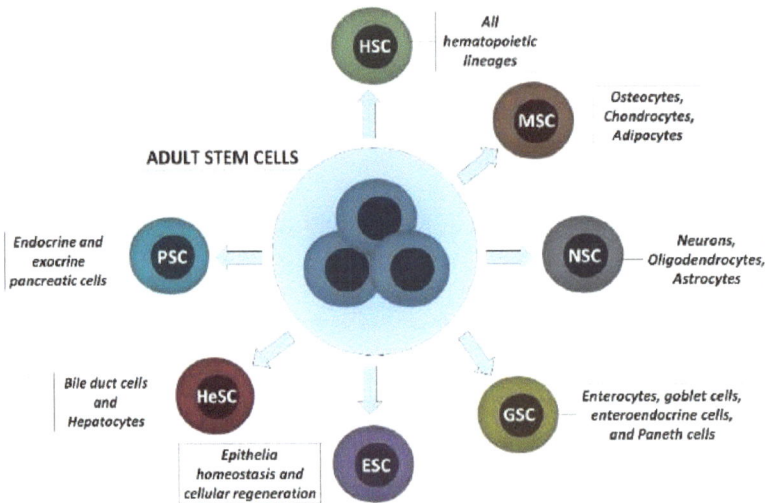

Fig. (1). Examples of adult stem cells, classified as their origin tissue: Hematopoietic stem cells (HSC), mesenchymal stem cells (MSC), neural stem cells (NSC), gastrointestinal stem cells (GSC), epidermal stem cells (ESC), hepatic stem cells (HSC), and pancreatic stem cells (PSC). All these SC populations are self-renewing but differentiate into different somatic lineages. For instance, HSCs are able to differentiate into all hematopoietic lineages, while MSCs can give rise to different cells of mesodermal germ layer origin such as osteocytes, chondrocytes, and adipocytes. NSCs can specialize into neurons, oligodendrocytes, and astrocytes; and GSC may differentiate into enterocytes, goblet cells, enteroendocrine cells, and Paneth cells. Noteworthy, homeostasis in labile cells is maintained by the regeneration potential of adult stem cells, which is pointed out by ESC in normal skin. Glandular tissue can also be maintained by specialized SC, whose HSC are able to differentiate into bile duct cells and hepatocytes; while PSCs differ into two major compromised cells, producing endocrine and exocrine pancreatic cells.

According to exceedingly fast epithelial repair, Rodini *et al.* (2017) reported that epithelial cells, from oral mucosae, proliferate in the basal layer in a period of 5-

40 days, depending on the region. These differences in proliferation rates and specialized cell lineages support the concept that only a small fraction of dividing cells have the stem property of infinitive division. Following that, adult SC slowly self-renew to produce equal daughter cells and produce cells committed to differentiation. These cells are called Transit-amplifying (TA) cells, which have a high proliferative rate but low self-renewal capacity. Thus, TA cells can enter into a specialized pathway and are not able to self-renew. The authors also reported that SC synergy in the oral epithelium is lost with cancer development and can be associated with tumor heterogeneity [29].

The SC field has been increasingly developed, and the discovery that specialized mature cells can be genetically reprogrammed to become pluripotent, *i.e.* capable of developing into all tissues of the body, rendered "The Nobel Prize in Physiology or Medicine" in 2012 to Gurdon and Yamanaka [30]. These genetically reprogrammed adult cells are named induced pluripotent stem cells (iPSC) and were first isolated from mouse embryonic cells and adult fibroblasts, with the induction of genes that are important for stem cell function (Oct3/4, Sox2, c-Myc, and Klf4) under embryonic stem cells conditions. The authors observed that iPSC exhibited the same morphology and growth properties as ES and were also positive for biomarkers associated with stemness [31]. It is important to know that new techniques and approaches focused on isolation, reprogramming, and activation of iPSC are currently ongoing [32], and iPSC can be a strategy to repair damaged tissues as well as to study drug development and modeling of diseases.

Finally, several models have been described to provide a better understanding of SC in the therapeutic field. Recently, a rodent middle carotid artery occlusion (MCAO) model demonstrated that MSC delivery to the surface of the ipsilateral cerebral cortex improves the neurological function after cerebral ischemia [33]. Likewise, another recent study observed that inflammatory stimulation could promote cell proliferation and mineralization of dental pulp SC; although this effect declines with age. Thus, despite SC properties, senescence is an important factor in tissue damage repair [34].

In summary, due to their unique biological properties, SCs are considered an important tool for cell therapy of several diseases and tissue regeneration. Recent research has focused on evaluating the potentialities of different sources of SCs, as well as biological safety, according to the desired clinical application.

Cancer Stem Cells

As discussed above, normal stem cells are able to self-renew and differentiate into several cell types. Self-renewal occurs by two different mechanisms, by which SC can give rise to either two identical daughter cells or one identical daughter cell and another that will differentiate into a specific specialized cell from a tissue [35]. Recent evidence suggests that tumor cells use a similar mechanism to proliferate and form a heterogeneous tumor mass. Tumoral heterogeneity has been supported by the presence and the maintenance of cancer cells with stemness ability – CSC. The CSC model is supported by the proposition that only one rare subpopulation of whole tumor cells is able to proliferate and initiate new tumor growth extensively [5]. The process of CSC self-renewal is not well understood and does not follow the pathways used by normal SC. Thus, this chapter will list some features and aspects of the CSC needed for cancer initiation, development, progression, and spread through metastasis, as well as its relation with patients' prognosis and therapeutic value.

The CSC subpopulation is the most migratory and highly metastatic cellular subpopulation within the tumor. CSCs appear to use features of cancer cells and stem cells, including self-renewal and resistance to apoptosis for survival and proliferation [6]. Several studies report that CSCs, despite being rare, are the major population responsible for tumor progression, since they present a higher rate of proliferation, migration and metastatic potential compared to other tumor cells [36 - 38].

The first study which reported the role of SC in cancer is from 1994, when Lapidot *et al.* (1994) identified an initiating population of tumor cells in acute myeloid leukemia (AML) after transplantation into severe combined immune-deficient (SCID) mice. Furthermore, the leukemia-initiating cells were found by the use of surface marker expression (CD34$^+$/CD38$^-$) [39]. The first concrete evidence for the presence of CSC in leukemia was from the studies of Bonnet & Dick (1997) [40], who identified these cells as (CD34^{++}/CD38$^-$). The series of subsequent studies on CSCs phenotype developed simultaneously with the search for surface markers to identify this rare subpopulation within the tumor cell mass. The first evidence of CSC in solid tumors occurred almost ten years after the first report on leukemia, specifically in 2003. This subpopulation was found in breast [41] and brain cancer [42], by the expression of CD44$^+$CD24$^{-/low}$ and CD133$^+$, respectively. The subsequent reports identified CD133$^+$ CSCs in a variety of other tumors, including colon [43], lung [44], and neuroblastoma [45].

Currently, many studies are evaluating the expression of several biomarkers to identify the CSC subpopulation in different types of human cancers, as well as to correlate them with valuable prognostic features (Table **1**), *e.g.* CD24, CD34, CD38, CD44, CD90 and CD133 and epithelial cell adhesion molecule (EpCAM) [46 - 49]. CD44 seems to be the most common CSC evaluated marker and it is overexpressed in various solid tumors, including breast [41], prostate [50], and colon cancers [51]. Some combined markers, such as aldehyde dehydrogenase ALDH1 and CD44, appear to be related to the CSC phenotype in several cancer tissues. For example, ALDH$^+$ ovarian cancer cells showed greater tumorigenicity and were more resistant to therapy [52]. Similarly, Ortiz *et al.* (2018) [53] found that cancer cells in oral squamous cell carcinoma (OSCC) samples with higher expression of ALDH1 and CD44 were associated with angiolymphatic invasion and metastasis, respectively [53].

Table 1. Cancer Stem Cell markers and tumors.

CSC Markers		Tumor Type	Results	References
CD34$^+$/CD38$^-$		Acute myeloid Leukemia; Leukemia	Tumorigenesis in immunocompromised mice	Lapidot *et al.* 1994; Bonnet & Dick 1997
CD133$^+$		Brain and Colon cancer	Tumor cell differentiation *in vitro*	Singh *et al.* 2003; Ricci-Vitiani *et al.* 2007
		Lung cancer	Tumorigenesis in immunocompromised mice	Eramo *et al.* 2008
		Neuroblastoma	Higher tumorigenic potential in I-type cells	Walton *et al.* 2004
CD44$^+$	CD24$^{-/low}$	Breast cancer	Tumorigenesis in immunocompromised mice	Al-Hajj *et al.* 2003
	CD133$^+$	Prostate cancer	Production of mixed populations of non-clonogenic cells	Collins *et al.* 2005
	EpCAM high	Colon cancer	Tumorigenesis in immunocompromised mice	Dalerba *et al.* 2007
	ALDH1$^+$	Ovarian and Oral cancers	Greater tumorigenicity, resistance to therapy in ovarian cancer cells; Angiolymphatic invasion and metastasis in OSCC	Yasuda *et al.* 2013; Ortiz *et al.* 2018
	ALDH1$^+$ Oct4$^+$	Breast cancer	Enhanced tumorsphere formation and chemoresistance *in vitro* and displayed strong tumorigenicity, metastatic potential and poor survival *in vivo*	Tan *et al.* 2019
OCT4$^+$ NANOG$^+$ SOX2$^+$ KLF4$^+$ c-MYC$^+$		Head and neck cancer	Found in tumor nests of head and neck squamous cell carcinoma	Koh *et al.* 2019
CD90		Malignant insulinoma	Malignant insulinoma cells showed increased tumor-initiating potential in athymic nude mice	Floryne *et al.* 2016

Considering that CSCs are thought to be responsible for cancer initiation, progression, and metastasis [54], as well as for recurrence of all cancers [55], they have become a potential therapeutic target for cancer elimination. As stated by Reya *et al.* (2001) [5], CSC "would be more resistant to chemotherapeutics than tumor cells with limited proliferative potential, and even therapies that cause complete regression of tumors might spare enough CSCs to allow regrowth of the tumors". CSC resistance to chemotherapy and radiotherapy, in comparison to other tumor cells, has been confirmed by several other studies [56 - 60]. As enumerated by Laplane (2016) [61], many cellular properties and biological processes have a role in CSC therapy resistance, such as overexpression of anti-apoptotic proteins [62, 63], quiescence [64 - 66], improved DNA damage response [67, 68], higher capacity for drug efflux [69 - 71], localization in a hypoxic niche [72], and a lower concentration of reactive oxygen species (ROS) that mediate cell death by radiation [73].

Recently, Tan *et al.* (2019) [74] isolated CSC from breast cancer by enrichment of CSC markers (CD44, ALDH1, and OCT4) and evaluated the interaction with hyaluronic acid from the extracellular matrix by CD44 binding. This study demonstrated that $CD44^+$ cancer cells, which exhibited a CSC phenotype, were adherent in hyaluronic acid hydrogel and that interaction could be useful in the future for anticancer strategies that target breast CSCs [74]. Other markers have been used for CSC isolation. Koh *et al.* (2019) [75] suggested the presence of an $OCT4^+/NANOG^+/SOX2^+/KLF4^+/c\text{-}MYC^+$ CSC subpopulation within the tumor nests of head and neck squamous cell carcinoma.

Additionally, metastatic cells appear to be more aggressive, more refractory to treatment, and responsible for decreased survival. Indeed, several studies associated metastasis and CSC phenotype with their ability to survive by upregulation of DNA repair mechanisms, redox capacity, drug efflux, and maintenance of dormancy [76]. For example, CSCs are susceptible to DNA damage from radiation when ROS exceeds the antioxidant capacity of the cell, which promotes a higher expression of ROS scavengers, such as glutathione (GSH). In fact, recent reports have shown that pharmacologic reduction of GSH results in greater radio-sensitivity in CSC [76, 77].

So far, classical cancer treatment strategies rely on the elimination of the tumor mass, regardless of its constitution or the cells that are targeted [78, 79]. However, the identification and understanding of CSC biological behavior have been extensively studied in recent research. Although all mechanisms that regulate CSC phenotype and contribute to poor prognosis in several types of cancer remain unclear, CSC-targeted therapy seems to be auspicious and of great value.

CANCER IMMUNOTHERAPY

The goal of cancer immunotherapy is to alert the host's immune system regarding the presence of tumor cells and successfully generate effector mechanisms, mainly tumor-specific CD8$^+$ T cells, to fight the tumor. Basically, the necessary physiological processes for a successful and powerful immune response against cancer need to be enhanced, while still keeping in mind the urgent necessity to minimize side effects. Immunotherapy is a type of treatment which does aim directly at tumor cells, recognizing the complexity of the tumor microenvironment and of the interactions among its various components. In this way, immunotherapy can be classified as *active*, which aims to activate the immune system to destroy tumors and prevent their recurrence (such as administration of antigen/adjuvant vaccine, dendritic cell (DC) vaccines and cytokines that activate APCs and T cells); or *adoptive,* which consists of passively transferring effector components of the immune response directly to the patient, and/or enhancing a pre-existing immune response, such as monoclonal antibodies administration and adoptive T cell therapy with, for example, genetically engineered T cells ([CAR]-T and [TCR]-T) [17, 80].

With evasion of the immune response being postulated as a hallmark feature of tumor cells [9], an array of different strategies presents itself as worthy of investigation. Immunotherapies based on monoclonal antibodies (mAb) are an attractive option since they have fewer and less severe adverse effects when compared to conventional chemotherapy [81]. The mAb is produced to specifically match a single relevant antigenic determinant, exerting direct effects on the target cell and/or relying on the immune system to effectively eradicate cells to which they bind, *via* antibody-dependent cellular cytotoxicity (ADCC) or complement [82]. In order to reduce side effects, Nobel Prize laureate Greg Winter developed humanized mAb, and improved the clinical benefits for human use [83, 84]. Epidermal growth factor receptor (EGFR) was the first target to which mAb was employed for the treatment of cancer [82]. EGFR is a tyrosine kinase receptor crucial for signal transduction in normal cells, but this pathway is specifically hijacked by cancer cells, with this receptor being overexpressed in several human cancers [82, 85]. Inhibition of EGFR signaling by mAb binding prevents receptor activation and downstream signaling and promotes its internalization and subsequent degradation [82]. Ultimately, this leads to reduced proliferation, cell cycle arrest, and cell death. Three different anti-EGFR mAb are currently approved by the U.S. Food and Drug Administration (FDA): cetuximab (humanized), necitumumab (humanized), and panitumumab (fully human), for the treatment of advanced colorectal cancer, non-small cell lung carcinoma and others [82, 86, 87]. Human epithelial growth factor receptor 2 (HER-2) is another tyrosine kinase that can be successfully inhibited by mAb, especially in advanced breast cancer. Similar to EGFR, HER-2 possesses proliferative and pro-survival properties and is overexpressed in about 20% of breast tumors [88]. Trastuzumab was the first anti-HER-2 mAb approved by the FDA for first-line treatment of advanced breast cancer in combination with cytotoxic agents such as paclitaxel [89].

Another recent, very promising approach for cancer immunotherapy is checkpoint inhibition. Checkpoints are the natural breaks of the immune system, exerting physiological effects during the contraction of an immune response and are pivotal for immune homeostasis and avoidance of autoimmunity. Cytotoxic T lymphocyte antigen 4 (CTLA-4) and programmed cell death protein 1 (PD-1) are two of these immune checkpoints to be blocked. CTLA-4 is expressed in the surface of activated $CD4^+$ and $CD8^+$ T cells and bind to costimulatory markers on APC to inhibit the immune response [90, 91]. During T cell activation, PD-1 is expressed especially on the surface of $CD8^+$ T cells causing T cell exhaustion [92]. Also, the upregulation of PD-L1 (PD-1 ligand) on tumor cells leads to T cell death, suppression of anti-tumor immunity, and deregulation of adaptive immune resistance to many cancer types [93 - 95]. In 2011, anti-CTLA-4 ipilimumab was approved by the FDA, and in 2014, two anti-PD-1 mAbs (pembrolizumab and nivolumab) were also approved for the treatment of melanoma [96]. Since then, another anti-PD-1, cemiplimab, as well as PD-L1 inhibitors, atezolizumab, avelumab, and durvalumab, have been approved for the treatment of head and neck squamous cell carcinoma (HNSCC), renal cell carcinoma, colorectal, lung and breast cancers, among others [97, 98].

Other checkpoint markers are currently under investigation regarding their feasibility as clinical targets or biomarkers, such as LAG3 (lymphocyte activation gene-3), TIM3 (T-cell immunoglobulin and mucin domain-3), and GITR (glucocorticoid induced TNF receptor). Limitations of passive immunotherapy include the fact that they require continuous research on the tumor/immune system relationship for the development of active immunotherapeutic interventions, once combination therapies of cytotoxic agents and targeted therapies are frequently followed by side events [99, 100]. In this aspect, one of the most promising proposals is the development of dendritic cell-based therapeutic vaccines, which aims for *in vivo* stimulation of the adaptive immune system to achieve tumor regression [101 - 103].

DC are found in most human tissues [104] and efficiently present antigens to naïve T cells, triggering a powerful immune response [105, 106]. Thus, they are considered the main professional APC, which support proposals for DC-based therapeutic antitumor vaccines [107 - 111]. Usually, DC process tumor antigens through the endocytic route for presenting peptides in association with MHC (major histocompatibility complex) class II molecules, however, they can also associate exogenous tumor peptides with MHC class I molecules through cross-priming or cross-presentation, hence their pivotal role in priming tumor-specific $CD8^+$ T cells [112, 113]. DC-based vaccines can be prepared by different protocols that range from the simple preparation of tumor cell lysates by rapid freezing and thawing [114] to the generation of hybrid cells by fusing DC to tumor cells [115] and DC transfection with tumor RNA [116, 117] (Fig. **2**). Recently, a small study involving a DC vaccination protocol increased neoantigen T cell response in melanoma patients, with no significant adverse effects [118]. Moreover, vaccination also revealed other neoepitopes to which an immune response was being launched. DC loaded with mRNA of HSP-70 (heat shock protein 70) produced complete responses in two patients with hepatocellular carcinoma and five presented with stable disease after vaccination [119].

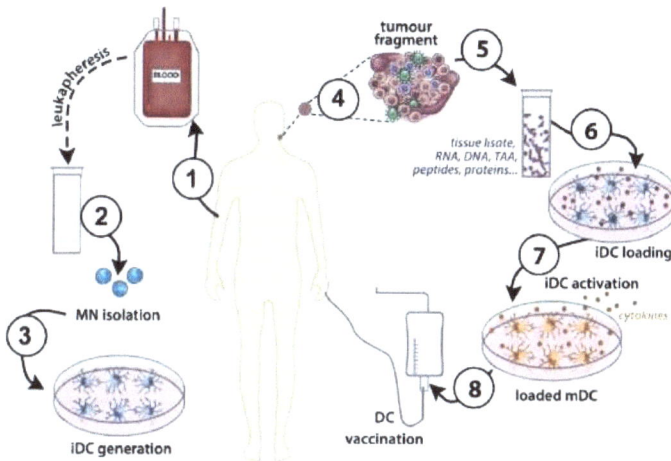

Fig. (2). General design of the production of autologous DC vaccines for cancer immunotherapy. **1)** Blood is collected from the patient and leukocytes are separated by means of leukapheresis. **2)** Monocytes are isolated and **3)** treated with specific cytokines (GM-CSF and IL-4) for the generation of monocyte-derived DC, which are still immature (iDC). **4)** Tumor fragments are isolated from the patient following surgical resection, and **5)** different products can be obtained from tumor (tissue lysate, RNA, DNA, peptides or antigens) according to the protocol of choice for **6)** iDC activation and loading *in vitro*. **7)** The final step of the process is DC activation/maturation, typically using a cocktail of activating cytokines. **8)** After usually two days in culture, the iDC becomes mature (mDC) and as a result, tumor antigen-presenting DC constitutes the vaccine that can be administered back to the patient, ready to start a strong specific immune response against cancer.

It is important to note that, although DC vaccine has shown modest effects on a subset of subjects over the years, they have yet to demonstrate their efficacy on a larger scale, especially for the treatment of advanced patients. A better understanding of the highly complex DC network *in vivo,* together with optimizing *ex vivo* activation by selecting relevant peptides and antigens, will possibly contribute to increasing the efficacy of this modality of immunotherapy.

Adoptive T cell therapy involves the extraction of Tumor-Infiltrating Lymphocytes (TIL) from surgical specimens, *ex vivo* expansion and activation, and then, delivery of the T cell product back to the patient (Fig. **3**). With easier access to neoantigen sequencing, adoptive T cell therapy using TIL has demonstrated durable antitumor activity in advanced melanoma patients, surpassing results obtained with cancer vaccines [120, 121]. There is also evidence to support the notion that, during checkpoint inhibition, the favorable clinical effects observed are due, at least partially, to neoepitope-reactive T cell clones [122]. Additionally, Rosenberg and colleagues have recently reported that neoepitope-targeted TIL therapy promoted tumor regression in two individual patients with metastatic cholangiocarcinoma and colorectal cancer [123, 124]. Human papillomavirus (HPV)-reactive TIL has also shown promise for the treatment of a cohort of cervical cancer patients [125].

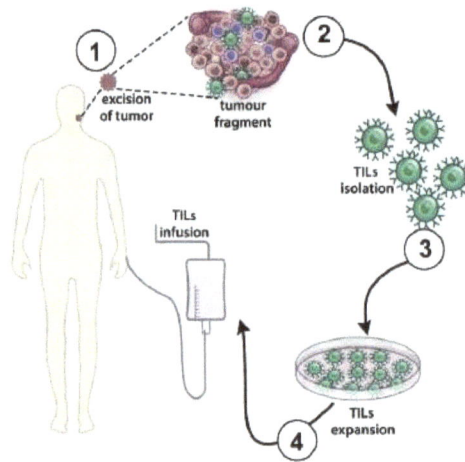

Fig. (3). Adoptive T cells therapy of Tumor-Infiltrating Lymphocytes (TILs). **1)** Excised tumor tissues are used as a source of TIL. **2)** TIL are isolated from excised tumor, and **3)** subsequently expanded by stimulating them *ex vivo* (in tissue culture) away from tumor's immunosuppressive environment. **4)** The highly activated, potent TIL are then infused back into the patient, without all the suppressive influences.

Genetically engineered T cells are also being explored in the context of adoptive cell transfer. Chimeric antigen receptor (CAR) T cells are engineered by fusing an antigen-specific antibody (scFv) with molecules of the T cell receptor (TCR)/CD3 complex, creating a structure similar to an antibody on the surface of T cells;

alternatively, TCR gene transfer can also be employed to generate T cells whose TCR have a high affinity for a relevant epitope [121, 126, 127]. CAR-T cells have been initially tested for hematological malignancies mainly focusing on targeting CD19 and CD20 [128], but have advanced into the solid tumor field, with significant challenges to overcome such as the selection of relevant yet safe tumor antigens, penetration into the tumor stroma, and resistance to exhaustion [129].

However, despite major advances in the field thus far, some cited therapies can exhibit toxicities, highlighting the need for new technology that promotes a better response and has fewer side effects, and CSC targeting is very promise. Several protocols are being tested and their side effects, as well as their immunotherapeutic efficacy, are inconclusive as of yet. Furthermore, the suppression of transferred activated T cells, when they find the tumor microenvironment, can be one of the reasons that adoptive cell therapy fails in some patients [17]. Cytotoxic agents and targeted therapies combined, especially EGFR inhibition by cetuximab or panitumumab, and vascular endothelial growth factor receptor (VEGFR) inhibition by bevacizumab administration, is frequently followed by side effects, such as erythema, acneiform dermatitis, pruritus, hypomagnesemia, skin exfoliation, fatigue, paronychia, abdominal pain, anorexia, nausea, diarrhea, skin rash and fissures [100, 130].

Cancer Stem Cell-Based Immunotherapy

Given the extensive knowledge built around the concepts of antitumor immunity and tumor heterogeneity in the recent years, as well as the substantial advances made with checkpoint inhibition and adoptive therapies, the moment is extremely favorable for the application of this newfound knowledge towards the development of CSC-targeted immunotherapies. Moreover, it is well known that the most popular anticancer treatments are chemotherapy and radiotherapy, and although these treatments have curative effects for some patients, in other cases, there is recurrence due to the repopulation of the tumor. One of the reasons that this occurs is the presence of CSC, which also have been proven to be less sensitive to conventional methods of cancer therapies, even molecular therapy [131 - 133]. During the quiescent phase of the cell cycle, CSCs express high levels of drug transporters and anti-apoptotic proteins, becoming resistant to DNA damage-induced death [134], and this CSC resistance to conventional treatments results in tumor relapse and metastasis, decreasing overall survival of patients in almost all cancer types. Therefore, ideal cancer treatment would be able to selectively target and kill CSCs, preventing tumor regrowth. This challenge has only recently started to be addressed, although the first identification of CSC was reported around 20 years ago [40]. Tumor stem cell research is still under development in different types of cancer, and immunotherapies involving CSCs are a very new target to be developed inside this promising scenario. Many types of studies have targeted different features of CSCs, including signaling pathways related to self-renewal mechanisms, cell surface antigens, stem cell niches, differentiation therapy, and transporters responsible for drug resistance [135 - 138]. However, there is still much to be unraveled before they are to be effectively applied in the clinic. Dendritic cells (DC), after being sensitized and injected in patients, migrate to draining lymph nodes and activate tumor-specific cytotoxic T cells, which are expanded and migrate into the tumor sites. NK cells, γδ T cells, and CTL can recognize CSC, but only effectors of adaptive immunity (T cells and antibodies) can develop a specific antitumor immune response [139] (Fig. **4**).

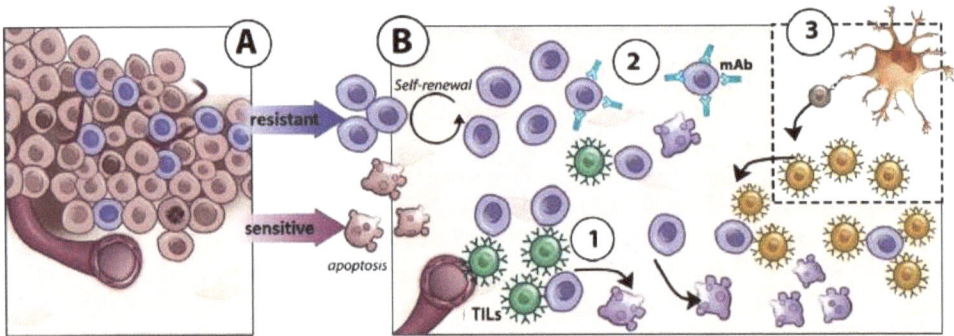

Fig. (4). A) Among the heterogeneous population of tumor cells, some are sensitive to traditional therapies (chemotherapy and radiotherapy) and undergo apoptosis, while a subset of cancer cells can be resistant and persists in the organism. **B)** Resistant cancer cells can be targeted by different modalities of CSC-focused immunotherapy, such as **1)** infusion of TIL, **2)** monoclonal antibody administration or **3)** vaccination with loaded mDC.

Monoclonal antibody has been proposed as an immunotherapy agent since the last decade, and Santamaria *et al.* (2017) [140] proposed strategies to directly target the CSC population, based on the following: (I) differences in surface marker expression; (II) interference with signaling pathways relevant to their function; (III) inhibition of their function; (IV) interference with metastasis formation; or (V) a combination of the above. Indeed, mAb are one of the most promising CSC-targeting immunotherapies and H90, a mouse IgG1 mAb against human CD44$^+$ cells, is the first mAb targeting CSCs (Vey 2016) [141]. H90 inhibited proliferation, induced terminal differentiation, and mediated apoptosis in human myeloid leukemia cell lines. Furthermore, the mAbs P245, H4C4, GV5, and RO5429083, also target CD44$^+$ cells and show important effects on eliminating CSC in different types of cancers [138]. A Phase I trial of a humanized IgG1 antibody against CD44, in heavily pre-treated patients with advanced CD44 expressing solid malignancies, proved to be safe but had only modest clinical effects [142]. However, CD44 also regulates the type 1 T helper (Th1) cell survival and its targeting may impair the anti-tumor immune responses that naturally occur in the system [143]. Radioiodinated mAb cocktail against both CD133 and CD44 inhibited tumor growth, prolonged mean survival, increased apoptosis, decreased proliferation and specific target expression (decreases in CSCs) in a xenografts mouse model [144]. More than surface markers, mAb can also target CSC niches like Bevacizumab [138], and target over-expressed antigens, demonstrating a very good response rate in a variety of cancers. According to Codd *et al.*, (2018) [143], over-expressed antigens can be: survivin (apoptosis-resistance genes), proto-oncogenes (HER-2), centrosomal protein 55 (CEP55), sex-determining region Y-box 2 (SOX-2), cytochrome C oxidase assembly factor 1 homologue (COA-1), stress-response related genes (HSP) or HOX genes. Recently, Wang *et al.* (2020) [145] summarized several mAb that have even more targets: Anti-LGR5 ADCs for colon cancer, B6H12 and Cirmtuzumab for breast cancer, Anti-CD36 neutralizing antibodies for oral carcinomas, BsAb-5 for non-small cell lung cancer and EpCAM/CD3-BsAb MT110 for pancreatic cancer. Additionally, the mAb Demcizumab (OMP-21M18) seems to be the most recently targeted therapy in clinical trials. It has been extensively tested in the latest clinical trials conducted against CSC (Table **2**). But more than that, it is very important to highlight that some of these antigens are also present in normal tissue but are overexpressed in cancer cells, especially in CSCs. Therefore, their blockade can possibly cause more collateral effects than other mAb targets [146 - 148].

DC-based immunotherapy against CSC has already been tried in mice and humans [149]. The use of professional APC, such as DC, to initiate a tumor-specific T cell response is considered one of the most encouraging strategies for cancer vaccination. Recently, studies showed that DC-based CSC vaccines lead to efficient antitumor immunity, bringing out both anti-CSC humoral and cellular immune responses [150 - 152]. This provides evidence that CSC can be recognized and eradicated by the immune system, and also supports the idea for new immunotherapeutic approaches targeting CSC. The generation of a DC vaccine based on ALDH^{high} CSC has demonstrated its efficiency for head and neck squamous cell carcinoma by pulsing autologous DC with ALDH^{high} CSC lysate isolated from cultured HNSCC cells. This vaccine shows to be more efficient against cancer than the same vaccine pulsed with non-CSC [153]. Accordingly, Ning *et al.* (2012) [154] demonstrated that DC vaccination based on CSC was significantly more effective in preventing lung metastasis in the D5 melanoma model, and also subcutaneous tumor growth in the SCC7 squamous cells carcinoma model when compared with control mice given DC pulsed with non-CSC. Interestingly, another CSC-DC vaccine significantly reduced ALDH^{high} CSC frequency in melanoma primary tumors by the specific binding of IgG, produced by vaccine primed B cells, resulting in lysis of the CSCs target in the presence of complement, suggesting that the use of CSC-DC as an adjuvant in local and systemic relapse could be useful in combination with conventional treatments of cancers [155]. Hu *et al.* (2016) [152] showed that vaccination of mice with an SCC7 tumor (ALDH[high])-based DC vaccine, after surgical excision of established SCC7 tumors, reduced local tumor relapse and prolonged animal survival, being even more effective in combination with anti-PD-L1, an immune checkpoint inhibitor. Indeed, the simultaneous administration of DC vaccine and immune checkpoint blockade is a recent development. Zheng *et al.* (2018) [156] showed that animals treated with CSC-DC vaccine and a dual blockade of PD- 1 and CTLA-4 presented significantly more tumor regression than the CSC-DC vaccine alone and moreover, triple combinatory treatment dramatically eliminated ALDH[high] CSC *in vivo* and enhanced CD8[+] T cell expansion and response against CSC. Similarly, Zhu *et al.* (2019) [157] showed that a combinatorial administration of anti-PD-L1 antibody and CSC lysate-pulsed DC vaccine, conferred greater survival advantage and decreased the Treg cell population in an orthotopic mouse model of glioma.

However, not only ALDH[high] CSC can be targeted, Wefers *et al.*, in 2018 [158] suggested that DC vaccine can also be loaded with transcription factors, such as NANOG, probably resulting in the stimulation of anti-tumor T cell responses in patients without chemotherapy or surgery. A CD44/CD24 CSC RNA-pulsed DC vaccine showed to be especially efficient in inducing a T cell response by increasing and activating CD8[+] T cells *in vitro*, which significantly induced breast cancer cell apoptosis [159]. An Ehrlich carcinoma cell line exposed to different concentrations of cisplatin, doxorubicin, or paclitaxel generates tumor cells with the highest expression of CSC markers (CD44[+]/CD24) that were selected to obtain enriched cell cultures with resistant CSC population. A DC vaccine, made with this subpopulation of cells, significantly reduced tumor size, prolonged overall survival, increased IFN-γ serum levels, and upregulated p53 gene expression *in vivo* [160]. More recently, the same group, El-Ashmawy *et al.* (2020) [161], demonstrated that the co-treatment with DC vaccine and cisplatin resulted in tumor growth inhibition, downregulation of MDR and Bcl-2 relative gene expression, enhanced apoptosis and absence of mitotic figures in tumor tissues. Finally, Integrin b4 (ITGB4) seems to be a new target to CSC, since it is significant for the regulation of these cells. Ruan *et al.* (2020) [162] demonstrated that its immune targeting might represent a novel pathway in cancer treatment showing two immunologic strategies to target ITGB4: ITGB4 protein–pulsed dendritic cells (ITGB4-DC) vaccine and adoptive transfer of anti-CD3/ant-
-ITGB4 bispecific antibody (ITGB4 BiAb).

Different therapeutic modalities are under investigation for the treatment of malignant tumors, and CTL plays an essential role in immune responses to cancers. CD8$^+$ T cells differentiate into CTL and undergo proliferation in the presence of appropriate stimulation. Once activated, CTL can migrate to peripheral tissues and directly mediate cytotoxicity and/or secrete effector cytokines leading to tumor elimination. CTL are able to recognize CSCs in an antigen-specific manner, once CSC express several tumor-associated antigens (TAA), becoming good sources for CSC-targeting immunotherapy [139]. Human CSC, derived from kidney, colon, prostate, lung, ovary, head and neck cancers and sarcomas, express several TAA, and CTL can recognize them both *in vitro* and *in vivo*, rendering TAA a very promising tool for next-generation cancer immunotherapy [163]. Visus *et al.*, (2007, 2011) reported tumor growth inhibition, metastasis inhibition, and increased survival of xenograft-bearing immunodeficient mice by generating CSC-specific CTL, using antigenic peptide from ALDH1A1, a pattern TAA of CSC from HNSCC [164, 165]. Also, based on ALDH1$^+$ cells, adoptive transfer of spleen T cells from pre-immunized mice inhibited tumor growth in näive tumor recipients without any side effects [166]. In a colorectal cancer model, Gao & Wang (2015) [167] demonstrated that CSCs are sensitive to CTL and that CEP55, another TAA of CSC, can be successfully used as a target for adoptive T cell immunotherapy for these resistant cells. More recently, Miyamoto *et al.* (2018) [168] showed that only colorectal CSCs express the ASB4 gene, another TAA. Because ASB4 was not expressed by normal tissues, its peptide epitope elicited CTL responses and the adoptive transfer of these CTL promoted CSC-specific eradication. These results suggest that T cell-based, CSC-targeted immunotherapy is getting highly specific, and, in the future, they can become increasingly efficient. Poncette *et al.* (2019) [169] showed that adoptive therapy with TCR from CD4$^+$T cells, exposed to nasopharyngeal cancer (NY-ESO-1) from a non-tolerant and non-human host, are of optimal affinity and that the combined use of MHC I– and II–restricted TCRs against NY-ESO-1 can make adoptive T cell therapy more effective. Besides that, another adoptive therapy, CAR-T cells targeting EpCAM, showed to be effective for local treatment of peritoneal carcinomatosis in mice, possibly being useful for clinical treatment of EpCAM-positive gastrointestinal and gynecological malignancies [170]. The first autologous CAR-T targeting CD133 immunotherapy reached a progression-free survival of 5 months and repeated cell infusions seemed to provide a longer period of disease stability, especially in patients who achieved tumor reduction after the first cell infusion [171]. However, in a clinical trial with advanced cholangiocarcinoma, the CAR-T cells developed against CD133 and EGFR receptors showed severe collateral effects [172]. Fig. (**5**) illustrates the different mechanisms of immunotherapies targeting cancer stem cells. In addition, clinical trials that have been conducted with different CSC-based immunotherapies are summarized in Table **2**.

Table 2. Cancer Stem Cells targets and immunotherapy in Clinical Trials.

Immunotherapy	Target	Tumor Treated	Clinical Phase	Reference or Website
Monoclonal antibody	CD44	Acute myeloid leukemia	Phase 1 Clinical trial	Vey N. *et al*, Oncotarget 2016
	CD44	Various solid tumors	Phase 1 Clinical trial	Menke-van der Houven C.W. *et al*, Oncotarget, 2016
	ALDH1	Breast cancer	Phase 2 Clinical trial	https://clinicaltrials.gov/ct2/show/NCT01190345
	CD44	Neoplasm	Phase 1 Clinical trial	https://clinicaltrials.gov/ct2/show/NCT01358903
	CD44/ALDH1/HER-2 (Trastuzumab)	HER2-positive Breast Cancer, Stage II Breast Cancer, Stage IIIA Breast Cancer	Phase 2 Clinical trial	https://clinicaltrials.gov/ct2/show/NCT01688609
	DLL4/VEGF	Ovaries, Peritoneal cancers, Fallopian Tube	Phase 1 Clinical trial	https://clinicaltrials.gov/ct2/show/NCT03030287
	DLL4/VEGF	Metastatic Colorectal Cancer	Phase 1 Clinical trial	https://clinicaltrials.gov/ct2/show/NCT03035253
	ROR1/Wnt5 (Cirmtuzumab)	Breast	Phase 1 Clinical trial	https://clinicaltrials.gov/ct2/show/NCT02776917
	ROR1/Wnt5/PD-1 (Demcizumab)	Locally Advanced or Metastatic Solid Tumors	Phase 1 Clinical trial	https://clinicaltrials.gov/ct2/show/NCT02722954
	ROR1/Wnt5 (Demcizumab)	Pancreas	Phase 1 Clinical trial	https://clinicaltrials.gov/ct2/show/NCT01189929
	ROR1/Wnt5 (Demcizumab)	Colorectal	Phase 1 Clinical trial	https://clinicaltrials.gov/ct2/show/NCT01189942
	ROR1/Wnt5 (Demcizumab)	Non-Small Cell Lung Cancer	Phase 1 Clinical trial	https://clinicaltrials.gov/ct2/show/NCT01189968

(Table 2) cont.....

Immunotherapy	Target	Tumor Treated	Clinical Phase	Reference or Website
DC Vaccine	Not specified	Glioblastoma	Phase 2 and 3 Clinical trial	https://clinicaltrials.gov/ct2/show/NCT03548571
	ALDH^{high}	Lung	Phase 1 and 2 Clinical trial	https://clinicaltrials.gov/ct2/show/NCT02115958
	ALDH^{high}	Colorectal	Phase 1 and 2 Clinical trial	https://clinicaltrials.gov/ct2/show/NCT02176746
	ALDH^{high}	Ovarian	Phase 1 and 2 Clinical trial	https://clinicaltrials.gov/ct2/show/NCT02178670
	Not specified	Recurrent Epithelial Ovarian Cancer	Phase 1 and 2 Clinical trial	https://clinicaltrials.gov/ct2/show/NCT01334047
	neurosphere-forming	Glioblastoma, Glioma, Astrocytoma, Brain tumor	Phase 1 Clinical trial	https://clinicaltrials.gov/ct2/show/NCT02010606
	CD133⁺	Glioblastoma Multiforme	Phase 1 Clinical trial	https://clinicaltrials.gov/ct2/show/NCT02049489
T cells	CD133	Various solid tumors	Phase 1 Clinical trial	Wang, Y. *et al.*, Oncoimmunology, 2018
	CD133	cholangiocarcinoma	Case report	Feng K. *et al*, JHO, 2017
	EGFR/IL-12	Metastatic colorectal cancer	Phase 1 Clinical trial	https://clinicaltrials.gov/ct2/show/NCT03542799
	MUC1/PD-1	Advanced Esophageal Cancer	Phase 1 and 2 Clinical trial	https://clinicaltrials.gov/ct2/show/NCT03706326
	CD133/EGRF/PD-1	Glioma, Malignant Glioma of Brain, Recurrence Tumor	Phase 1 Clinical trial	https://clinicaltrials.gov/ct2/show/NCT03423992
	EpCAM	Malignant Neoplasm of Nasopharynx TNM Staging Distant Metastasis (M), Breast Cancer Recurrent	Phase 1 Clinical trial	https://clinicaltrials.gov/ct2/show/NCT02915445

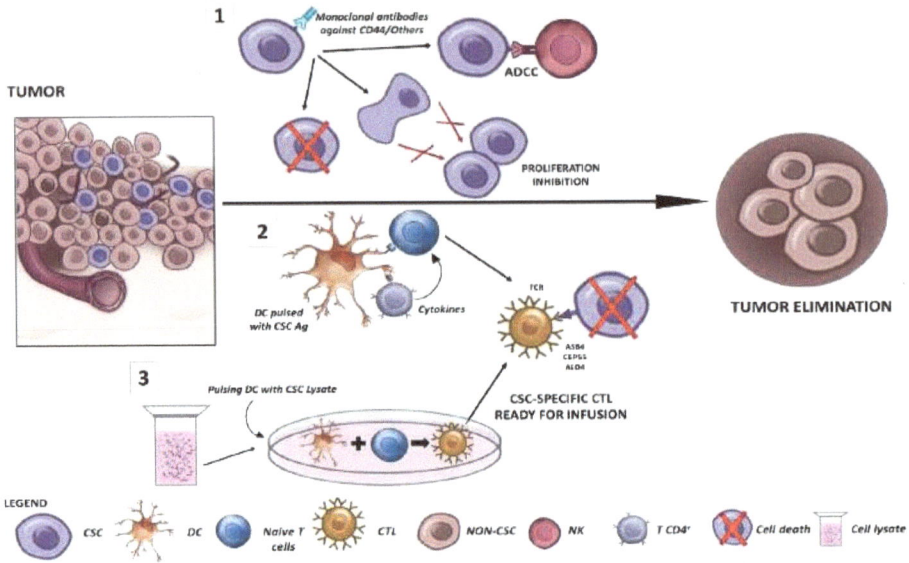

Fig. (5). Schematic representation of the different underlying mechanisms of various immunotherapies targeting cancer stem cells. Among the heterogeneous population of tumor cells, resistant cancer stem cells can be targeted by different modalities of CSC-focused immunotherapy to bring tumor elimination. **1)** monoclonal antibody administration against specific CSC surface markers, stem cell niche markers, or overexpressed antigens can lead to cell death, inhibit proliferation, or increase ADCC recognition. **2)** DC pulsed with CSC antigens can be delivered to patients and stimulate cellular immune response; CD8$^+$ T cells recognize CSC information and become a specific CSC CTL; CD4$^+$ T cells produce cytokines that help CD8$^+$ T cells to fight tumor *in vivo*. **3)** DC can be pulsed with CSC lysate from a patient, co-cultured with autologous T cells *in vitro* to generate CSC specific CTL, ready for infusion *in vivo*. Also, CSC specific CTL ready for infusion can be generated by genetically engineered T cells (CAR-T).

CONCLUSION

Several techniques have been developed aiming at CSC, such as monoclonal antibodies, adoptive T cell therapy, and also DC vaccines. These techniques can be associated with checkpoint blockade in different manners; all of them improve the immune response and efficiently eliminate CSCs. These approaches still need to be extensively tested, but it is believed that, since the combination of immunotherapeutic approaches with more conventional treatments has shown success, the association of CSC-focused immunotherapy can be another weapon in the arsenal of oncologists.

CONSENT FOR PUBLICATION

Not applicable.

CONFLICT OF INTEREST

The author declares that there is no conflict of interest in this chapter.

ACKNOWLEDGEMENTS

The authors would like to thank FAPESP (São Paulo Research Foundation, Grant #2017/01212-2) for financial support, Coordination for the Improvement of Higher Education Personnel - CAPES (Finance Code 001) and the National Council for Scientific and Technological Development - CNPq (process number 307603/2018-0). We are also thankful to Dr. Carolina Vieira de Almeida for the opportunity and confidence, to Dr. Cláudia Cristina Biguetti for her excellent artwork and Pedro Vannini for prompt help anytime.

LIST OF ABBREVIATION

ADCC	antibody-dependent cellular cytotoxicity
AML	acute myeloid leukemia
ALDH1	aldehyde dehydrogenase
APC	antigen-presenting cells
CAR-T	chimeric antigen receptor (car) T-cell therapy
CSC	cancer stem cells
CTLA-4	Cytotoxic T lymphocyte antigen 4
DC	dendritic cells
EGFR	epidermal growth factor receptor
EpCAM	epithelial cell adhesion molecule
ESC	epidermal stem cells
GSC	gastrointestinal stem cells
GSH	glutathione
HER-2	Human epithelial growth factor receptor 2
HNSCC	head and neck squamous cell carcinoma
HSC	hematopoietic stem cells
HSC	hepatic stem cells
iDC	imature dendritic cells
IgG	immunoglobulin G
iPSC	induced pluripotent stem cells
MCAO	middle carotid artery occlusion
MDR	multi drug resistance
MHC	major histocompatibility complex

MSC	mesenchymal stem cells
MTD	maximum tolerated dose
NK	natural killer cells
NSC	neural stem cells
OSCC	oral squamous cell carcinoma
PD-1	programmed cell death protein 1
PD-L1	programmed cell death protein 1 ligand
PSC	pancreatic stem cells
ROS	reactive oxygen species
SC	stem cells
SCID	severe combined immune-deficient mice
TA	transit-amplifying
TAA	tumor associated antigen
TCR	T cell receptor
Th1	type 1_T helper cell
TIL	Tumor-Infiltrating Lymphocytes
TME	tumor microenvironment
VEGF	vascular endothelial growth factor receptor

REFERENCES

[1]   International Association for Research on Cancer - World Health Organization. Latest global cancer data: Cancer burden rises to 18.1 million new cases and 9.6 million cancer deaths in 2018. Geneva 2018 2018. Press Release no 263.

[2]   D'Angelica M, Gonen M, Brennan MF, Turnbull AD, Bains M, Karpeh MS. Patterns of initial recurrence in completely resected gastric adenocarcinoma. Ann Surg 2004; 240(5): 808-16.
[http://dx.doi.org/10.1097/01.sla.0000143245.28656.15] [PMID: 15492562]

[3]   Macdonald JS, Smalley SR, Benedetti J, *et al.* Chemoradiotherapy after surgery compared with surgery alone for adenocarcinoma of the stomach or gastroesophageal junction. N Engl J Med 2001; 345(10): 725-30.
[http://dx.doi.org/10.1056/NEJMoa010187] [PMID: 11547741]

[4]   Shurin MRNH, Naiditch H, Gutkin DW, Umansky V, Shurin GV. ChemoImmunoModulation: immune regulation by the antineoplastic chemotherapeutic agents. Curr Med Chem 2012; 19(12): 1792-803.
[http://dx.doi.org/10.2174/092986712800099785] [PMID: 22414087]

[5]   Reya T, Morrison SJ, Clarke MF, Weissman IL. Stem cells, cancer, and cancer stem cells. Nature 2001; 414(6859): 105-11.
[http://dx.doi.org/10.1038/35102167] [PMID: 11689955]

[6]   Yu Z, Pestell TG, Lisanti MP, Pestell RG. Cancer stem cells. Int J Biochem Cell Biol 2012; 44(12): 2144-51.
[http://dx.doi.org/10.1016/j.biocel.2012.08.022] [PMID: 22981632]

[7]   Hobson-Gutierrez SA, Carmona-Fontaine C. The metabolic axis of macrophage and immune cell

polarization. Dis Model Mech 2018; 11(8): dmm034462.
[http://dx.doi.org/10.1242/dmm.034462] [PMID: 29991530]

[8]   Peddareddigari VG, Wang D, Dubois RN. The tumor microenvironment in colorectal carcinogenesis. Cancer Microenviron 2010; 3(1): 149-66.
[http://dx.doi.org/10.1007/s12307-010-0038-3] [PMID: 21209781]

[9]   Hanahan D, Weinberg RA. Hallmarks of cancer: the next generation. Cell 2011; 144(5): 646-74.
[http://dx.doi.org/10.1016/j.cell.2011.02.013] [PMID: 21376230]

[10]   O'Toole A, Michielsen AJ, Nolan B, *et al.* Tumour microenvironment of both early- and late-stage colorectal cancer is equally immunosuppressive. Br J Cancer 2014; 111(5): 927-32.
[http://dx.doi.org/10.1038/bjc.2014.367] [PMID: 25058349]

[11]   O'Neill LA, Hardie DG. Metabolism of inflammation limited by AMPK and pseudo-starvation. Nature 2013; 493(7432): 346-55.
[http://dx.doi.org/10.1038/nature11862] [PMID: 23325217]

[12]   Ganeshan K, Chawla A. Metabolic regulation of immune responses. Annu Rev Immunol 2014; 32: 609-34.
[http://dx.doi.org/10.1146/annurev-immunol-032713-120236] [PMID: 24655299]

[13]   Olenchock BA, Rathmell JC, Vander Heiden MG. Biochemical Underpinnings of Immune Cell Metabolic Phenotypes. Immunity 2017; 46(5): 703-13.
[http://dx.doi.org/10.1016/j.immuni.2017.04.013] [PMID: 28514672]

[14]   Mantovani A, Allavena P, Sica A, Balkwill F. Cancer-related inflammation. Nature 2008; 454(7203): 436-44.
[http://dx.doi.org/10.1038/nature07205] [PMID: 18650914]

[15]   Ferrone C, Dranoff G. Dual roles for immunity in gastrointestinal cancers. J Clin Oncol 2010; 28(26): 4045-51.
[http://dx.doi.org/10.1200/JCO.2010.27.9992] [PMID: 20644090]

[16]   Agüera-González S, Burton OT, Vázquez-Chávez E, *et al.* Adenomatous Polyposis Coli Defines Treg Differentiation and Anti-inflammatory Function through Microtubule-Mediated NFAT Localization. Cell Rep 2017; 21(1): 181-94.
[http://dx.doi.org/10.1016/j.celrep.2017.09.020] [PMID: 28978472]

[17]   Sanmamed MF, Chen L. A Paradigm Shift in Cancer Immunotherapy: From Enhancement to Normalization. Cell 2018; 175(2): 313-26.
[http://dx.doi.org/10.1016/j.cell.2018.09.035] [PMID: 30290139]

[18]   Hall PA, Watt FM. Stem cells: the generation and maintenance of cellular diversity. Development 1989; 106(4): 619-33.
[PMID: 2562658]

[19]   Swift ME, Kleinman HK, DiPietro LA. Impaired wound repair and delayed angiogenesis in aged mice. Lab Invest 1999; 79(12): 1479-87.

[20]   Weissman IL. Stem cells: units of development, units of regeneration, and units in evolution. Cell 2000; 100(1): 157-68.
[http://dx.doi.org/10.1016/S0092-8674(00)81692-X] [PMID: 10647940]

[21]   He S, Nakada D, Morrison SJ. Mechanisms of stem cell self-renewal. Annu Rev Cell Dev Biol 2009; 25: 377-406.
[http://dx.doi.org/10.1146/annurev.cellbio.042308.113248] [PMID: 19575646]

[22]   Wagers AJ, Weissman IL. Plasticity of adult stem cells. Cell 2004; 116(5): 639-48.
[http://dx.doi.org/10.1016/S0092-8674(04)00208-9] [PMID: 15006347]

[23]   Jaenisch R, Young R. Stem cells, the molecular circuitry of pluripotency and nuclear reprogramming. Cell 2008; 132(4): 567-82.

[http://dx.doi.org/10.1016/j.cell.2008.01.015] [PMID: 18295576]

[24]   Bryder D, Rossi DJ, Weissman IL. Hematopoietic stem cells: the paradigmatic tissue-specific stem cell. Am J Pathol 2006; 169(2): 338-46.
       [http://dx.doi.org/10.2353/ajpath.2006.060312] [PMID: 16877336]

[25]   Molofsky AV, Pardal R, Morrison SJ. Diverse mechanisms regulate stem cell self-renewal. Curr Opin Cell Biol 2004; 16(6): 700-7.
       [http://dx.doi.org/10.1016/j.ceb.2004.09.004] [PMID: 15530784]

[26]   Pittenger MF, Mackay AM, Beck SC, Jaiswal RK, Douglas R, Mosca JD, *et al.* Multilineage potential of adult human mesenchymal stem cells. Science 1999; 284(5411): 143-7.
       [http://dx.doi.org/10.1126/science.284.5411.143]

[27]   EL-Barky AR, Ehab MMA, Mohamed TM. Stem cells, classifications and their clinical applications. Am J Pharmacol Ther 2017; 1: 1-7.

[28]   Bianco P, Riminucci M, Gronthos S, Robey PG. Bone marrow stromal stem cells: nature, biology, and potential applications. Stem Cells 2001; 19(3): 180-92.
       [http://dx.doi.org/10.1634/stemcells.19-3-180] [PMID: 11359943]

[29]   Rodini CO, Lopes NM, Lara VS, Mackenzie IC. Oral cancer stem cells - properties and consequences. J Appl Oral Sci 2017; 25(6): 708-15.
       [http://dx.doi.org/10.1590/1678-7757-2016-0665] [PMID: 29211293]

[30]   Gurdon JB. The developmental capacity of nuclei taken from intestinal epithelium cells of feeding tadpoles. J Embryol Exp Morphol 1962; 10: 622-40.
       [PMID: 13951335]

[31]   Takahashi K, Yamanaka S. Induction of pluripotent stem cells from mouse embryonic and adult fibroblast cultures by defined factors. Cell 2006; 126(4): 663-76.
       [http://dx.doi.org/10.1016/j.cell.2006.07.024] [PMID: 16904174]

[32]   Seki T, Fukuda K. Methods of induced pluripotent stem cells for clinical application. World J Stem Cells 2015; 7(1): 116-25.
       [http://dx.doi.org/10.4252/wjsc.v7.i1.116] [PMID: 25621111]

[33]   Lam PK, Wang KKW, Chin DWC, *et al.* Topically applied adipose-derived mesenchymal stem cell treatment in experimental focal cerebral ischemia. J Clin Neurosci 2020; 71: 226-33.
       [PMID: 31431402]

[34]   Ning T, Shao J, Zhang X, *et al.* Aging affects the proliferation and mineralization of rat dental pulp stem cells under inflammatory conditions. Int Endod J 2020; 53(1): 72-83.

[35]   National Institutes of Health resource for stem cell research. [July 21, 2019]; The stem cell information Stem Cell Basics page. Available at: http://stemcells.nih.gov/info/basics/defaultpage.asp

[36]   Visvader JE. Cells of origin in cancer. Nature 2011; 469(7330): 314-22.
       [http://dx.doi.org/10.1038/nature09781] [PMID: 21248838]

[37]   Aguilar-Gallardo C, Simón C. Cells, stem cells, and cancer stem cells. Semin Reprod Med 2013; 31(1): 5-13.
       [http://dx.doi.org/10.1055/s-0032-1331792] [PMID: 23329631]

[38]   Prasetyanti PR, Medema JP. Intra-tumor heterogeneity from a cancer stem cell perspective. Mol Cancer 2017; 16(1): 41.
       [http://dx.doi.org/10.1186/s12943-017-0600-4] [PMID: 28209166]

[39]   Lapidot T, Sirard C, Vormoor J, *et al.* A cell initiating human acute myeloid leukaemia after transplantation into SCID mice. Nature 1994; 367(6464): 645-8.
       [http://dx.doi.org/10.1038/367645a0] [PMID: 7509044]

[40]   Bonnet D, Dick JE. Human acute myeloid leukemia is organized as a hierarchy that originates from a primitive hematopoietic cell. Nat Med 1997; 3(7): 730-7.

[http://dx.doi.org/10.1038/nm0797-730] [PMID: 9212098]

[41]   Al-Hajj M, Wicha MS, Benito-Hernandez A, Morrison SJ, Clarke MF. Prospective identification of tumorigenic breast cancer cells. Proc Natl Acad Sci USA 2003; 100(7): 3983-8.
[http://dx.doi.org/10.1073/pnas.0530291100] [PMID: 12629218]

[42]   Singh SK, Clarke ID, Terasaki M, *et al.* Identification of a cancer stem cell in human brain tumors. Cancer Res 2003; 63(18): 5821-8.
[PMID: 14522905]

[43]   Ricci-Vitiani L, Lombardi DG, Pilozzi E, *et al.* Identification and expansion of human colon-cance-
-initiating cells. Nat 2007; 445(7123): 111-5.

[44]   Eramo A, Lotti F, Sette G, *et al.* Identification and expansion of the tumorigenic lung cancer stem cell population. Cell Death Differ 2008; 15(3): 504-14.
[http://dx.doi.org/10.1038/sj.cdd.4402283] [PMID: 18049477]

[45]   Walton JD, Kattan DR, Thomas SK, *et al.* Characteristics of stem cells from human neuroblastoma cell lines and in tumors. Neoplasia 2004; 6(6): 838-45.
[http://dx.doi.org/10.1593/neo.04310] [PMID: 15720811]

[46]   Visvader JE, Lindeman GJ. Cancer stem cells in solid tumours: accumulating evidence and unresolved questions. Nat Rev Cancer 2008; 8(10): 755-68.
[http://dx.doi.org/10.1038/nrc2499] [PMID: 18784658]

[47]   Buishand FO, Arkesteijn GJ, Feenstra LR, *et al.* Identification of CD90 as putative cancer stem cell marker and therapeutic target in insulinomas. Stem Cells Dev 2016; 25(11): 826-35.
[http://dx.doi.org/10.1089/scd.2016.0032] [PMID: 27049037]

[48]   Zöller M. CD44: can a cancer-initiating cell profit from an abundantly expressed molecule? Nat Rev Cancer 2011; 11(4): 254-67.
[http://dx.doi.org/10.1038/nrc3023] [PMID: 21390059]

[49]   Pattabiraman DR, Weinberg RA. Tackling the cancer stem cells - what challenges do they pose? Nat Rev Drug Discov 2014; 13(7): 497-512.
[http://dx.doi.org/10.1038/nrd4253] [PMID: 24981363]

[50]   Collins AT, Berry PA, Hyde C, Stower MJ, Maitland NJ. Prospective identification of tumorigenic prostate cancer stem cells. Cancer Res 2005; 65(23): 10946-51.
[http://dx.doi.org/10.1158/0008-5472.CAN-05-2018] [PMID: 16322242]

[51]   Dalerba P, Dylla SJ, Park IK, *et al.* Phenotypic characterization of human colorectal cancer stem cells. Proc Natl Acad Sci USA 2007; 104(24): 10158-63.
[http://dx.doi.org/10.1073/pnas.0703478104] [PMID: 17548814]

[52]   Yasuda K, Torigoe T, Morita R, *et al.* Ovarian cancer stem cells are enriched in side population and aldehyde dehydrogenase bright overlapping population. PLoS One 2013; 8(8): e68187.
[http://dx.doi.org/10.1371/journal.pone.0068187] [PMID: 23967051]

[53]   Ortiz RC, Lopes NM, Amôr NG, *et al.* CD44 and ALDH1 immunoexpression as prognostic indicators of invasion and metastasis in oral squamous cell carcinoma. J Oral Pathol Med 2018; 47(8): 740-7.
[http://dx.doi.org/10.1111/jop.12734] [PMID: 29791975]

[54]   Chen K, Huang YH, Chen JL. Understanding and targeting cancer stem cells: therapeutic implications and challenges. Acta Pharmacol Sin 2013; 34(6): 732-40.
[http://dx.doi.org/10.1038/aps.2013.27] [PMID: 23685952]

[55]   Kasai T, Chen L, Mizutani A, *et al.* Cancer stem cells converted from pluripotent stem cells and the cancerous niche. J Stem Cells Regen Med 2014; 10(1): 2-7.
[http://dx.doi.org/10.46582/jsrm.1001002] [PMID: 25075155]

[56]   Elrick LJ, Jorgensen HG, Mountford JC, Holyoake TL. Punish the parent not the progeny. Blood 2005; 105(5): 1862-6.

[http://dx.doi.org/10.1182/blood-2004-08-3373] [PMID: 15528314]

[57]   Vlashi E, Kim K, Lagadec C, *et al. In vivo* imaging, tracking, and targeting of cancer stem cells. J Natl Cancer Inst 2009; 101(5): 350-9.
[http://dx.doi.org/10.1093/jnci/djn509] [PMID: 19244169]

[58]   Kiyohara MH, Dillard C, Tsui J, *et al.* EMP2 is a novel therapeutic target for endometrial cancer stem cells. Oncogene 2017; 36(42): 5793-807.
[http://dx.doi.org/10.1038/onc.2017.142] [PMID: 28604744]

[59]   Shlush LI, Mitchell A, Heisler L, *et al.* Tracing the origins of relapse in acute myeloid leukaemia to stem cells. Nature 2017; 547(7661): 104-8.
[http://dx.doi.org/10.1038/nature22993] [PMID: 28658204]

[60]   Fang D, Kitamura H. Cancer stem cells and epithelial-mesenchymal transition in urothelial carcinoma: Possible pathways and potential therapeutic approaches. Int J Urol 2018; 25(1): 7-17.
[http://dx.doi.org/10.1111/iju.13404] [PMID: 28697535]

[61]   Laplane L. Cancer stem cells: philosophy and therapies. Cambridge: Harvard University Press 2016.
[http://dx.doi.org/10.4159/9780674969582]

[62]   Liu G, Yuan X, Zeng Z, *et al.* Analysis of gene expression and chemoresistance of CD133+ cancer stem cells in glioblastoma. Mol Cancer 2006; 5: 67.
[http://dx.doi.org/10.1186/1476-4598-5-67] [PMID: 17140455]

[63]   Hambardzumyan D, Becher OJ, Rosenblum MK, Pandolfi PP, Manova-Todorova K, Holland EC. PI3K pathway regulates survival of cancer stem cells residing in the perivascular niche following radiation in medulloblastoma *in vivo.* Genes Dev 2008; 22(4): 436-48.
[http://dx.doi.org/10.1101/gad.1627008] [PMID: 18281460]

[64]   Graham SM, Jørgensen HG, Allan E, *et al.* Primitive, quiescent, Philadelphia-positive stem cells from patients with chronic myeloid leukemia are insensitive to STI571 in vitro. Blood 2002; 99(1): 319-25.
[http://dx.doi.org/10.1182/blood.V99.1.319] [PMID: 11756187]

[65]   Holtz MS, Forman SJ, Bhatia R. Nonproliferating CML CD34+ progenitors are resistant to apoptosis induced by a wide range of proapoptotic stimuli. Leukemia 2005; 19(6): 1034-41.
[http://dx.doi.org/10.1038/sj.leu.2403724] [PMID: 15815728]

[66]   Copland M, Hamilton A, Elrick LJ, *et al.* Dasatinib (BMS-354825) targets an earlier progenitor population than imatinib in primary CML but does not eliminate the quiescent fraction. Blood 2006; 107(11): 4532-9.
[http://dx.doi.org/10.1182/blood-2005-07-2947] [PMID: 16469872]

[67]   Bao S, Wu Q, McLendon RE, *et al.* Glioma stem cells promote radioresistance by preferential activation of the DNA damage response. Nature 2006; 444(7120): 756-60.
[http://dx.doi.org/10.1038/nature05236] [PMID: 17051156]

[68]   Zhang M, Atkinson RL, Rosen JM. Selective targeting of radiation-resistant tumor-initiating cells. Proc Natl Acad Sci USA 2010; 107(8): 3522-7.
[http://dx.doi.org/10.1073/pnas.0910179107] [PMID: 20133717]

[69]   Hirschmann-Jax C, Foster AE, Wulf GG, *et al.* A distinct "side population" of cells with high drug efflux capacity in human tumor cells. Proc Natl Acad Sci USA 2004; 101(39): 14228-33.
[http://dx.doi.org/10.1073/pnas.0400067101] [PMID: 15381773]

[70]   Huss WJ, Gray DR, Greenberg NM, Mohler JL, Smith GJ. Breast cancer resistance protein-mediated efflux of androgen in putative benign and malignant prostate stem cells. Cancer Res 2005; 65(15): 6640-50.
[http://dx.doi.org/10.1158/0008-5472.CAN-04-2548] [PMID: 16061644]

[71]   Abbott BL. ABCG2 (BCRP): a cytoprotectant in normal and malignant stem cells. Clin Adv Hematol Oncol 2006; 4(1): 63-72.
[PMID: 16562373]

[72]   Calabrese C, Poppleton H, Kocak M, *et al.* A perivascular niche for brain tumor stem cells. Cancer Cell 2007; 11(1): 69-82.
       [http://dx.doi.org/10.1016/j.ccr.2006.11.020] [PMID: 17222791]

[73]   Diehn M, Cho RW, Lobo NA, *et al.* Association of reactive oxygen species levels and radioresistance in cancer stem cells. Nature 2009; 458(7239): 780-3.
       [http://dx.doi.org/10.1038/nature07733] [PMID: 19194462]

[74]   Tan S, Yamashita A, Gao SJ, Kurisawa M. Hyaluronic acid hydrogels with defined crosslink density for the efficient enrichment of breast cancer stem cells. Acta Biomater 2019; 94: 320-9.
       [http://dx.doi.org/10.1016/j.actbio.2019.05.040] [PMID: 31125725]

[75]   Koh SP, Brasch HD, de Jongh J, Itinteang T, Tan ST. Cancer stem cell subpopulations in moderately differentiated head and neck cutaneous squamous cell carcinoma. Heliyon 2019; 5(8): e02257.
       [http://dx.doi.org/10.1016/j.heliyon.2019.e02257] [PMID: 31463389]

[76]   Caparosa EM, Stem J, Snook AE, Waldman SA. Biomarker targeting of colorectal cancer stem cells. Biomark Med 2019; 13(11): 891-4.
       [http://dx.doi.org/10.2217/bmm-2019-0227]

[77]   Chatterjee A. Reduced glutathione: a radioprotector or a modulator of DNA-repair activity? Nutrients 2013; 5(2): 525-42.
       [http://dx.doi.org/10.3390/nu5020525] [PMID: 23434907]

[78]   Therasse P, Arbuck SG, Eisenhauer EA, *et al.* New guidelines to evaluate the response to treatment in solid tumors. J Natl Cancer Inst 2000; 92(3): 205-16.
       [http://dx.doi.org/10.1093/jnci/92.3.205] [PMID: 10655437]

[79]   Eisenhauer EA, Therasse P, Bogaerts J, *et al.* New response evaluation criteria in solid tumours: revised RECIST guideline (version 1.1). Eur J Cancer 2009; 45(2): 228-47.
       [http://dx.doi.org/10.1016/j.ejca.2008.10.026] [PMID: 19097774]

[80]   Farkona S, Diamandis EP, Blasutig IM. Cancer immunotherapy: the beginning of the end of cancer? BMC Med 2016; 14: 73.
       [http://dx.doi.org/10.1186/s12916-016-0623-5] [PMID: 27151159]

[81]   Toomey PG, Vohra NA, Ghansah T, Sarnaik AA, Pilon-Thomas SA. Immunotherapy for gastrointestinal malignancies. Cancer Contr 2013; 20(1): 32-42.
       [http://dx.doi.org/10.1177/107327481302000106] [PMID: 23302905]

[82]   Martinelli E, De Palma R, Orditura M, De Vita F, Ciardiello F. Anti-epidermal growth factor receptor monoclonal antibodies in cancer therapy. Clin Exp Immunol 2009; 158(1): 1-9.
       [http://dx.doi.org/10.1111/j.1365-2249.2009.03992.x] [PMID: 19737224]

[83]   Riechmann L, Clark M, Waldmann H, Winter G. Reshaping human antibodies for therapy. Nature 1988; 332(6162): 323-7.
       [http://dx.doi.org/10.1038/332323a0] [PMID: 3127726]

[84]   Gura T. Therapeutic antibodies: magic bullets hit the target. Nature 2002; 417(6889): 584-6.
       [http://dx.doi.org/10.1038/417584a] [PMID: 12050630]

[85]   Woodburn JR. The epidermal growth factor receptor and its inhibition in cancer therapy. Pharmacol Ther 1999; 82(2-3): 241-50.
       [http://dx.doi.org/10.1016/S0163-7258(98)00045-X] [PMID: 10454201]

[86]   Díaz-Serrano A, Sánchez-Torre A, Paz-Ares L. Necitumumab for the treatment of advanced non-small-cell lung cancer. Future Oncol 2019; 15(7): 705-16.
       [http://dx.doi.org/10.2217/fon-2018-0594] [PMID: 30501503]

[87]   Qiu W, Zhang C, Wang S, *et al.* A novel anti-egfr mab ame55 with lower toxicity and better efficacy than cetuximab when combined with irinotecan. J Immunol Res 2019; 2019: 3017360.
       [http://dx.doi.org/10.1155/2019/3017360] [PMID: 30733972]

[88]   Gutierrez C, Schiff R. HER2: biology, detection, and clinical implications. Arch Pathol Lab Med 2011; 135(1): 55-62.
[PMID: 21204711]

[89]   Yao M, Fu P. Advances in anti-HER2 therapy in metastatic breast cancer. Linchuang Zhongliuxue Zazhi 2018; 7(3): 27.
[http://dx.doi.org/10.21037/cco.2018.05.04] [PMID: 30056729]

[90]   Pardoll DM. The blockade of immune checkpoints in cancer immunotherapy. Nat Rev Cancer 2012; 12(4): 252-64.
[http://dx.doi.org/10.1038/nrc3239] [PMID: 22437870]

[91]   Rezaeeyan H, Hassani SN, Barati M, Shahjahani M, Saki N. PD-1/PD-L1 as a prognostic factor in leukemia. J Hematop 2017; 10: 17-24.
[http://dx.doi.org/10.1007/s12308-017-0293-z]

[92]   Gianchecchi E, Delfino DV, Fierabracci A. Recent insights into the role of the PD-1/PD-L1 pathway in immunological tolerance and autoimmunity. Autoimmun Rev 2013; 12(11): 1091-100.
[http://dx.doi.org/10.1016/j.autrev.2013.05.003] [PMID: 23792703]

[93]   Geller A, Yan J. The role of membrane bound complement regulatory proteins in tumor development and cancer immunotherapy. Front Immunol 2019; 10: 1074.
[http://dx.doi.org/10.3389/fimmu.2019.01074] [PMID: 31164885]

[94]   Mariotti FR, Quatrini L, Munari E, Vacca P, Moretta L. Innate lymphoid cells: expression of PD-1 and other checkpoints in normal and pathological conditions. Front Immunol 2019; 10: 910.
[http://dx.doi.org/10.3389/fimmu.2019.00910] [PMID: 31105707]

[95]   Juneja VR, McGuire KA, Manguso RT, *et al.* PD-L1 on tumor cells is sufficient for immune evasion in immunogenic tumors and inhibits CD8 T cell cytotoxicity. J Exp Med 2017; 214(4): 895-904.
[http://dx.doi.org/10.1084/jem.20160801] [PMID: 28302645]

[96]   Sharma P, Allison JP. The future of immune checkpoint therapy. Science 2015; 348(6230): 56-61.
[http://dx.doi.org/10.1126/science.aaa8172] [PMID: 25838373]

[97]   Passardi A, Canale M, Valgiusti M, Ulivi P. Immune checkpoints as a target for colorectal cancer treatment. Int J Mol Sci 2017; 18(6): 1324.
[http://dx.doi.org/10.3390/ijms18061324] [PMID: 28635639]

[98]   Vaddepally RK, Kharel P, Pandey R, Garje R, Chandra AB. Review of indications of fda-approved immune checkpoint inhibitors per NCCN guidelines with the level of evidence. Cancers (Basel) 2020; 12(3): E738.
[http://dx.doi.org/10.3390/cancers12030738] [PMID: 32245016]

[99]   Ferris RL, Lenz HJ, Trotta AM, *et al.* Rationale for combination of therapeutic antibodies targeting tumor cells and immune checkpoint receptors: Harnessing innate and adaptive immunity through IgG1 isotype immune effector stimulation. Cancer Treat Rev 2018; 63: 48-60.
[http://dx.doi.org/10.1016/j.ctrv.2017.11.008] [PMID: 29223828]

[100]   López-Gómez M, Merino M, Casado E. Long-term treatment of metastatic colorectal cancer with panitumumab. Clin Med Insights Oncol 2012; 6: 125-35.
[http://dx.doi.org/10.4137/CMO.S5055] [PMID: 22408376]

[101]   Kalinski P, Okada H. Polarized dendritic cells as cancer vaccines: directing effector-type T cells to tumors. Semin Immunol 2010; 22(3): 173-82.
[http://dx.doi.org/10.1016/j.smim.2010.03.002] [PMID: 20409732]

[102]   Lee HJ, Hong CY, Kim MH, *et al. In vitro* induction of anterior gradient-2-specific cytotoxic T lymphocytes by dendritic cells transduced with recombinant adenoviruses as a potential therapy for colorectal cancer. Exp Mol Med 2012; 44(1): 60-7.
[http://dx.doi.org/10.3858/emm.2012.44.1.006] [PMID: 22089087]

[103]   Steinman RM. Decisions about dendritic cells: past, present, and future. Annu Rev Immunol 2012; 30: 1-22.
[http://dx.doi.org/10.1146/annurev-immunol-100311-102839] [PMID: 22136168]

[104]   Banchereau J, Steinman RM. Dendritic cells and the control of immunity. Nature 1998; 392(6673): 245-52.
[http://dx.doi.org/10.1038/32588] [PMID: 9521319]

[105]   Mitchell EP, Piperdi B, Lacouture ME, *et al.* The efficacy and safety of panitumumab administered concomitantly with FOLFIRI or Irinotecan in second-line therapy for metastatic colorectal cancer: the secondary analysis from STEPP (Skin Toxicity Evaluation Protocol With Panitumumab) by KRAS status. Clin Colorectal Cancer 2011; 10(4): 333-9.
[http://dx.doi.org/10.1016/j.clcc.2011.06.004] [PMID: 22000810]

[106]   Lipscomb MF, Masten BJ. Dendritic cells: immune regulators in health and disease. Physiol Rev 2002; 82(1): 97-130.
[http://dx.doi.org/10.1152/physrev.00023.2001] [PMID: 11773610]

[107]   Palucka AK, Ueno H, Fay J, Banchereau J. Dendritic cells: a critical player in cancer therapy? J Immunother 2008; 31(9): 793-805.
[http://dx.doi.org/10.1097/CJI.0b013e31818403bc] [PMID: 18833008]

[108]   Grabbe S, Beissert S, Schwarz T, Granstein RD. Dendritic cells as initiators of tumor immune responses: a possible strategy for tumor immunotherapy? Immunol Today 1995; 16(3): 117-21.
[http://dx.doi.org/10.1016/0167-5699(95)80125-1] [PMID: 7718082]

[109]   Gilboa E. DC-based cancer vaccines. J Clin Invest 2007; 117(5): 1195-203.
[http://dx.doi.org/10.1172/JCI31205] [PMID: 17476349]

[110]   Shurin MR. Dendritic cells presenting tumor antigen. Cancer Immunol Immunother 1996; 43(3): 158-64.
[http://dx.doi.org/10.1007/s002620050317] [PMID: 9001569]

[111]   Steinman RM. The dendritic cell system and its role in immunogenicity. Annu Rev Immunol 1991; 9: 271-96.
[http://dx.doi.org/10.1146/annurev.iy.09.040191.001415] [PMID: 1910679]

[112]   Arina A, Tirapu I, Alfaro C, *et al.* Clinical implications of antigen transfer mechanisms from malignant to dendritic cells. exploiting cross-priming. Exp Hematol 2002; 30(12): 1355-64.
[http://dx.doi.org/10.1016/S0301-472X(02)00956-6] [PMID: 12482496]

[113]   Amado RG, Wolf M, Peeters M, *et al.* Wild-type KRAS is required for panitumumab efficacy in patients with metastatic colorectal cancer. J Clin Oncol 2008; 26(10): 1626-34.
[http://dx.doi.org/10.1200/JCO.2007.14.7116] [PMID: 18316791]

[114]   Reyes D, Salazar L, Espinoza E, *et al.* Tumour cell lysate-loaded dendritic cell vaccine induces biochemical and memory immune response in castration-resistant prostate cancer patients. Br J Cancer 2013; 109(6): 1488-97.
[http://dx.doi.org/10.1038/bjc.2013.494] [PMID: 23989944]

[115]   Koido S, Homma S, Okamoto M, *et al.* Strategies to improve the immunogenicity of anticancer vaccines based on dendritic cell/malignant cell fusions. OncoImmunology 2013; 2(9): e25994.
[http://dx.doi.org/10.4161/onci.25994] [PMID: 24228229]

[116]   Nencioni A, Müller MR, Grünebach F, *et al.* Dendritic cells transfected with tumor RNA for the induction of antitumor CTL in colorectal cancer. Cancer Gene Ther 2003; 10(3): 209-14.
[http://dx.doi.org/10.1038/sj.cgt.7700557] [PMID: 12637942]

[117]   de Camargo MR, Gorgulho CM, Rodrigues CP, *et al.* Low Concentration of 5-Fluorouracil Increases the Effectiveness of Tumor RNA to Activate Murine Dendritic Cells. Cancer Biother Radiopharm 2017; 32(8): 302-8.
[http://dx.doi.org/10.1089/cbr.2017.2259] [PMID: 29053415]

[118] Carreno BM, Magrini V, Becker-Hapak M, *et al.* Cancer immunotherapy. A dendritic cell vaccine increases the breadth and diversity of melanoma neoantigen-specific T cells. Science 2015; 348(6236): 803-8.
[http://dx.doi.org/10.1126/science.aaa3828] [PMID: 25837513]

[119] Maeda Y, Yoshimura K, Matsui H, *et al.* Dendritic cells transfected with heat-shock protein 70 messenger RNA for patients with hepatitis C virus-related hepatocellular carcinoma: a phase 1 dose escalation clinical trial. Cancer Immunol Immunother 2015; 64(8): 1047-56.
[http://dx.doi.org/10.1007/s00262-015-1709-1] [PMID: 25982372]

[120] Rosenberg SA, Yang JC, Sherry RM, *et al.* Durable complete responses in heavily pretreated patients with metastatic melanoma using T-cell transfer immunotherapy. Clin Cancer Res 2011; 17(13): 4550-7.
[http://dx.doi.org/10.1158/1078-0432.CCR-11-0116] [PMID: 21498393]

[121] Ott PA, Dotti G, Yee C, Goff SL. An Update on Adoptive T-Cell Therapy and Neoantigen Vaccines. Am Soc Clin Oncol Educ Book 2019; 39: e70-8.
[http://dx.doi.org/10.1200/EDBK_238001] [PMID: 31099621]

[122] van Rooij N, van Buuren MM, Philips D, *et al.* Tumor exome analysis reveals neoantigen-specific T-cell reactivity in an ipilimumab-responsive melanoma. J Clin Oncol 2013; 31(32): e439-42.
[http://dx.doi.org/10.1200/JCO.2012.47.7521] [PMID: 24043743]

[123] Tran E, Robbins PF, Lu YC, *et al.* T-Cell Transfer Therapy Targeting Mutant KRAS in Cancer. N Engl J Med 2016; 375(23): 2255-62.
[http://dx.doi.org/10.1056/NEJMoa1609279] [PMID: 27959684]

[124] Tran E, Turcotte S, Gros A, *et al.* Cancer immunotherapy based on mutation-specific CD4+ T cells in a patient with epithelial cancer. Science 2014; 344(6184): 641-5.
[http://dx.doi.org/10.1126/science.1251102] [PMID: 24812403]

[125] Stevanović S, Helman SR, Wunderlich JR, *et al.* A phase II study of tumor-infiltrating lymphocyte therapy for human papillomavirus-associated epithelial cancers. Clin Cancer Res 2019; 25(5): 1486-93.
[http://dx.doi.org/10.1158/1078-0432.CCR-18-2722] [PMID: 30518633]

[126] Klaver Y, Kunert A, Sleijfer S, Debets R, Lamers CH. Adoptive T-cell therapy: a need for standard immune monitoring. Immunotherapy 2015; 7(5): 513-33.
[http://dx.doi.org/10.2217/imt.15.23] [PMID: 26065477]

[127] Jafferji MS, Yang JC. Adoptive t-cell therapy for solid malignancies. Surg Oncol Clin N Am 2019; 28(3): 465-79.
[http://dx.doi.org/10.1016/j.soc.2019.02.012] [PMID: 31079800]

[128] Maus MV, Grupp SA, Porter DL, June CH. Antibody-modified T cells: CARs take the front seat for hematologic malignancies. Blood 2014; 123(17): 2625-35.
[http://dx.doi.org/10.1182/blood-2013-11-492231] [PMID: 24578504]

[129] Ramakrishna S, Barsan V, Mackall C. Prospects and challenges for use of CAR T cell therapies in solid tumors. Expert Opin Biol Ther 2020; 20(5): 503-16.
[http://dx.doi.org/10.1080/14712598.2020.1738378] [PMID: 32125191]

[130] Pozzi C, Cuomo A, Spadoni I, *et al.* The EGFR-specific antibody cetuximab combined with chemotherapy triggers immunogenic cell death. Nat Med 2016; 22(6): 624-31.
[http://dx.doi.org/10.1038/nm.4078] [PMID: 27135741]

[131] Gemenetzidis E, Gammon L, Biddle A, Emich H, Mackenzie IC. Invasive oral cancer stem cells display resistance to ionising radiation. Oncotarget 2015; 6(41): 43964-77.
[http://dx.doi.org/10.18632/oncotarget.6268] [PMID: 26540568]

[132] Naik PP, Das DN, Panda PK, *et al.* Implications of cancer stem cells in developing therapeutic resistance in oral cancer. Oral Oncol 2016; 62: 122-35.

[http://dx.doi.org/10.1016/j.oraloncology.2016.10.008] [PMID: 27865365]

[133]   Shibue T, Weinberg RA. EMT, CSCs, and drug resistance: the mechanistic link and clinical implications. Nat Rev Clin Oncol 2017; 14(10): 611-29.
[http://dx.doi.org/10.1038/nrclinonc.2017.44] [PMID: 28397828]

[134]   Ola MS, Nawaz M, Ahsan H. Role of Bcl-2 family proteins and caspases in the regulation of apoptosis. Mol Cell Biochem 2011; 351(1-2): 41-58.
[http://dx.doi.org/10.1007/s11010-010-0709-x] [PMID: 21210296]

[135]   Roesler R, Cornelio DB, Abujamra AL, Schwartsmann G. HER2 as a cancer stem-cell target. Lancet Oncol 2010; 11(3): 225-6.
[http://dx.doi.org/10.1016/S1470-2045(09)70404-8] [PMID: 20202610]

[136]   Katayama R, Koike S, Sato S, Sugimoto Y, Tsuruo T, Fujita N. Dofequidar fumarate sensitizes cancer stem-like side population cells to chemotherapeutic drugs by inhibiting ABCG2/BCRP-mediated drug export. Cancer Sci 2009; 100(11): 2060-8.
[http://dx.doi.org/10.1111/j.1349-7006.2009.01288.x] [PMID: 19673889]

[137]   Takahashi-Yanaga F, Kahn M. Targeting Wnt signaling: can we safely eradicate cancer stem cells? Clin Cancer Res 2010; 16(12): 3153-62.
[http://dx.doi.org/10.1158/1078-0432.CCR-09-2943] [PMID: 20530697]

[138]   Pan Y, Ma S, Cao K, *et al.* Therapeutic approaches targeting cancer stem cells. J Cancer Res Ther 2018; 14(7): 1469-75.
[http://dx.doi.org/10.4103/jcrt.JCRT_976_17] [PMID: 30589025]

[139]   Hirohashi Y, Torigoe T, Inoda S, *et al.* Immune response against tumor antigens expressed on human cancer stem-like cells/tumor-initiating cells. Immunotherapy 2010; 2(2): 201-11.
[http://dx.doi.org/10.2217/imt.10.10] [PMID: 20635928]

[140]   Santamaria S, Delgado M, Kremer L, Garcia-Sanz JA. Will a mAb-Based Immunotherapy Directed against Cancer Stem Cells Be Feasible? Front Immunol 2017; 8: 1509.
[http://dx.doi.org/10.3389/fimmu.2017.01509] [PMID: 29170667]

[141]   Vey N, Delaunay J, Martinelli G, *et al.* Phase I clinical study of RG7356, an anti-CD44 humanized antibody, in patients with acute myeloid leukemia. Oncotarget 2016; 7(22): 32532-42.
[http://dx.doi.org/10.18632/oncotarget.8687] [PMID: 27081038]

[142]   Menke-van der Houven van Oordt CW, Gomez-Roca C, van Herpen C, *et al.* First-in-human phase I clinical trial of RG7356, an anti-CD44 humanized antibody, in patients with advanced, CD44-expressing solid tumors. Oncotarget 2016; 7(48): 80046-58.
[http://dx.doi.org/10.18632/oncotarget.11098] [PMID: 27507056]

[143]   Codd AS, Kanaseki T, Torigo T, Tabi Z. Cancer stem cells as targets for immunotherapy. Immunology 2018; 153(3): 304-14.
[http://dx.doi.org/10.1111/imm.12866] [PMID: 29150846]

[144]   She X, Qin S, Jing B, *et al.* Radiotheranostic Targeting Cancer Stem Cells in Human Colorectal Cancer Xenografts. Mol Imaging Biol 2020; 22(4): 1043-53.
[http://dx.doi.org/10.1007/s11307-019-01467-7] [PMID: 32125599]

[145]   Wang W, Bai L, Xu D, Li W, Cui J. Immunotherapy: A Potential Approach to Targeting Cancer Stem Cells. Curr Cancer Drug Targets 2020.
[http://dx.doi.org/10.2174/1568009620666200504111914] [PMID: 32364076]

[146]   Pivot X, Verma S, Fallowfield L, *et al.* PrefHer Study Group. Efficacy and safety of subcutaneous trastuzumab and intravenous trastuzumab as part of adjuvant therapy for HER2-positive early breast cancer: Final analysis of the randomised, two-cohort PrefHer study. Eur J Cancer 2017; 86: 82-90.
[http://dx.doi.org/10.1016/j.ejca.2017.08.019] [PMID: 28963915]

[147]   Baker JHE, Kyle AH, Reinsberg SA, *et al.* Heterogeneous distribution of trastuzumab in HER2-positive xenografts and metastases: role of the tumor microenvironment. Clin Exp Metastasis 2018;

35(7): 691-705.
[http://dx.doi.org/10.1007/s10585-018-9929-3] [PMID: 30196384]

[148] Menderes G, Lopez S, Han C, *et al.* Mechanisms of resistance to HER2-targeted therapies in HER2-amplified uterine serous carcinoma, and strategies to overcome it. Discov Med 2018; 26(141): 39-50.
[PMID: 30265854]

[149] Dashti A, Ebrahimi M, Hadjati J, Memarnejadian A, Moazzeni SM. Dendritic cell based immunotherapy using tumor stem cells mediates potent antitumor immune responses. Cancer Lett 2016; 374(1): 175-85.
[http://dx.doi.org/10.1016/j.canlet.2016.01.021] [PMID: 26803056]

[150] Teitz-Tennenbaum S, Wicha MS, Chang AE, Li Q. Targeting cancer stem cells *via* dendritic-cell vaccination. OncoImmunology 2012; 1(8): 1401-3.
[http://dx.doi.org/10.4161/onci.21026] [PMID: 23243607]

[151] Xu Q, Liu G, Yuan X, *et al.* Antigen-specific T-cell response from dendritic cell vaccination using cancer stem-like cell-associated antigens. Stem Cells 2009; 27(8): 1734-40.
[http://dx.doi.org/10.1002/stem.102] [PMID: 19536809]

[152] Hu Y, Lu L, Xia Y, *et al.* Therapeutic Efficacy of Cancer Stem Cell Vaccines in the Adjuvant Setting. Cancer Res 2016; 76(16): 4661-72.
[http://dx.doi.org/10.1158/0008-5472.CAN-15-2664] [PMID: 27325649]

[153] Prince MEP, Zhou L, Moyer JS, *et al.* Evaluation of the immunogenicity of ALDH(high) human head and neck squamous cell carcinoma cancer stem cells *in vitro*. Oral Oncol 2016; 59: 30-42.
[http://dx.doi.org/10.1016/j.oraloncology.2016.05.013] [PMID: 27424180]

[154] Ning N, Pan Q, Zheng F, *et al.* Cancer stem cell vaccination confers significant antitumor immunity. Cancer Res 2012; 72(7): 1853-64.
[http://dx.doi.org/10.1158/0008-5472.CAN-11-1400] [PMID: 22473314]

[155] Lu L, Tao H, Chang AE, *et al.* Cancer stem cell vaccine inhibits metastases of primary tumors and induces humoral immune responses against cancer stem cells. OncoImmunology 2015; 4(3): e990767.
[http://dx.doi.org/10.4161/2162402X.2014.990767] [PMID: 25949905]

[156] Zheng F, Dang J, Zhang H, *et al.* Cancer Stem Cell Vaccination With PD-L1 and CTLA-4 Blockades Enhances the Eradication of Melanoma Stem Cells in a Mouse Tumor Model. J Immunother 2018; 41(8): 361-8.
[http://dx.doi.org/10.1097/CJI.0000000000000242] [PMID: 30063587]

[157] Zhu S, Lv X, Zhang X, *et al.* An effective dendritic cell-based vaccine containing glioma stem-like cell lysate and CpG adjuvant for an orthotopic mouse model of glioma. Int J Cancer 2019; 144(11): 2867-79.
[http://dx.doi.org/10.1002/ijc.32008] [PMID: 30565657]

[158] Wefers C, Schreibelt G, Massuger LFAG, de Vries IJM, Torensma R. immune Curbing of Cancer stem Cells by CtLs directed to nanog. Front Immunol 2018; 9: 1412.
[http://dx.doi.org/10.3389/fimmu.2018.01412] [PMID: 29971070]

[159] Sumransub N, Jirapongwattana N, Jamjuntra P, *et al.* Breast cancer stem cell RNA-pulsed dendritic cells enhance tumor cell killing by effector T cells. Oncol Lett 2020; 19(3): 2422-30.
[http://dx.doi.org/10.3892/ol.2020.11338] [PMID: 32194742]

[160] El-Ashmawy NE, El-Zamarany EA, Salem ML, Khedr EG, Ibrahim AO. A new strategy for enhancing antitumor immune response using dendritic cells loaded with chemo-resistant cancer stem-like cells in experimental mice model. Mol Immunol 2019; 111: 106-17.
[http://dx.doi.org/10.1016/j.molimm.2019.04.001] [PMID: 31051312]

[161] El-Ashmawy NE, Salem ML, Khedr EG, El-Zamarany EA, Ibrahim AO. Dual-targeted therapeutic strategy combining CSC-DC-based vaccine and cisplatin overcomes chemo-resistance in experimental mice model. Clin Transl Oncol 2020; 22(7): 1155-65.

[http://dx.doi.org/10.1007/s12094-019-02242-4] [PMID: 31748959]

[162] Ruan S, Lin M, Zhu Y, *et al.* Integrin β4-Targeted Cancer Immunotherapies Inhibit Tumor Growth and Decrease Metastasis. Cancer Res 2020; 80(4): 771-83.
[http://dx.doi.org/10.1158/0008-5472.CAN-19-1145] [PMID: 31843981]

[163] Hirohashi Y, Torigoe T, Tsukahara T, Kanaseki T, Kochin V, Sato N. Immune responses to human cancer stem-like cells/cancer-initiating cells. Cancer Sci 2016; 107(1): 12-7.
[http://dx.doi.org/10.1111/cas.12830] [PMID: 26440127]

[164] Visus C, Ito D, Amoscato A, *et al.* Identification of human aldehyde dehydrogenase 1 family member A1 as a novel CD8+ T-cell-defined tumor antigen in squamous cell carcinoma of the head and neck. Cancer Res 2007; 67(21): 10538-45.
[http://dx.doi.org/10.1158/0008-5472.CAN-07-1346] [PMID: 17974998]

[165] Visus C, Wang Y, Lozano-Leon A, *et al.* Targeting ALDH(bright) human carcinoma-initiating cells with ALDH1A1-specific CD8+ T cells. Clin Cancer Res 2011; 17(19): 6174-84.
[http://dx.doi.org/10.1158/1078-0432.CCR-11-1111] [PMID: 21856769]

[166] Wang J, Shao L, Wu L, *et al.* Expression levels of a gene signature in hiPSC associated with lung adenocarcinoma stem cells and its capability in eliciting specific antitumor immune-response in a humanized mice model. Thorac Cancer 2020; 11(6): 1603-12.
[http://dx.doi.org/10.1111/1759-7714.13440] [PMID: 32314522]

[167] Gao XY, Wang XL. An adoptive T cell immunotherapy targeting cancer stem cells in a colon cancer model. J BUON 2015; 20(6): 1456-63.
[PMID: 26854441]

[168] Miyamoto S, Kochin V, Kanaseki T, *et al.* The Antigen ASB4 on Cancer Stem Cells Serves as a Target for CTL Immunotherapy of Colorectal Cancer. Cancer Immunol Res 2018; 6(3): 358-69.
[http://dx.doi.org/10.1158/2326-6066.CIR-17-0518] [PMID: 29371260]

[169] Poncette L, Chen X, Lorenz FKM, Blankenstein T. Effective NY-ESO-1-specific MHC II-restricted T cell receptors from antigen-negative hosts enhance tumor regression. J Clin Invest 2019; 129(1): 324-35.
[http://dx.doi.org/10.1172/JCI120391] [PMID: 30530988]

[170] Ang WX, Li Z, Chi Z, *et al.* Intraperitoneal immunotherapy with T cells stably and transiently expressing anti-EpCAM CAR in xenograft models of peritoneal carcinomatosis. Oncotarget 2017; 8(8): 13545-59.
[http://dx.doi.org/10.18632/oncotarget.14592] [PMID: 28088790]

[171] Wang Y, Chen M, Wu Z, *et al.* CD133-directed CAR T cells for advanced metastasis malignancies: A phase I trial. OncoImmunology 2018; 7(7): e1440169.
[http://dx.doi.org/10.1080/2162402X.2018.1440169] [PMID: 29900044]

[172] Feng KC, Guo YL, Liu Y, *et al.* Cocktail treatment with EGFR-specific and CD133-specific chimeric antigen receptor-modified T cells in a patient with advanced cholangiocarcinoma. J Hematol Oncol 2017; 10(1): 4.
[http://dx.doi.org/10.1186/s13045-016-0378-7] [PMID: 28057014]

CHAPTER 4

Immunotherapy for the Treatment of Hepatocellular Carcinoma

Stepan M. Esagian[1], Ioannis A. Ziogas[2] and Georgios Tsoulfas[2,*]

[1] *Faculty of Medicine, Democritus University of Thrace, Alexandroupoulis, Greece*

[2] *First Department of Surgery, Aristotle University of Thessaloniki, Thessaloniki, Greece*

Abstract: This chapter will present the most recent advances in the management of hepatocellular carcinoma (HCC) with immune checkpoint inhibitors (ICIs). Immunotherapy is a rapidly developing and promising field of cancer treatment with many applications, including HCC. In this chapter, we will explain the rationale behind the use of ICIs in the management of HCC by highlighting their molecular mechanisms of action and interactions with the tumor microenvironment. We will also present the most recent data for their safety and efficacy in the resectable, unresectable and post-transplantation setting. Furthermore, we will assess their current status according to the most recent HCC management guidelines and how they compare with other available treatments. The proposed synergy of ICIs with other molecular targeted agents, such as vascular endothelial growth factor inhibitors, will also be analyzed. Finally, we will discuss the current limitations and challenges of ICIs and explore future research perspectives that may solidify their role as a standard HCC therapeutic option, in an era of personalized cancer treatment.

Keywords: Anti-CTLA4, Anti-VEGF, Atezolizumab, Bevacizumab, Camlerizumab, Durvalumab, Hepatocellular carcinoma, Immune checkpoint inhibitors, Ipilimumab, Nivolumab, PD-1 inhibitor, PD-L1 inhibitor, Pembrolizumab, Ramucirumab.

INTRODUCTION

Epidemiology

According to the World Health Organization, hepatocellular carcinoma (HCC) represents the sixth most common malignancy and the third most common cause of cancer-related mortality worldwide, with an estimated 905,977 new cases and 830,180 HCC-related deaths in 2020 [1]. Both incidence and mortality are expected to increase by over 50% in the following two decades [2].

---
[*] **Corresponding author Georgios Tsoulfas:** First Department of Surgery, Aristotle University of Thessaloniki, Thessaloniki, Greece; Tel: (30)6971895190; Fax: (30)2310332022; E-mail: tsoulfasg@gmail.com

Atta-ur-Rahman & M. Iqbal Choudhary (Eds.)
All rights reserved-© 2021 Bentham Science Publishers

The geographic distribution of HCC varies widely; Eastern Asia, Western Africa, and certain parts of Oceania have the highest incidence rates, as infection-related cancers tend to be more common in low- and middle-income countries [1, 3]. Up to 78% of cases worldwide can be attributed to chronic HBV and HCV infection, while the majority of the remaining cases can be attributed to alcohol [4, 5]. Cirrhosis confers up to a 31-fold risk increase for HCC and constitutes the primary pathway through which both viral hepatitis and alcohol lead to cancer development; 80-90% of patients with HCC are cirrhotic [6, 7]. Non-alcoholic fatty liver disease (NAFLD) is another important etiology with rapidly growing proportions, particularly in Western countries [8, 9]. The mean age of diagnosis and gender distribution vary significantly, mainly because of differences in the epidemiology and transmission of viral hepatitis. Countries with higher incidence tend to have a lower mean age of diagnosis and stronger male predominance [7].

Management

Early and Intermediate Hepatocellular Carcinoma

The most widely used classification system for HCC is the Barcelona Clinic Liver Cancer (BCLC) staging system [10]. Surgical resection is preferred for early-stage (BCLC stage 0 and A) patients that have single tumors without any evidence of extrahepatic spread or vascular invasion, good performance status, adequate baseline liver function, and no clinical signs of portal hypertension [11]. Liver transplantation is an alternative for non-surgical BCLC stage A candidates, with the added benefit of treating the underlying liver disease; the Milan criteria define ideal transplant candidates as those with a single tumor ≤ 5cm in diameter or up to three tumors ≤ 3cm each [12]. Those with BCLC Stage 0 and surgery/transplant-ineligible BCLC stage A HCC may receive locoregional ablation therapies. These include thermal ablation (radiofrequency, microwave, or laser), cryoablation, and ablation with percutaneous ethanol injection. Transarterial procedures are the preferred management option for patients with intermediate stage (BCLC stage B); these include transarterial chemoembolization (TACE) and selective internal radiation therapy (SIRT). Both locoregional ablation therapies and transarterial procedures may also be used as a neoadjuvant treatment in patients awaiting liver transplantation, either to prevent progression in those within the Milan criteria [13] or to downstage those outside the Milan criteria [14, 15].

Advanced Hepatocellular Carcinoma Management

Sorafenib and Other Targeted Molecular Agents

Advanced (BCLC Stage C) HCC is primarily managed with systemic therapy, yet no effective regimen existed for many decades, due to HCC's significant chemoresistance and increased systemic toxicity in patients with impaired liver function. In 2007, the United States Food and Drug Administration (FDA) approved sorafenib, a targeted agent inhibiting multiple kinases involved in the tumor's angiogenic and proliferative molecular pathways [16, 17]. Following the approval of sorafenib, many other tyrosine kinase inhibitors (TKIs) were tested in phase III randomized controlled trials (RCTs), but failed to provide evidence of superiority or non-inferiority to sorafenib. These include brivanib, sunitinib, and linifanib [18 - 20]. Similarly, combination regimens of sorafenib with doxorubicin [21, 22], erlotinib [23], cisplatin and fluorouracil hepatic arterial infusion [24] resulted in increased toxicity without any survival benefit. For more than a decade, sorafenib remained the only effective first-line option for advanced HCC, until the multikinase inhibitor lenvatinib gained FDA approval as a first-line therapy in 2018, following the results of a phase III non-inferiority trial [25]. Since then, the TKI cabozantinib and the monoclonal antibody ramucirumab have also been approved as second-line treatments for patients progressing on sorafenib [26, 27].

Immunotherapy

History

Cancer immunotherapy is an umbrella term and includes all forms of cancer treatment that elicit an anti-tumor response through (re)activation of the immune system's ability to recognize and eliminate cancer cells. The concept of utilizing the immune system against tumor cells existed for many centuries, but it was not until recently that immunotherapy was established as the fourth pillar of oncology, along with surgery, chemotherapy, and radiotherapy. Many different forms of cancer immunotherapy exist, and they can primarily be divided into cytokine-based (*e.g.*, interferon-a, interleukin-2), cell-based (*e.g.*, chimeric antigen receptor T-cell therapy, dendritic cell therapy), and antibody-based (*e.g.*, immune checkpoint inhibitors [ICIs]) immunotherapies.

In particular, antibody-based immunotherapy with ICIs has shown rapid success over the last decade. Ipilimumab was the first ICI to gain FDA approval for metastatic melanoma in 2011 [28]. Since then, six other ICIs have been approved by the FDA for more than ten different cancer types, including HCC [29]. All ICIs are monoclonal antibodies directed against cell surface proteins, which normally downregulate the immune response. By inhibiting these immunosuppressory signals, ICIs promote activation of the immune system against tumor cells [29].

Immunotherapy in the Context of Hepatocellular Carcinoma

As of 2020, there are currently four FDA-approved ICI regimens for advanced HCC. Nivolumab is a monoclonal antibody directed against programmed cell death protein 1 (PD-1) and was the first ICI to receive FDA approval as a second-line treatment for HCC in 2017, following the results of the CheckMate 040 phase I/II trial [30]. The results of cohort 4 from the same trial investigating nivolumab together with ipilimumab, a cytotoxic T-lymphocyte associated protein 4 (CTLA-4) inhibitor, also led to FDA approval of this combination as second-line treatment 3 years later [31]. Pembrolizumab became the second PD-1 inhibitor to be approved in 2018 as a second-line treatment following the results of the KEYNOTE-224 phase II trial [32]. In May 2020, the programmed cell death ligand 1 (PD-L1) inhibitor, atezolizumab, in combination with bevacizumab, an anti-vascular endothelial growth factor (VEGF) monoclonal antibody, became the fourth FDA-approved ICI regimen for advanced HCC following the results of the IMbrave150 phase III trial [33]. Notably, this was the first systemic therapy to show superior efficacy to sorafenib since the establishment of the latter as first-line treatment 13 years prior, creating a paradigm shift in the management of advanced HCC and showing the great future potential of immunotherapy.

This chapter will focus on the mechanisms of action, efficacy, and safety of current first- and second-line ICI regimens and will highlight current challenges and future perspectives in their use for HCC management.

MECHANISMS OF ACTION

Immune Checkpoints and Cancer Immunoediting

Immune checkpoints represent physiologic pathways that act as molecular switches that downregulate the immune response following its activation, thus preventing excess tissue damage from overt inflammation [34]. Many tumors have gained the ability to exploit these pathways to avoid detection by the immune system, thus creating a localized immunosuppressive microenvironment that favors tumor proliferation. This event occurs as part of a three-phase process entailing the interactions between tumor cells and immune cells, termed cancer immunoediting. The immune system is actively involved in the recognition and elimination of cancer cells, *via* both innate and adaptive immunity. This active immunosurveillance phase, however, is often incomplete; certain tumor cells are able to survive and because of the selection pressure exerted by the immune system, they make adaptations that enable them to evade immune recognition. As such, tumor cells reach an equilibrium (equilibrium phase) and eventually overpower the immune system (escape phase), resulting in uncontrolled cell proliferation that manifest clinically as active disease [35].

The PD-1/PD-L1 Pathway

The PD-1 cell surface receptor is normally found in a variety of immune cells, namely T-cells, B-cells, tumor-infiltrating lymphocytes, and dendritic cells. Its main ligand, PD-L1 (also known as B7-H1 and CD274), is expressed in numerous normal tissues, but may also be overexpressed in tumor cells [30, 32]. PD-L2 (also known as B7-DC and CD273) is another ligand to PD-1. Activation of the PD-1 receptor by either of its ligands results in downregulation of T-cell activity through inhibition of kinases involved in T-cell activation [36, 37]. In addition, PD-1 is highly expressed on Treg cells, and activation of the receptor results in Treg proliferation. Both of these mechanisms act to suppress physiologic immune responses, thus preventing tissue damage and autoimmunity. Overactivation of the PD-1/PD-L1 pathway in the setting of malignancy represents a major mechanism through which cancer cells are able to evade immune responses against them. This is mediated by both PD-1 in tumor-infiltrating T-lymphocytes, as well as PD-L1 overexpression in the tumor microenvironment. PD-1 overexpression is primarily mediated by chronic exposure to cancer antigens, inducing a state of anergy similar to chronic viral infections. On the other hand, PD-L1 upregulation in tumor cells occurs through two main pathways. In some cancer cells, this may be the result of constitutive oncogenic molecular signaling, thus representing an innate resistance to immunity. In contrast, other cancer cells upregulate PD-L1 as a response to immune signals like INF-γ, similar to normal tissues, a process termed adaptive resistance to immunity [36]. Blockade of the PD-1/PD-L1 interaction serves to eliminate these immunosuppressor signals in the tumor microenvironment and reconstitute immune antitumor activity, primarily through T-cells, but also through NK-cells and B-cells, as they also express PD-1 [36]. Nivolumab and pembrolizumab are examples of PD-1 inhibitors, while atezolizumab and durvalumab are examples of PD-L1 inhibitors.

The CTLA-4 Pathway

CTLA-4 belongs to the immunoglobulin superfamily expressed by activated T cells and in contrast to its homologous stimulatory molecule, CD28, CTLA-4 plays an inhibitory role. Both CTLA-4 and CD28 bind to B7-1 (CD80) and B7-2 (CD86) on antigen presenting cells, however, CTLA-4 does so with greater affinity than CD28 [38 - 41]. CTLA-4 exerts its inhibitory effects by counteracting kinases involved in T-cell activation pathways, as well as by preventing the interaction of CD80 and CD86 with CD28, or even removing CD80 and CD86 from antigen-presenting cells entirely. CTLA-4 exerts its immunosuppressive effects by suppressing the T-helper cells and simultaneously enhancing the inhibitory effect of Treg cells. As a result, blocking the interaction of CTLA-4 with CD80 and CD86 through a monoclonal antibody that binds to it results in anti-tumor activity through T-helper cell activation and Treg downregulation [36]. Ipilimumab and tremelimumab are examples of CTLA-4 inhibitors. A summary of the major immune checkpoints involved in the regulation of T-cell activity is presented in Fig. (**1**).

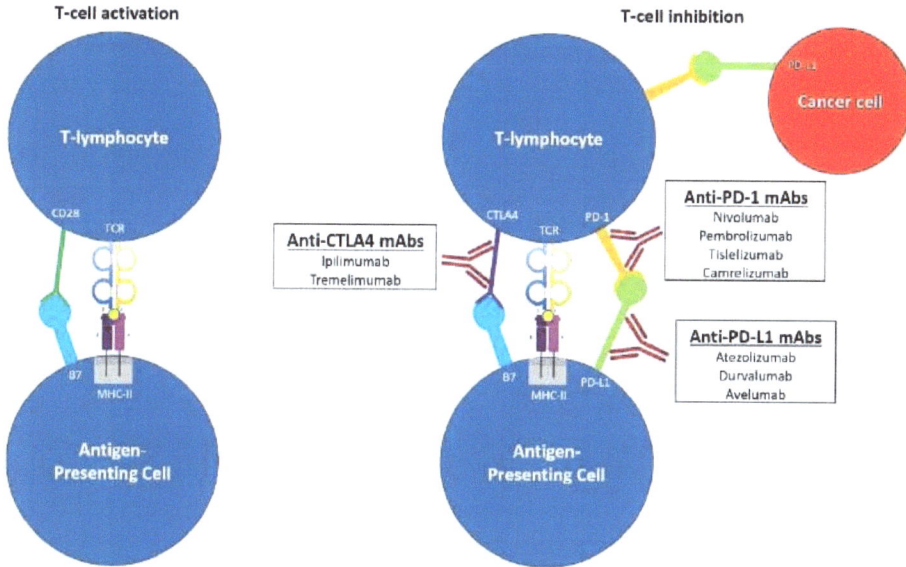

Fig. (1). Regulation of T-cell activation *via* immune checkpoints that serve as actionable targets to immune checkpoint inhibitors. mAbs = monoclonal antibodies.

Combination to Enhance Anti-tumor Immune Responses

ICIs are often combined together (dual checkpoint blockade), with other systemic agents, or with locoregional therapies, as data suggest that they may have an additive or synergistic effect through their distinct immunomodulatory effects [42]. The addition of an agent directed vascular endothelial growth factor (VEGF) may lead to the formation of high endothelial venules that enhance tumor infiltration by lymphocytes [43]. In addition, antiangiogenic therapy results in tumor hypoxia, which upregulates OX40, a costimulatory molecule on CD8+ T-cells which promotes T-cell activation and survival [44]. On the other hand, locoregional therapies, such as TACE and radiofrequency ablation (RFA), induce a localized immunomodulatory effect through immunogenic cell death that may further enhance the immune-activating effect of ICIs [45].

FDA-APPROVED IMMUNOTHERAPY REGIMENS FOR HCC

Single-agent Immune Checkpoint Inhibitors

Nivolumab

Nivolumab is a fully humanized immunoglobulin G (IgG) 4 monoclonal antibody that inhibits PD-1. CheckMate 040 was a phase I/II trial on the safety and efficacy of nivolumab and the first ICI clinical trial for HCC. Eligibility criteria included histologically-confirmed HCC with well-preserved liver function (Child-Pugh score ≤7 and ≤6 for the dose escalation and dose expansion phases, respectively), adequate baseline performance status (Eastern Cooperative Oncology Group [ECOG] performance status ≤1), and antiviral treatment in case of HBV infection. During the dose escalation phase, 48 patients across four countries, divided among three cohorts according to their viral hepatitis status, received escalating doses of nivolumab ranging from 0.1 mg/kg to 10 mg/kg every two weeks. Subsequently, 214 patients across 11 countries were included in the dose expansion phase, receiving a dose of 3 mg/kg every two weeks based on the results of the dose expansion phase. Both treatment-naive (expansion phase: n = 11, escalation phase: n = 69) and sorafenib-progressors were included (expansion phase: n = 37, escalation phase: n = 145).

The objective response rate (ORR) was 20% (95% confidence interval [CI]: 15 to 26), including 3 patients with a complete response (CR), with a median duration of response (DoR) of 9.9 months (95% CI: 8.3 to not reached [NR]), and was similar between sorafenib-naive patients and sorafenib progressors. The disease control rate (DCR) was 64% (95% CI: 58 to 71); 83% of patients were alive at 6 months and 74% at 9 months. The safety and tolerability profile of nivolumab was considered acceptable and similar to that of other trials, with fatigue, pruritus, rash, and diarrhea being the most common clinical symptoms, and elevations of hepatic enzymes, bilirubin, and lipase being the most common laboratory findings; grade 3 or 4 treatment-related serious adverse events occurred in just 4% of patients during both phases; 6% of patients in the dose escalation phase and 11% in the dose expansion phase discontinued therapy due to adverse events of any grade. No deaths directly related to nivolumab occurred [30]. Based on the acceptable efficacy and safety data from the CheckMate 040 trial, nivolumab subsequently received FDA approval in September 2017 as a second-line therapy for patients previously treated with sorafenib [46].

The comparable efficacy between patients with and without prior sorafenib treatment also prompted further investigation of nivolumab as a first-line treatment. In the multicenter phase III clinical trial CheckMate 459, 743 patients with advanced HCC were randomized to receive 240 mg of nivolumab every two weeks (n=371) or 400 mg of sorafenib twice a day (n=372). Preliminary results were presented at the European Society of Medical Oncology (ESMO) 2019 Congress in September 2019. With overall survival (OS) as a primary endpoint, nivolumab showed marginal but not statistically significant improvements, with a median OS of 16.4 months (95% CI: 13.9 to 18.4) *vs.* 14.7 months (95% CI: 11.9 to 17.2) with sorafenib, a 1-year OS rate of 59.7% (95% CI: 54.4 to 64.6) *vs.* 55.1% (95% CI: 49.8 to 60.1), and a 2-year OS rate of 36.8% (95% CI: 31.8 to 41.8) *vs.* 33.1% (95% CI: 28.3 to 38.0). In contrast, the median PFS of the two agents were similar, with a median PFS of 3.7 months (95% CI: 3.1 to 3.9) in the nivolumab group and 3.8 months (95% CI: 3.7 to 4.5) in the sorafenib group. The ORR to nivolumab was 15% (*vs.* 7%) and was higher in patients with PD-L1 expression ≥1% (28%) compared to those with <1% (12%). The safety profile was favorable compared to CheckMate 040, with a rate of discontinuation of 4% in the nivolumab group and 8% in the sorafenib group [47].

Additional results from the CheckMate 459 trial were presented at the ESMO World Congress on Gastrointestinal Cancer in July 2020. Using a minimum follow-up period of 33.6 months, the median OS with nivolumab was 16.4 months (95% CI: 14.0 to 18.5) *vs.* 14.8 months (95% CI: 12.1 to 17.3) with sorafenib (HR: 0.85, 95% CI: 0.72-1.00), and 29% of patients were alive at 33 months (95% CI: 25-34) *vs.* 21% (95% CI: 17-25) with sorafenib. Subgroup analyses showed a clinically meaningful OS advantage with nivolumab over sorafenib in patients with PD-L1 expression ≥1% (16.1 months, 95% CI: 8.4 to 22.3 *vs.* 8.6 months, 95% CI: 5.7 to 16.3), HCV (17.5 *vs.* 12.7 months, HR: 0.72, 95% CI: 0.51 to 1.02), HBV (16.1 *vs.* 10.4 months, HR: 0.79, 95% CI: 0.59 to 1.07). Nivolumab also led to better liver function preservation (as evidenced by albumin/bilirubin levels and Child-Pugh scores) and fewer grade 3/4 adverse events (22.3% *vs.* 49.6%) [48]. The final results of CheckMate 459 were recently posted in clinicaltrials.gov. The ORR of nivolumab was 15.4% (95% CI: 11.8 to 19.4) and was significantly higher *versus* that of sorafenib (7.0%, 95% CI: 4.6 to 10.1). In contrast, there was no clinically meaningful OS benefit (median OS - nivolumab: 16.4 months, 95% CI: 13.9 to 18.4; sorafenib: 14.7 months, 95% CI: 11.9 to 17.2; HR: 0.85, 95% CI 0.71 to 1.02, *p* = 0.0752). The median PFS was similar between the two groups (nivolumab: 3.7 months, 95%: 3.1 to 3.9; sorafenib: 3.8, 95% CI: 3.7 to 4.5; HR: 0.93, 95% CI: 0.79 to 1.10).

Meanwhile, numerous observational studies using real-world data have had similar findings. In an international multicenter retrospective study by Fessas *et al.*, 233 patients with advanced HCC received standard dose nivolumab. The ORR was 22.4%, while the DCR was 52.1%. The median OS was 12.2 months (95% CI: 8.4 to 16.0), with a 6-month-OS rate of 57.5%, and a 1-year-OS rate of

32.6%; those with a complete and partial response had a median OS of 30.6 (95% CI: 26.5 to 34.7) and 18.7 months (95% CI 13.7 to 23.7), respectively. The safety profile was comparable to that demonstrated in previous studies, with a reported adverse event rate leading to discontinuation of 3.4% [49]. In a retrospective study conducted in Korea, Choi *et al.* investigated the outcomes of 203 patients with advanced HCC treated with nivolumab. The ORR of 11.3% was somewhat lower compared to previous studies. Their study population included a significant proportion of patients with Child Pugh B liver function and stratification of the patient population according to Child-Pugh class revealed statistically significant differences between patients with Child-Pugh A and B liver function; the former achieved an ORR and DCR of 15.9% and 42.4%, respectively, while the latter had an ORR of just 2.8% ($p = 0.010$) and a DCR of 22.5% ($p = 0.008$). These differences translated into superior OS for the Child-Pugh A group, with a median OS of 42.9 weeks (95% CI: 34.1 to 54.3) *vs.* 11.3 weeks (95% CI: 7.7 to 15.4) (adjusted HR: 2.10, 95% CI: 1.38 to 3.19; $p <0.001$) in the Child-Pugh B group, and a multivariable regression analysis adjusting for other prognostic factors showed a definitive association between Child-Pugh class and survival with nivolumab therapy (hazard ratio [HR]: 1.93, 95% confidence interval [CI]: 1.11–3.35). However, progression-free survival (PFS) and time-to-treatment failure (TTF) were not significantly different between the two groups. The authors attributed these findings to earlier treatment discontinuation, mainly due to death from hepatic decompensation, as well as immune impairment resulting from cirrhosis [50]. The lower rate of immune-related adverse events in the Child-Pugh B group was consistent with this explanation.

Similarly, smaller scale retrospective studies have shown that Child-Pugh B stage is significantly associated with shorter OS. Examples include a study of 34 patients in three German centers by Finkelmeier *et al.* (HR: 7.72, 95% CI: 2.62–22.78) [51], as well as a single-center study of 76 patients in Korea by Yu *et al.* (HR: 7.27, 95% CI: 3.72 to 14.20) [52]. In contrast, results of the Child-Pugh B cohort from the CheckMate 040 trial presented at the Liver Meeting 2018 hosted by the American Association for the Study of Liver Diseases (AASLD) showed more promising outcomes for this patient group, with an on ORR of 10.2% and a DCR of 55.1%, albeit a median OS of 7.6 months. However, patients a Child-Pugh score of B9 were excluded from the CheckMate 040 trial, which may account for this ORR and DCR difference [53].

CheckMate 9DX is a large, global, double-blind, phase III RCT that will evaluate nivolumab as an adjuvant therapy in patients undergoing curative resection or ablation, with recurrence-free survival (RFS) as the primary endpoint, and is currently in the recruitment phase [54]. TACE-3 is a single-center phase II/III trial in the UK that will evaluate the combination of nivolumab and TACE/transarterial embolization (TAE) *vs.* TACE/TAE alone and is also in the recruiting phase [55]. Multiple other ongoing or recruitment phase II trials are also evaluating the combination of nivolumab with other agents, including sorafenib [56], regorafenib [57, 58], the cycline-dependent kinase inhibitor abemaciclib [59], relatlimab (a monoclonal antibody against lymphocyte-activation gene 3) [60], and pexastimogene devacirepvec (an oncolytic virus) [61]. The combination of nivolumab and ipilimumab is discussed separately below.

Pembrolizumab

Pembrolizumab is a humanized IgG4 monoclonal antibody directed against PD-1. Following the success of nivolumab that paved the road for other ICIs in the management of advanced HCC, the efficacy and safety of pembrolizumab were first assessed in the phase II KEYNOTE-224 trial conducted in 47 different centers across 10 countries. The study sample was limited to patients with histologically- or cytologically-confirmed advanced HCC that were intolerant to or had progressed on prior sorafenib treatment and had well-preserved baseline liver function (Child-Pugh A) and adequate baseline performance status (ECOG ≤1). A total of 104 patients received pembrolizumab 200 mg every three weeks, achieving an ORR of 17% (95% CI: 11 to 26) and a DCR of 62% (95% CI: 52 to 71). At 1 year, the OS rate was 54% (95% CI: 44 to 63) and the PFS was 28% (95% CI: 19 to 37). Although tumor PD-L1 expression was not significantly correlated with survival, a combined immunohistochemistry score that assessed PD-L1 expression in both tumor and immune cells showed a significant association with both OS and PFS. The safety profile of pembrolizumab was similar to that reported in previous studies of other malignancies, with the most common treatment-related adverse events occurring in ≥10% of patients being fatigue, diarrhea, pruritus, rash, and hepatic enzyme elevation; immune-related adverse events such as hypothyroidism and adrenal insufficiency were relatively uncommon [32]. Serious treatment-related adverse events occurred in 15% of patients, including one death due to ulcerative esophagitis that was considered potentially treatment-related. The satisfactory efficacy and safety results from the KEYNOTE-224 trial prompted the FDA to grant pembrolizumab accelerated approval for advanced HCC in the post-sorafenib setting in November 2018 [62].

A smaller scale single-center phase II clinical trial was conducted in parallel, testing the efficacy of pembrolizumab 200mg every three weeks in 29 advanced HCC patients with a Child-Pugh score ≤7 and ECOG performance status ≤1. Nine patients achieved a response, resulting in an ORR of 32.2% (95% CI: 15.9 to 52.4), including one CR, while 13 patients achieved disease control, resulting in a DCR of 46.4%. The median OS was 13 months (95% CI: 7 to NR), while the median PFS was 4.5 months (95% CI: 2 to 7). Three patients (10%) developed serious treatment-related adverse events. Interestingly, the study revealed that circulating TGF-b levels were potentially associated with response to pembrolizumab [63].

Building on the success of KEYNOTE-224, the KEYNOTE-240 trial was a double-blind, phase III, randomized controlled trial conducted across 119 centers in 27 countries. Using the same eligibility criteria as KEYNOTE-224, a total of 413 patients were included and were subsequently randomized to receive pembrolizumab 200 mg every three weeks or placebo, in a 2:1 fashion. The primary endpoints of KEYNOTE-240 focused on OS and PFS. Pembrolizumab resulted in superior long-term outcomes, with a median OS of 13.9 months (*vs.* 10.6 months; HR: 0.781, 95% CI: 0.611 to 0.998; $p = 0.0238$) and a median PFS of 3.0 months (*vs.* 2.8 months; HR: 0.718, 95% CI: 0.570 to 0.904; $p = 0.0022$). Despite these improvements, statistical significance was not reached, as the prespecified goals of $p = 0.0174$ for OS and $p = 0.002$ for PFS resulting from the α distribution strategy that was followed, were not reached. The failure to reach statistical significance in OS was partly attributed to the approval of second-line agents, such as nivolumab and regorafenib, after KEYNOTE-240 was initiated; 47.6% of in the placebo group (*vs.* 41.7% in the pembrolizumab group) received systemic therapies following progression, which may have had an impact on their post-progression survival. A post-hoc analysis accounting for these treatment switches showed a significant improvement in OS, with a median OS of 13.9 months in the pembrolizumab group, compared to 9.3 months in the placebo group (HR: 0.67, 95% CI: 0.48 to 0.92; $p = 0.0066$). The ORR to pembrolizumab was 18.3% (95% CI: 14.0 to 23.4), with 2.2% experiencing a CR, and was significantly higher compared to that of sorafenib (4.4, 95% CI: 1.6 to 9.4, p = 0.00007), while the DCR was 62.2% (*vs.* 53.3%). One death was attributed to pembrolizumab [64].

Two more ongoing phase III studies are currently assessing pembrolizumab for HCC. KEYNOTE-394 is an ongoing multinational, double-blind RCT that will evaluate pembrolizumab against placebo as a second-line advanced HCC treatment specifically in the Asian population, with OS as the primary endpoint [65]. KEYNOTE-937 is a global, double-blind RCT that will compare pembrolizumab against placebo as an adjuvant treatment following resection or ablation therapy. The primary endpoints will be OS and RFS [66].

Multiple ongoing or recruiting phase II trials are also evaluating the efficacy of pembrolizumab together with sorafenib [67], regorafenib [68], elbasvir/grazoprevir and ribavirin in HCV-positive patients [69], TACE [70] or other ablation therapies [71], stereotactic body radiotherapy [72], the GNOS-PV02 and INO-9012 anti-cancer vaccines [73], the oncolytic virus talimogene laherparepvec [74], and radioembolization [75]. The combination of pembrolizumab and lenvatinib is discussed separately.

Double Immune Checkpoint Inhibitor Combination

Nivolumab and Ipilimumab

The success of combining nivolumab and ipilimumab, a CTLA-4 inhibitor, in various other malignancies, such as melanoma, renal cell carcinoma, and colorectal cancer [76 - 78], led to the concurrent investigation of this ICI combination in a separate cohort of CheckMate 040. The patients were divided into 3 study arms: i) arm A received nivolumab 1 mg/kg and ipilimumab 3 mg/kg every three weeks for a total of four doses, followed by 240 mg nivolumab every two weeks ii) arm B received nivolumab 3 mg/kg and ipilimumab 1 mg/kg every three weeks for a total of four doses, followed by 240 mg nivolumab every two weeks, and iii) arm C received nivolumab 3 mg/kg every two weeks and ipilimumab 1 mg/kg every 6 weeks. Interim results from this cohort presented at the American Society of Clinical Oncology (ASCO) 2019 annual meeting were very promising, with an ORR of 32%, 31%, and 31% and median OS of 23 (95% CI: 9 to NR), 12 (95% CI: 8 to 15), and 13 months (95% CI: 7 to 33), for arms A, B, and C, respectively [79]. The significant improvements in the ORR and OS of patients receiving the combination of nivolumab and ipilimumab compared to nivolumab monotherapy, led to the accelerated approval of this combination with the dosage scheme of that used in arm A of CheckMate 040, due to its superior OS [80]. The final results of CheckMate 040 for this cohort were published in October 2020 and were overall consistent with the interim results presented the previous year. Arm A achieved an ORR of 32% (95% CI: 20 to 47), a DCR of 54%, and a median DoR of 17.5 months (range: 4.6 to 30.5+). In comparison, arm B had an ORR of 31% (95% CI: 18 to 45), a DCR of 43%, and median DoR of 22.2 months (range: 4.2 to 29.9+), while arm C had an ORR of 31% (95% CI: 18 to 45), a DCR of 49%, and a median DoR of 16.6 months (range: 4.1+ to 32.0+). In terms of overall survival, arm A had a median OS of 22.8 months (95% CI: 9.4 to NR), arm B 12.5 months (95% CI: 7.6 to 16.4), and arm C 12.7 months (95% CI: 7.4 to 33.0). The safety profile of nivolumab and ipilimumab was similar to that of nivolumab monotherapy. Most adverse events were immune-mediated and had a higher incidence compared to nivolumab monotherapy. Pruritus, rash, diarrhea, fatigue, hepatic enzyme elevation, hypothyroidism, and adrenal insufficiency were the most common adverse events. The incidence of grade ≥3 treatment-related adverse events was 53% in arm A, 29% in arm B, and 31% in arm C. The rate of discontinuation due to adverse events was 16.3% in arm A, 6.3% in arm B, and 4.2% in arm C. Nonetheless, these results were consistent with those of previous studies on the same regimen used for other malignancies and were considered acceptable, given the survival benefit [31].

Two large global phase III trials are evaluating nivolumab and ipilimumab and are currently in the recruitment phase. CheckMate 9DW is an open-label RCT that will compare nivolumab plus ipilimumab against sorafenib plus lenvatinib, with OS as the primary endpoint. Treatment-naive advanced HCC patients with well-preserved liver function (Child-Pugh A) and adequate performance status (ECOG ≤1) are currently being enrolled. The study is expected to be completed in September 2023 [81]. Similarly, CheckMate 74W is a double-blind RCT that will compare nivolumab plus ipilimumab plus TACE in two different dosing schemes against TACE plus placebo in patients with intermediate-stage HCC. Time to TACE progression and OS are the primary endpoints [82]. Other experimental combinations that will be tested in phase I and II trials include nivolumab and ipilimumab together with stereotactic body radiotherapy [83] or cabozantinib and TACE [84]. PRIME-HCC is a clinical trial that will evaluate the combination of nivolumab and ipilimumab in the resectable setting as neoadjuvant therapy [85].

Immune Checkpoint Inhibitor and anti-VEGF Monoclonal Antibody Combination

Atezolizumab and Bevacizumab

Atezolizumab is a fully humanized IgG1 monoclonal antibody directed against PD-L1. Bevacizumab is a monoclonal antibody directed against VEGF. Previous phase III clinical trials on non-small cell lung carcinoma and renal-cell carcinoma testing this regimen had proven successful and resulted in remarkable improvements in survival compared to the respective first-line treatments [86, 87]. The GO30140 phase Ib trial was the first to assess atezolizumab for advanced HCC. Eligible patients with advanced HCC who had not received prior systemic therapy were split into two groups: group A included 104 patients who received atezolizumab 1200 mg and bevacizumab 15 mg/kg every three weeks and was designed to assess the ORR, while patients in group F were randomized 1:1 to receive either the same treatment as group A (n = 60) or atezolizumab 1200mg every three weeks as monotherapy (n = 59), with a primary objective of assessing a potential PFS benefit of the combination regimen over atezolizumab monotherapy. The ORR in group A was 36% (95% CI: 26 to 46), with 12% showing a CR, while the DCR was 71%. Of interest, a significant minority of patients (19%) experienced response after five months of treatment. The median OS was 17.1 months and the median PFS was 7.3 months (95% CI: 5.4 to 9.9). In group F, the atezolizumab-bevacizumab combination resulted in an ORR of 20% (95% CI: 11 to 32), with 2% showing a CR, a DCR of 67%, and a median PFS of

5.6 months (95% CI: 3.6 to 7.4). In comparison, atezolizumab monotherapy had an ORR of 17% (95% CI: 8 to 29), with 5% showing a CR, a DCR of 68% and a median PFS of 3.4 months (95% CI: 1.9 to 5.2). The difference in PFS was statistically significant in favor of the combination regimen (HR:0.55, 80% CI: 0.40 to 0.74). Subgroup analyses of the ORR in group A patients with certain high-risk features relating to high tumor burden, such as bile duct invasion, main portal vein invasion, and ≥50% liver occupancy did not significantly affect this outcome. Other features such as the lack of extrahepatic disease or macrovascular invasion, as well hepatitis C-related HCC showed increased response rates, albeit the size of the samples was too small to conclude if the response differs significantly in these subgroups compared to the general population. In general, the combination of atezolizumab and bevacizumab had an acceptable safety profile, with most adverse events being mild, manageable, and did not differ compared to previous clinical trials with other malignancies. Serious treatment-related adverse events were observed in 24% of patients of group A, including upper gastrointestinal hemorrhage, pneumonitis, and colitis. In group F, severe treatment-related adverse events were noted in 12% receiving atezolizumab and bevacizumab, and 3% of patients receiving bevacizumab only, including hypertension and proteinuria, although a direct comparison could not be made due to difference in the treatment duration between the subgroups [88].

Following the success of atezolizumab and bevacizumab in the GO30140 phase Ib trial, the IMBrave150 phase III trial was initiated to compare the efficacy of this regimen against sorafenib, which had been the first-line standard of care since 2007. Patients with advanced HCC, well-preserved liver function (Child-Pugh A), adequate baseline performance status (ECOG ≤1), and no prior systemic therapy were considered eligible and were enrolled across 111 study centers in 17 countries. A total 501 patients were randomized in a 2:1 fashion to receive either atezolizumab 1200 mg plus bevacizumab 15 mg/kg every three weeks (n = 336) or sorafenib 400 mg twice daily (n = 165). The primary endpoints were OS and PFS, with the combination of atezolizumab and bevacizumab proving superior in both outcomes. Specifically, the 1-year and 2-year OS rates were 84.8% (*vs.* 72.2%) and 67.2% (*vs.* 54.6%), respectively, and the overall risk of death was significantly lower (stratified HR: 0.58, 95% CI: 0.42 to 0.79, *p* <0.001). Similarly, atezolizumab and bevacizumab resulted in a significantly longer median PFS (6.8 months, 95% CI: 5.7 to 8.3 *vs.* 4.3 months, 95% CI: 4.0 to 5.6), superior 6-month PFS rate (54.5% *vs.* 37.2%), and a lower overall risk of progression or death (stratified HR: 0.59; 95% CI, 0.47 to 0.76; *p* <0.001). The significant difference in the PFS of the two groups meant that patients in the sorafenib group received additional systemic therapies, including second-line ICI therapy that had been approved at that point, yet the OS advantage of atezolizumab and bevacizumab persisted despite this imbalance. The secondary endpoints again favored atezolizumab and bevacizumab, with an ORR of 27.3% (95% CI: 22.5 to 32.5) *vs.* 11.9% (95% CI: 7.4 to 18.0) with sorafenib, including CR in 5.5% of patients (*vs.* 0%), a DCR of 73.6% (*vs.* 55.3%), a durable response rate exceeding 6 months of 87.6% (59.1%). These results largely persisted in subgroup analyses based on clinically relevant characteristics. The safety profile of atezolizumab and bevacizumab was similar to that of the GO30140 phase Ib trial; 15.5% of patients experience an adverse event that led to treatment discontinuation (*vs.* 10.3% of patients receiving sorafenib). An important caveat regarding the safety of bevacizumab is that patients had to be evaluated and treated for esophageal varices regardless of size before enrollment. Bleeding is an important adverse event of bevacizumab with the possibility of being fatal, and thus its incidence (7.6%) might have been underestimated; nonetheless, it was not significantly lower than the rate reported in clinical trials on bevacizumab monotherapy for advanced HCC [33, 89, 90].

The results of the IMBrave150 were a significant breakthrough in the management of advanced HCC. Since its FDA approval in 2007, sorafenib remained the only available first-line treatment option for over a decade. Eleven years later, the multi-kinase inhibitor lenvatinib gained approval after the results of the REFLECT phase III clinical trial showed that it was non-inferior to sorafenib [25, 91]. No regimen had proven superior to sorafenib and no other immunotherapy regimen had gained approval in the first-line setting, until the arrival of atezolizumab and bevacizumab. In May 2020, the FDA granted atezolizumab and bevacizumab its approval for patients with previously untreated advanced HCC, marking a turning point in the management of advanced HCC [92].

IMBrave050 is a large, global, open-label, phase III RCT that will compare the efficacy of atezolizumab plus bevacizumab against active surveillance only in the adjuvant setting following curative resection or ablation. The trial is currently recruiting patients, and the inclusion criteria include well-preserved liver function (Child Pugh A), adequate baseline performance status (ECOG ≤1), and eligibility for curative resection or ablation. The primary endpoint is RFS and the study is estimated to be completed in September 2027 [93, 94]. In addition, two other phase II trials will evaluate the efficacy of atezolizumab and bevacizumab together with ^{90}Y transcatheter arterial radioembolization [95] and TACE [96].

A summary of the results of all phase III clinical trials on FDA-approved ICIs is presented in Table **1**.

Table 1. Summary of phase III clinical trials on FDA-approved immune checkpoint inhibitors.

Trial	Agent	Setting	Control Group	ORR (%)	mOS	OS HR	mPFS	PFS HR
Checkmate 459	Nivolumab	Treatment-naive	Sorafenib	15.4 (11.8-19.4)	16.4 (13.9-18.4)	0.85 (0.71-1.02)	3.7 (3.1-3.9)	0.93 (0.79 1.10)
KEYNOTE-240	Pembrolizumab	Post-sorafenib	Placebo	18.3 (14.0-23.4)	13.9 (11.6-16.0)	0.78 (0.61-0.99)	3.0 (2.8-4.1)	0.72 (0.57-0.90)
IMBrave150	Atezolizumab/ Bevacizumab	Treatment-naive	Sorafenib	27.3 (22.5-32.5)	NE	0.58 (0.42-0.79)	6.8 (5.7-8.3)	0.59 (0.47-0.76)

ORR: objective response rate; mOS: median overall survival (in months); HR: hazard ratio; mPFS: median progression-free survival (in months); NE: not estimated.

NON-FDA APPROVED IMMUNOTHERAPY UNDER INVESTIGATION

Single-agent Immune Checkpoint Inhibitors

Tislelizumab

Tislelizumab (BGB-A317) is a humanized immunoglobulin G4 monoclonal antibody directed against PD-1. It was specifically engineered with the goal of minimizing the affinity of its Fc region to the macrophage Fc receptor IA [97]. Although this interaction naturally serves a crucial role in the immune system by enabling antibody-dependent phagocytosis, it may also act as mechanism of resistance to anti-PD-1 therapy by triggering the elimination of activated intratumoral T-cells, to which the anti-PD-1 agent is bound [98]. In addition, tislelizumab's affinity to PD-1 is much higher, with a dissociation rate almost 100 slower than pembrolizumab and 50 times slower than nivolumab [99].

The safety and preliminary efficacy of tislelizumab was first assessed in a multicenter phase Ia/Ib trial which enrolled patients from Australia, Korea, New Zealand, and Taiwan on patients with various advanced solid malignancies that had received prior treatment. In the phase Ia component of the trial, 116 patients were enrolled and were subsequently spread into three different cohorts, including a dose escalation cohort of dosages ranging from 0.5 to 10 mg/kg every two weeks, a schedule expansion cohort with either 2 mg/kg or 5 mg/kg every two or three weeks, and a fixed dose expansion cohort with 200 mg every three weeks. In the phase Ib component of the trial, 335 patients spread across nine different study arms were enrolled and were administered a dosage of 5 mg/kg every two weeks, including arm 4 with advanced HCC patients (n = 50). Tislelizumab was considered to be safe, with treatment-related serious adverse events and discontinuation rates of 7.8% and 5.3%, respectively. Fatigue (13.1%) was the only treatment-related adverse event occurring in ≥10% of patients. Based on the pharmacokinetic and safety profile of tislelizumab, a fixed dosage of 200 mg every three weeks was selected for its evaluation in future clinical trials. In the overall study population, preliminary efficacy data showed an ORR of 13.3% (95% CI: 10.3 to 16.8), including 1.3% CR, a DCR of 44.6% (95% CI: 39.9 to 49.3), a median DoR of 16.0 months (95% CI: 11.1 to 25.6), a median OS of 10.3 months (95% CI: 8.5 to 11.6), and a median PFS of 2.1 months (95% CI: 2.1 to 2.7). In the HCC arm of phase IB, the ORR was 12.0%. A subgroup analysis of HCC patients with a PD-1 expression ≥1% revealed an ORR of 23.1% (95% CI: 9.0 to 43.7) [97].

A phase I/II trial was conducted shortly after across 16 centers in China, with 300 participants with advanced pre-treated solid malignances receiving tislelizumab 200 mg every three weeks. In phase I, 20 patients were enrolled in the dose expansion cohort to assess the safety and tolerability of tislelizumab, and 57 patients were enrolled in the pharmacokinetics cohort run in parallel. In phase II, 223 patients were enrolled and divided in 11 study arms, including arm 11 with 20 advanced HCC patients with well-preserved liver function (Child-Pugh A). The most common treatment-related adverse events were anemia, liver enzyme elevation, and proteinuria and 8% of patients discontinued treatment due to treatment-related adverse events. In the overall population, the ORR was 18% (although no patient achieved a CR), with a median OS of 11.5 months and a median PFS of 2.6 months. In the HCC subgroup of 18 patients with an evaluable response, three patients achieved a response (17%, 95% CI: 3.6 to 41.4) and 10 patients achieved disease control (56%, 95% CI: 30.8 to 78.5). The 1-year OS rate of HCC was 60% (95% CI: 40 to 80) and their median PFS was 4.0 months (95% CI: 2.7 to NR). Notably, all patients in the HCC subgroup were PD-L1 negative [100].

Tislelizumab as a first-line treatment is currently being evaluated in the global, randomized, open-label multicenter, phase III RATIONALE 301 trial. Approximately 640 patients will be enrolled across 100 study centers and will be randomized to receive tislelizumab 200 mg every three weeks or sorafenib 400 mg twice a day. Eligibility criteria include treatment-naive advanced HCC with well-preserved liver function (Child-Pugh A) and adequate baseline performance status (ECOG ≤1). Overall survival is the primary endpoint, while ORR, PFS, DoR, and TTP are the secondary endpoint. The study is currently ongoing and is expected to be completed in May 2022 [101, 102].

Multiple phase II trials are also investigating the efficacy of tislelizumab in combination with TKIs [68, 103, 104], locoregional therapies in the advanced setting [105, 106], and as neoadjuvant therapy in the resectable setting [107].

Camrelizumab

Camrelizumab (SHR-1210) is another humanized monoclonal IgG4 antibody that binds to the PD-1 receptor with high affinity using a different epitope compared to nivolumab and pembrolizumab [108, 109]. Its safety profile and pharmacokinetics were first assessed in a phase I trial of 36 patients with pre-treated advanced solid malignancies, including four HCC patients. Three different dosages (60, 100, and 200 mg) were tested in three groups of 12 patients. The most common treatment-related events were reactive capillary hemangiomas, pruritus, and fatigue; two patients (5.6%) experienced a treatment-related serious adverse event and one patient (2.8%) had to discontinue camrelizumab due to a treatment-related adverse event. Notably, this was the first time that capillary hemangiomas were reported as a side effect with an anti-PD-1 agent in this frequency. However, they did not result in treatment discontinuation in any patient. One out of the two patients with HCC demonstrated an objective response. Overall, camrelizumab was considered to be safe and tolerable, and a fixed dosage of 200 mg was selected for future clinical trials [109].

The efficacy of camrelizumab for HCC was first assessed in phase II trial conducted across 13 study centers in China. Eligible patients had advanced HCC, well-preserved liver function (Child-Pugh score ≤7), adequate baseline performance status (ECOG ≤1), and had progressed on prior sorafenib treatment. A total of 220 patients were randomized to receive camrelizumab 3 mg/kg every two weeks (n = 111) or three weeks (n = 109). The prevalence of HBV infection in the total cohort (83%) was much higher compared to other multinational clinical trials, which was expected as the study was geographically restricted to China. The group receiving the agent every two weeks had an ORR of 11.9% (95% CI: 6.5 to 19.5), a DCR of 47.7% (95% CI: 38.1 to 57.5), a 1-year OS rate of 59.6% (95% CI: 49.6 to 58.2), a median OS of 14.2 months (95% CI: 11.5 to NR), and a median PFS of 2.3 months (95% CI: 1.9 to 3.2). Similarly, the group receiving the agent every three weeks had an ORR of 17.6% (95% CI: 10.9 to 26.1), a DCR of 40.7% (95% CI: 31.4 to 50.6), a 1-year OS rate of 52.2% (95% CI: 42.3 to 61.2), a median OS of 13.2 months (95% CI: 9.4 to 17.0 months), and a median PFS of 2.0 months (95% CI: 2.0 to 3.2). No CRs were noted in either treatment group. In regards to safety and tolerability, treatment-related adverse events occurred in 7.6% of patients and resulted in camrelizumab discontinuation in 3.7% of patients. Similar to the previous phase I trial, reactive capillary hemangioma formation was again one of the most common adverse events. The hemangiomas mainly affected the skin in the face and trunk (and more rarely the oral and nasal mucosa), and were self-limited; the authors hypothesized that the different PD-1 epitope that camrelizumab binds to may create small differences in the immune response compared to other anti-PD-1 agents that may in turn result in an imbalance of proangiogenic and anti-angiogenic factors [109].

In a Chinese single-center retrospective study assessing the efficacy of camrelizumab, among other anti-PD-1 monoclonal antibodies, in a real-world setting, 33 HBV-associated advanced HCC patients were administered camrelizumab 200 mg every two to three weeks and achieved an ORR of 36.4% (including a CR of 6.1%) and a DCR of 81.8%. The 1-year OS rate was 83.1% (95% CI: 66.2 to 100.0) and the 1-year PFS-rate was 60.7% (95% CI: 33.5 to 87.9). The safety analysis revealed common treatment-related adverse effects like rash, diarrhea, fatigue, and nausea, but interestingly no reactive capillary hemangiomas were recorded. The authors attributed this finding to the addition of other treatment agents, such as chemotherapeutic molecular targeted agents, to camrelizumab monotherapy in many patients. In the same study, two other anti-PD-1 monoclonal antibodies were also evaluated, including the humanized monoclonal antibody toripalimab and the fully human sintilimab, with both agents showing comparable safety and efficacy to camrelizumab [110].

A large, double-blind, phase III RCT involving 81 Chinese study centers will evaluate camrelizumab in combination with FOLFOX4 against FOLFOX4 plus placebo in the first-line setting of advanced HCC [111]. The primary endpoint is OS. Other combinations under evaluation in phase I/II trials include lenvatinib in the first-line setting [112] and TACE [113]. The combination of camrelizumab and apatinib is discussed separately.

Durvalumab

Durvalumab is a humanized IgG1 monoclonal antibody against PD-L1. Preliminary safety and efficacy data from a phase I/II clinical trial were presented in the annual ASCO 2017 Conference. Forty advanced HCC patients with well-preserved liver function (Child-Pugh A) received durvalumab 10 mg/kg every two weeks, achieving an ORR of 10.3% and a DCR of 33.3%. The median OS was 13.2 months and the 1-year OS rate was 56.4%. The most common side effects were fatigue, pruritus, and elevated liver enzymes, with no treatment-related adverse events leading to discontinuation [114].

Study arms in clinical trials evaluating the efficacy and safety of durvalumab monotherapy are included in the phase II Study 22 trial and the ongoing phase III HIMALAYA trial, which will be discussed in more extent in the subsection regarding non-FDA approved double ICI combinations.

Tremelimumab

Tremelimumab is a fully human IgG2 monoclonal antibody directed against CTLA-4 and was the first ICI to be tested in a clinical trial for advanced HCC. Twenty-one HCV-positive patients with advanced HCC, good performance status (ECOG ≤1), and baseline liver function ranging from well-preserved to impaired (Child Pugh A or B) were enrolled in a single Spanish study center and received up to four cycles of tremelimumab 15 mg/kg every 90 days. The ORR was 17.6%, with no CRs, while the DCR was 76.4%. The median OS was 8.2 months and the 1-year OS rate was 43%. Almost half of the patients (45%) experienced severe elevation (grade ≥3) in their liver enzymes. However, this elevation was transient, did not correlate with a viral load increase, did not reappear in subsequent treatment cycles, and was thus attributed to an immune reaction mediated by proinflammatory cytokines rather than direct hepatotoxicity or HCV reactivation. Other than that, the most common treatment-related adverse events were rash, fatigue, and diarrhea, with only one serious adverse event (immune-mediated colitis) attributed to the treatment. Notably, patients experienced a transient HCV viral load decrease, consistent with the enhanced T-cell immune response of tremelimumab as its primary mechanism of action [115].

Study arms in clinical trials evaluating the efficacy and safety of tremelimumab monotherapy are included in the phase II Study 22 trial and the on-going phase III HIMALAYA trial, which will be discussed in more extent in the subsection regarding non-FDA approved double ICI combinations.

Atezolizumab

A study arm of atezolizumab monotherapy was included in the GO30140 phase Ib trial and is discussed more extensively in the subsection regarding FDA-approved ICI and anti-VEGF combinations [88]. Atezoliumab monotherapy showed inferior results compared to the combination of atezolizumab and bevacizumab and thus only the latter was evaluated against sorafenib in subsequent phase III trials such as IMBrave150 and IMBrave050.

Immune Checkpoint Inhibitor and Tyrosine Kinase Inhibitor Combination

Pembrolizumab and Lenvatinib

The combination of pembrolizumab and lenvatinib was evaluated in Study 116, a multicenter phase Ib trial clinical trial. A total of 104 patients with unresectable HCC without any prior systemic therapy, well-preserved liver function (Child Pugh A), and adequate baseline performance status (ECOG ≤1) were enrolled and received lenvatinib 8 or 12 mg once daily (if bodyweight was <60 kg or ≥60 kg, respectively) and pembrolizumab 200 mg every three weeks. The study consisted of a dose-limiting toxicity phase with a 3+3 design, and a subsequent dose expansion phase. The results were very promising; pembrolizumab and lenvatinib achieved an ORR of 36% (including a 1% CR), a DCR of 88% and a median DoR of 12.6 months. The median OS was 22.0 months, the median PFS was 8.6 months and the 12-month PFS rate was 27.4%. No new toxicities emerged from the combination of the two agents, and the most common adverse events were hypertension, diarrhea, fatigue, decreased appetite, and hypothyroidism. Adverse events related to treatment that were deemed serious or led to treatment discontinuation of both agents were reported in 36% and 6% of patients, respectively. Three treatment-related deaths occurred due to intestinal perforation, acute respiratory distress syndrome, and liver failure.

The success of Study 116 prompted the further evaluation of pembrolizumab and lenvatinib in two large phase III trials. LEAP-002 is an active randomized double-blind global phase III trial which will compare standard dose pembrolizumab and lenvatinib (as in Study 116) to lenvatinib monotherapy in treatment-naive advanced HCC patients, with long-term outcomes (PFS, OS) as the primary endpoints [116]. Similarly, LEAP-012 is another randomized quadruple-blind global phase III trial (currently in the recruitment phase) that will compare lenvatinib plus pembrolizumab plus TACE against TACE only plus placebo using the same active primary endpoints [117].

Atezolizumab and Cabozantinib

Cabozantinib is a TKI that was approved by the FDA in January 2019 as a second-line therapy for advanced HCC, after it demonstrated superior survival *versus* placebo in the randomized double-blind phase III CELESTIAL trial [26, 118]. Two global multicenter trials are currently evaluating the combination of cabozantinib with atezolizumab. A phase I/II trial that is currently recruiting will evaluate its safety and preliminary efficacy in a large cohort made up of patients with various solid malignancies, including HCC. In the dose escalation phase, patients will receive daily cabozantinib at varying daily doses (20, 40, and 60 mg) plus atezolizumab 1200 mg every three weeks using a 3+3 design. The dose expansion phase will include 24 cohorts and cohort 14 will specifically include HCC patients with well-preserved liver function (Child-Pugh A) [119]. COSMIC-312 is a phase III evaluating the efficacy of atezolizumab 1200 mg every three weeks and cabozantinib 40 mg daily (experimental arm) *versus* cabozantinib 40 mg daily monotherapy (cabozantinib arm) and sorafenib 400 mg twice daily monotherapy. Eligible patients will include treatment-naive advanced HCC patients with well-preserved liver function (Child-Pugh A), and adequate baseline performance status (ECOG ≤1) and the primary outcome measures will be OS and PFS [120, 121].

Avelumab and Axitinib

Avelumab is a fully humanized IgG1 monoclonal antibody against PD-L1. Axitinib is a tyrosine kinase inhibitor with primarily antiangiogenic action through inhibition of VEGF receptors 1-3, platelet derived growth factor receptor (PDGFR), and c-KIT [122]. The combination of avelumab and axitinib has shown great success in the treatment of renal cell carcinoma and has already been approved by the FDA following the results of the JAVELIN Renal 101 phase III trial [123, 124]. The VEGF Liver 100 phase Ib trial was conducted in seven Japanese centers and was the first to assess the safety and preliminary efficacy of this combination for advanced HCC. Twenty-two treatment-naive patients with well-preserved liver function (Child-Pugh A) and adequate baseline performance status (ECOG ≤1) were enrolled and subsequently received avelumab 10 mg/kg every two weeks plus axitinib 5 mg twice daily. Treatment-related adverse events that were grade 3 or higher occurred in a significant proportion of patients (17/22, 77.2%), with hypertension and hand-foot syndrome being the most common of them. The ORR was 13.6% (95% CI: 2.9 to 34.9), the DCR was 68.2% (95% CI: 45.1 to 86.1), and the median DoR was 7.3 months (95% CI: 3.7 to 12.9). The median OS was 14.1 months (95% CI: 8.0 to NR) and the median PFS was 5.5 months (95% CI: 1.9 to 7.4) [125].

Camrelizumab and Apatinib

Apatinib is a TKI that selectively inhibits the VEGF receptor 2. The safety of its combination with camrelizumab was first assessed in a single center phase I study in China. Their sample included 43 patients with advanced HCC, gastric cancer, and esophagogastric cancer that had progressed on first-line treatment. In the dose escalation (Ia) phase of the trial, 15 patients were divided into 3 cohorts of 5 patients and received camrelizumab 200 mg and axitinib 125, 250, or 500 mg. Based on the results of phase Ia, 250 mg was determined to be the recommended dose of axitinib; 28 patients were enrolled in the dose expansion (Ib) phase of the trial. The most common grade ≥3 treatment-related adverse events were hypertension and elevated liver enzymes and resulted in two treatment discontinuations in the entire cohort. Of the 43 patients enrolled in the study, 18 patients had advanced HCC and those evaluable for efficacy achieved an ORR of 50.0% (95% CI: 24.7 to 75.4), with no CRs, and a DCR of 93.8% (95% CI: 69.8 to 99.8). During a median follow-up of 7.9 months, the median DoR and OS were NR, while the median PFS was 5.8 months (95% CI: 2.6 months to NR) [126].

These promising results prompted the further evaluation of camrelizumab and apatinib in the multicenter Chinese RESCUE phase II trial. Patients with advanced HCC, well-preserved liver function (Child-Pugh A), adequate baseline performance status (ECOG ≤1) were eligible; both treatment-naive (n = 70; first-line cohort) and first-line progressors (n = 120; second-line cohort) were included. All patients received camrelizumab 200 mg (bodyweight ≥50 kg) or 3 mg/kg (for bodyweight <50 kg) every two weeks and apatinib 250 mg daily. In the first-line cohort, the ORR was 34.3% (95% CI: 23.3 to 46.6), including one CR, the DCR was 77.1% (95% CI: 65.6 to 86.3), and the median DoR was 14.8 months (95% CI: 5.5 months to NR). In comparison, the second-line cohort achieved an ORR of 22.5% (95% CI: 15.4 to 31.0), a DCR of 75.8% (95% CI: 67.2 to 83.2), while the median DoR was NR. A subgroup analysis according to PD-L1 expression did not find any significant differences in the ORR of patients expressing PD-L1 in ≥1% or <1% of their tumor cells. In terms of long-term outcomes, the 1-year OS rate and median PFS were 74.7% (95% CI 62.5 to 83.5) and 5.7 months (95% CI 5.4 to 7.4) in the first-line cohort, and 68.2% (95% CI: 59.0 to 75.7) and 5.5 months (95% CI: 3.7 to 5.6) in the second-line cohort. The incidence of grade ≥3 treatment-related adverse events was 77.4% and 28.9% of patients experienced a treatment-related adverse event that was considered serious and led to treatment discontinuation in 12.1% of patients. Two patients died due to pneumonitis and liver failure as a result of the treatment. Upper gastrointestinal haemorrhage occurred in 1.6% of patients in the first-line cohort and 1.4% of the patients in the second-line cohort, which was comparatively lower to that of the IMBrave150 trial on atezolizumab and bevacizumab. Reactive capillary hemangiomas, which occurred with uniquely high incidence in prior camrelizumab trials, occurred in a significant proportion of patients (29.5%), albeit much lower compared to that previously reported with camrelizumab monotherapy [127].

A retrospective Chinese study from 5 study centers also evaluated the safety and efficacy of camrelizumab and apatinib in a real-world setting. Their sample was restricted to 63 patients with HBV-related HCC and concurrent portal vein tumor thrombosis (PVTT), with varying baseline liver function (Child-Pugh A and B). All patients received camrelizumab 200 mg every three weeks plus apatinib 250 mg daily. The ORR was 44%, including one CR, and the DCR was 75%. The median OS was 14.8 months (95% CI: 12.3 to 17.3), and the median PFS was 11.8 months (95% CI: 6.4 to 17.2). Subgroup analyses according to PVTT type revealed that absence of main PVTT (types B and C) was associated with significantly better OS and PFS. The incidence of upper gastrointestinal bleeding was 3.2% [128].

A number of other trials are currently evaluating this combination in various settings, including the perioperative setting for resectable HCC [129, 130], the transplantation setting as downstaging/bridging therapy [131], and the advanced setting in combination with localized therapies like TACE and hepatic artery infusion chemotherapy (HAIC) [132 - 134].

Immune Checkpoint Inhibitor and anti-VEGF Monoclonal Antibody Combination

Durvalumab and Ramucirumab

Ramucirumab is a fully human IgG1 monoclonal antibody directed against VEGF receptor 2 [135]. JVDJ is a multinational phase I trial that evaluated the safety and preliminary efficacy of ramucirumab combined with durvalumab in patients. A total of 85 patients were enrolled across 25 study centers. All eligible patients had advanced solid malignancies, including non-small cell lung cancer (n = 28), gastric/gastroesophageal junction cancer (n = 29), and HCC (n = 28), and had progressed on prior systemic therapies (except for ramucirumab monotherapy). For HCC specifically, patients had well-preserved liver function (Child-Pugh A). The study consisted of dose-escalation (Ia) phase with a 6+3 design, and a dose expansion (Ib) phase. In the HCC cohort, patients received ramucirumab 8 mg/kg and durvalumab 750 mg intravenously every two weeks and achieved an ORR of 11% with no CRs and a DCR of 61%. The median OS was 10.7 months (95% CI: 5.1 to 18.4) and the 1-year OS rate was 50% (95% CI: 29 to 67). The median PFS was 4.4 months (95% CI: 1.6 to 5.7) and the 1-year PFS rate was 16% (95% CI: 5 to 35). Diarrhea and fatigue were the most common adverse events and 42.9% of HCC patients experienced a grade $\geq$3 adverse event that was treatment-related. Hemorrhagic events (including epistaxis and gingival hemorrhage) occurred in 39.3% of HCC patients and were grade $\geq$3 in 10.7% of them.

EMERALD-2 is a global, double-blind, phase III RCT that is currently recruiting HCC patients with well-preserved liver function (Child-Pugh A) and adequate performance status (ECOG $\leq$1). The trial will compare the combination of durvalumab 1120 mg every three weeks and bevacizumab 15 mg/kg every three weeks against either durvalumab monotherapy or placebo in the adjuvant setting following curative resection or ablation. The primary endpoint is RFS and the trial is estimated to be completed in September 2023 [136].

Double Immune Checkpoint Inhibitor Combination

Tremelimumab and Durvalumab

The efficacy and safety of tremelimumab combined with durvalumab as a second-line treatment (post-sorafenib or sorafenib intolerant) advanced HCC is currently being assessed in the global phase II Study 22 trial. Eligible patients were randomized into four study arms, including two arms receiving combination ICI therapy and two-arms receiving single-agent therapy: the first arm received one dose of tremelimumab 300 mg plus durvalumab 1500 mg, followed by durvalumab 75 mg every four weeks; the second arm received tremelimumab 75 mg every four weeks plus durvalumab 1500 mg every four weeks for the first 4 doses, followed by the same dose of durvalumab only every four weeks only; the third arm received durvalumab 1500 mg monotherapy every four weeks; and the fourth arm received tremelimumab 750 mg monotherapy every four weeks. Preliminary results were presented in the annual ASCO 2020 conference. A total of 332 patients had been enrolled (arm 1, n = 75; arm 2, n = 84; arm 3, n = 104; arm 4, n = 69). Arm 1 showed the highest efficacy, with an ORR of 22.7% (*vs.* 9.5%, 9.6%, and 7.5%), a median DoR that had not been reached after a median follow-up of 11.7 months (*vs.* 13.2, 14.8, and 24.0 months), and a median OS of 18.7 months (*vs.* 11.3, 11.7, and 17.1 months). Arms 1, 2, and 3 had comparable toxicity with a rate of serious (grade ≥3 adverse events) of 13.5%, 11.0%, and 10.9%, and a treatment-related discontinuation rate of 10.8%, 6.1%, and 7.9%, respectively. In comparison, tremelimumab monotherapy (arm 4) resulted in increased toxicity, with a 21.7% rate of serious treatment-related adverse events, and a treatment-related discontinuation rate of 11.6%. Evaluation of the peripheral blood of patients achieving a response among all study arms revealed an increased circulating CD8+ lymphocyte count in patients receiving combined tremelimumab and durvalumab. This finding together with the superior efficacy and long-term outcomes of arm 1 suggest an additive pharmacodynamic interaction between the two agents [137].

The efficacy of tremelimumab combined with durvalumab is currently being evaluated in the randomized phase III HIMALAYA, clinical trial. Patients with advanced HCC, well-preserved liver function (Child Pugh A) and good performance status (ECOG ≤1) are currently being recruited. The trial will include four study arms, including two study arms with combined tremelimumab and durvalumab therapy, one study arm with durvalumab monotherapy, and one arm with sorafenib, the current standard of care, to serve as the control group. The primary endpoint will be OS, while the secondary endpoints will be time to progression, PFS, ORR, DCR, and DoR [138].

Immune Checkpoint Inhibitor and Locoregional Therapy Combination

Tremelimumab and Ablation

A phase I/II study evaluated the combination of tremelimumab together with TACE, RFA, or cryoablation (CA). Thirty-two patients with advanced HCC, Child-Pugh score ≤7, and ECOG performance status ≤2 that had progressed on or were intolerant to sorafenib were included. They were split into two dosage groups, with one group receiving tremelimumab 3.5 mg/kg (n = 6), and another group receiving tremelimumab 10 mg/kg (n = 26). The ORR was 26% (95% CI: 9.1 to 51.2). The median OS was 12.3 months (95% CI: 9.3 to 15.4) and the 1-year OS rate was 50.8% (95% CI: 29.1 to 68.9). The median time to progression was 7.4 months (95% CI: 4.7 to 19.4) and the 1-year PFS rate was 33.1% (95% CI: 16.2 to 51.2). Fifteen patients (47%) developed an adverse event that was grade ≥3 and 4 patients (13%) had to discontinue treatment due to an adverse event. Notably, there was a significant reduction in the viral load in the majority of patients who HCV-positive [139].

Multiple trials are currently evaluating the efficacy of tremelimumab either alone or together with durvalumab in combination with locoregional therapies [140, 141] and hypofractionated radiotherapy [142].

A summary of all ongoing phase III trials on ICIs for HCC is presented below in Table **2**.

Table **2**. Summary of ongoing phase III clinical trials on immune checkpoint inhibitors for hepatocellular carcinoma.

Trial	Agent	Setting	Control Group	Primary Endpoint
ICI Monotherapy				
CheckMate 9DX	Nivolumab	Adjuvant to curative resection or ablation	Placebo	RFS
KEYNOTE-394	Pembrolizumab	Post-sorafenib	Placebo	OS
KEYNOTE-937	Pembrolizumab	Adjuvant to curative resection or ablation	Placebo	OS, RFS
RATIONALE 301	Tislelizumab	Treatment-naive	Sorafenib	ORR, PFS, DoR, TTP
Double ICI Combination				
CheckMate 9DW	Nivolumab/ Ipilimumab	Treatment-naive	Sorafenib plus Lenvatinib	OS
CheckMate 74W	Nivolumab/ Ipilimumab plus TACE	Intermediate stage HCC	TACE plus placebo	Time to TACE progression, OS
HIMALAYA	Tremelimumab/ Durvalumab	Treatment-naive	Durvalumab, Sorafenib	OS
ICI Plus anti-VEGF Monoclonal Antibody				
IMBrave050	Atezolizumab/ Bevacizumab	Adjuvant to curative resection or ablation	Placebo	RFS

(Table 2) cont.....

Trial	Agent	Setting	Control Group	Primary Endpoint
EMERALD-2	Durvalumab/ Bevacizumab	Adjuvant to curative resection or ablation	Durvalumab, Placebo	RFS
ICI Plus Tyrosine Kinase Inhibitor				
LEAP-002	Pembrolizumab/ Lenvatinib	Treatment-naive	Lenvatinib	OS, PFS
LEAP-012	Pembrolizumab/ Lenvatinib Plus TACE	N/A	TACE Plus placebo	OS, PFS
COSMIC-312	Atezolizumab/ Cabozantinib	Treatment-naive	Cabozantinib, Sorafenib	OS, PFS
ICI Plus Chemotherapy				
NCT03605706	Camrelizumab/ FOLFOX4	Treatment-naive	FOLFOX4 plus placebo	OS

ICI: immune checkpoint inhibitor; RFS: recurrence-free survival; OS: overall survival; PFS: progression-free survival; DoR: duration of response; TTP: time-to-progression; TACE: transarterial chemoembolization; HCC: hepatocellular carcinoma; VEGF: vascular endothelial growth factor; N/A: not available; FOLFOX4: 5-fluorouracil, leucovorin, and oxaliplatin

IMMUNOTHERAPY IN THE SETTING OF LIVER TRANSPLANTATION

According to a recent systematic review of the literature [143], 10 studies reporting on 15 patients have reported the use of ICIs in the setting of liver transplantation (1 pre-LT, 14 post-LT) [144 - 153]. The one patient receiving ICI in the pre-LT setting, had HCC beyond the Milan criteria, received nivolumab as a bridge to LT, and was able to undergo LT after successful downstaging. Nevertheless, the patient succumbed post-LT due to fatal graft rejection.

In the post-LT setting, 14 patients with a mean age of 50.8±17.2 years have received ICIs for the management of HCC recurrence (10 nivolumab, 2 pembrolizumab, 2 ipilimumab) [143]. Twelve of them (85.7%) had received sorafenib before ICI initiation. Disease recurrence occurred in these 14 LT recipients over a median time of 34.2 (interquartile range: 14.4 to 62.0) months. The median OS and PFS periods after ICI initiation were 1.1 months (interquartile range: 1.0 to 1.3) and 1.3 months (interquartile range: 0.7 to 2.2), respectively. Overall, 78.6% (n = 11/14) experienced death and the cause of death was graft rejection in five, and disease progression or multiorgan failure in six. The remaining three patients were still alive at 29, 20, and 10 months of follow-up after ICI initiation and had functional grafts [143].

Graft rejection occurred at an overall rate of 40% (n = 6/15, one patient receiving ICI pre-LT and five post-LT) [143]. This high graft rejection rate, despite the limited available evidence, generates further questions regarding the safety of ICIs for the treatment of disease recurrence after LT for HCC. Nevertheless, they have demonstrated promising antitumor efficacy and acceptable tolerability. Therefore, future research should focus on the mechanisms that are potentially associated with ICI-related graft rejection in an attempt to broaden their indications in the setting of LT.

CONCLUSION

In conclusion, immunotherapy has led to a paradigm shift in the treatment of advanced HCC. Over the past few years, numerous ICIs have been established as an effective and safe therapeutic option in both the first-line and second-line setting. The goal has now shifted to increasing the efficacy of these agents through combinations with other ICIs, TKIs, anti-VEGF monoclonal antibodies, and locoregional therapies, while also maintaining their toxicity to tolerable levels and improving quality of life. As numerous ongoing phase II and phase III clinical trials are currently testing these new combinations, the landscape of systemic therapy for advanced HCC is still evolving.

CONSENT FOR PUBLICATION

Not applicable.

CONFLICT OF INTEREST

The authors declare no conflict of interest, financial or otherwise.

ACKNOWLEDGEMENTS

Declared none.

REFERENCES

[1]   Cancer Today [Internet]. [cited 2020 Dec 21]. Available from. https://gco.iarc.fr/today/home

[2]   Cancer Tomorrow [Internet]. [cited 2020 Dec 21]. Available from. https://gco.iarc.fr/tomorrow/en

[3]   Bray F, Soerjomataram I. The Changing Global Burden of Cancer: Transitions in Human Development and Implications for Cancer Prevention and Control. In: Disease Control Priorities, Third Edition (Volume 3): Cancer. The World Bank; 2015. p. 23–44.

[4]   Perz JF, Armstrong GL, Farrington LA, Hutin YJF, Bell BP. The contributions of hepatitis B virus and hepatitis C virus infections to cirrhosis and primary liver cancer worldwide. J Hepatol 2006; 45(4): 529-38.
[http://dx.doi.org/10.1016/j.jhep.2006.05.013] [PMID: 16879891]

[5]   Rehm J, Room R, Graham K, Monteiro M, Gmel G, Sempos CT. The relationship of average volume

of alcohol consumption and patterns of drinking to burden of disease: an overview. Addiction 2003; 98(9): 1209-28.
[http://dx.doi.org/10.1046/j.1360-0443.2003.00467.x] [PMID: 12930209]

[6]   Thiele M, Gluud LL, Fialla AD, Dahl EK, Krag A. Large variations in risk of hepatocellular carcinoma and mortality in treatment Naïve hepatitis B patients: Systematic Review with Meta-analyses. In: Chemin IA, Ed. PLoS ONE. Public Library of Science 2014; 9: p. e107177.

[7]   El-Serag HB. Epidemiology of viral hepatitis and hepatocellular carcinoma. Gastroenterology 2012; 142(6): 1264-1273.e1.
[http://dx.doi.org/10.1053/j.gastro.2011.12.061] [PMID: 22537432]

[8]   Younossi Z, Stepanova M, Ong JP, *et al.* Global Nonalcoholic Steatohepatitis Council. Nonalcoholic steatohepatitis is the fastest growing cause of hepatocellular carcinoma in liver transplant candidates. Clin Gastroenterol Hepatol 2019; 17(4): 748-755.e3.
[http://dx.doi.org/10.1016/j.cgh.2018.05.057] [PMID: 29908364]

[9]   Ziogas IA, Zapsalis K, Giannis D, Tsoulfas G. Metabolic syndrome and liver disease in the era of bariatric surgery: What you need to know! World J Hepatol 2020; 12(10): 709-21.
[http://dx.doi.org/10.4254/wjh.v12.i10.709] [PMID: 33200011]

[10]   Llovet JM, Brú C, Bruix J. Prognosis of hepatocellular carcinoma: the BCLC staging classification. Semin Liver Dis 1999; 19(3): 329-38.
[http://dx.doi.org/10.1055/s-2007-1007122] [PMID: 10518312]

[11]   Roayaie S, Jibara G, Tabrizian P, *et al.* The role of hepatic resection in the treatment of hepatocellular cancer. Hepatology 2015; 62(2): 440-51.
[http://dx.doi.org/10.1002/hep.27745] [PMID: 25678263]

[12]   Mazzaferro V, Regalia E, Doci R, *et al.* Liver transplantation for the treatment of small hepatocellular carcinomas in patients with cirrhosis. N Engl J Med 1996; 334(11): 693-9.
[http://dx.doi.org/10.1056/NEJM199603143341104] [PMID: 8594428]

[13]   Tsochatzis E, Garcovich M, Marelli L, *et al.* Transarterial embolization as neo-adjuvant therapy pretransplantation in patients with hepatocellular carcinoma. Liver Int 2013; 33(6): 944-9.
[http://dx.doi.org/10.1111/liv.12144] [PMID: 23530918]

[14]   Ibrahim SM, Kulik L, Baker T, *et al.* Treating and downstaging hepatocellular carcinoma in the caudate lobe with yttrium-90 radioembolization. Cardiovasc Intervent Radiol 2012; 35(5): 1094-101.
[http://dx.doi.org/10.1007/s00270-011-0292-x] [PMID: 22069121]

[15]   Yao FY, Mehta N, Flemming J, *et al.* Downstaging of hepatocellular cancer before liver transplant: long-term outcome compared to tumors within Milan criteria. Hepatology 2015; 61(6): 1968-77.
[http://dx.doi.org/10.1002/hep.27752] [PMID: 25689978]

[16]   Llovet JM, Ricci S, Mazzaferro V, *et al.* Sorafenib in advanced hepatocellular carcinoma. N Engl J Med 2008; 359(4): 378-90.
[http://dx.doi.org/10.1056/NEJMoa0708857] [PMID: 18650514]

[17]   Cheng AL, Kang YK, Chen Z, *et al.* Efficacy and safety of sorafenib in patients in the Asia-Pacific region with advanced hepatocellular carcinoma: a phase III randomised, double-blind, placebo-controlled trial. Lancet Oncol 2009; 10(1): 25-34.
[http://dx.doi.org/10.1016/S1470-2045(08)70285-7] [PMID: 19095497]

[18]   Johnson PJ, Qin S, Park JW, *et al.* Brivanib *versus* sorafenib as first-line therapy in patients with unresectable, advanced hepatocellular carcinoma: results from the randomized phase III BRISK-FL study. J Clin Oncol 2013; 31(28): 3517-24.
[http://dx.doi.org/10.1200/JCO.2012.48.4410] [PMID: 23980084]

[19]   Cheng AL, Kang YK, Lin DY, *et al.* Sunitinib *versus* sorafenib in advanced hepatocellular cancer: results of a randomized phase III trial. J Clin Oncol 2013; 31(32): 4067-75.
[http://dx.doi.org/10.1200/JCO.2012.45.8372] [PMID: 24081937]

[20]   Cainap C, Qin S, Huang WT, *et al.* Linifanib *versus* Sorafenib in patients with advanced hepatocellular carcinoma: results of a randomized phase III trial. J Clin Oncol 2015; 33(2): 172-9.
[http://dx.doi.org/10.1200/JCO.2013.54.3298] [PMID: 25488963]

[21]   Abou-Alfa GK, Johnson P, Knox JJ, *et al.* Doxorubicin plus sorafenib vs doxorubicin alone in patients with advanced hepatocellular carcinoma: a randomized trial. JAMA 2010; 304(19): 2154-60.
[http://dx.doi.org/10.1001/jama.2010.1672] [PMID: 21081728]

[22]   Abou-Alfa GK, Niedzwieski D, Knox JJ, Kaubisch A, Posey J, Tan BR, *et al.* Phase III randomized study of sorafenib plus doxorubicin *versus* sorafenib in patients with advanced hepatocellular carcinoma (HCC): CALGB 80802 (Alliance). J Clin Oncol 2016; 34(4_suppl): 192-2.

[23]   Zhu AX, Rosmorduc O, Evans TRJ, *et al.* SEARCH: a phase III, randomized, double-blind, placebo-controlled trial of sorafenib plus erlotinib in patients with advanced hepatocellular carcinoma. J Clin Oncol 2015; 33(6): 559-66.
[http://dx.doi.org/10.1200/JCO.2013.53.7746] [PMID: 25547503]

[24]   Kudo M, Ueshima K, Yokosuka O, *et al.* Sorafenib plus low-dose cisplatin and fluorouracil hepatic arterial infusion chemotherapy *versus* sorafenib alone in patients with advanced hepatocellular carcinoma (SILIUS): a randomised, open label, phase 3 trial. Lancet Gastroenterol Hepatol 2018; 3(6): 424-32.
[http://dx.doi.org/10.1016/S2468-1253(18)30078-5] [PMID: 29631810]

[25]   Kudo M, Finn RS, Qin S, *et al.* Lenvatinib *versus* sorafenib in first-line treatment of patients with unresectable hepatocellular carcinoma: a randomised phase 3 non-inferiority trial. Lancet 2018; 391(10126): 1163-73.
[http://dx.doi.org/10.1016/S0140-6736(18)30207-1] [PMID: 29433850]

[26]   Abou-Alfa GK, Meyer T, Cheng A-L, *et al.* Cabozantinib in patients with advanced and progressing hepatocellular carcinoma. N Engl J Med 2018; 379(1): 54-63.
[http://dx.doi.org/10.1056/NEJMoa1717002] [PMID: 29972759]

[27]   Zhu AX, Kang YK, Yen CJ, *et al.* REACH-2 study investigators. Ramucirumab after sorafenib in patients with advanced hepatocellular carcinoma and increased α-fetoprotein concentrations (REACH-2): a randomised, double-blind, placebo-controlled, phase 3 trial. Lancet Oncol 2019; 20(2): 282-96.
[http://dx.doi.org/10.1016/S1470-2045(18)30937-9] [PMID: 30665869]

[28]   Robert C, Thomas L, Bondarenko I, *et al.* Ipilimumab plus dacarbazine for previously untreated metastatic melanoma. N Engl J Med 2011; 364(26): 2517-26.
[http://dx.doi.org/10.1056/NEJMoa1104621] [PMID: 21639810]

[29]   Filin IY, Solovyeva VV, Kitaeva KV, Rutland CS, Rizvanov AA. Current trends in cancer immunotherapy. Biomedicines 2020; 8(12): 621.
[http://dx.doi.org/10.3390/biomedicines8120621] [PMID: 33348704]

[30]   El-Khoueiry AB, Sangro B, Yau T, *et al.* Nivolumab in patients with advanced hepatocellular carcinoma (CheckMate 040): an open-label, non-comparative, phase 1/2 dose escalation and expansion trial. Lancet 2017; 389(10088): 2492-502.
[http://dx.doi.org/10.1016/S0140-6736(17)31046-2] [PMID: 28434648]

[31]   Yau T, Kang YK, Kim TY, *et al.* Efficacy and safety of nivolumab plus ipilimumab in patients with advanced hepatocellular carcinoma previously treated with sorafenib: the checkmate 040 randomized clinical trial. JAMA Oncol 2020; 6(11): e204564-4.
[http://dx.doi.org/10.1001/jamaoncol.2020.4564] [PMID: 33001135]

[32]   Zhu AX, Finn RS, Edeline J, *et al.* KEYNOTE-224 investigators. Pembrolizumab in patients with advanced hepatocellular carcinoma previously treated with sorafenib (KEYNOTE-224): a non-randomised, open-label phase 2 trial. Lancet Oncol 2018; 19(7): 940-52.
[http://dx.doi.org/10.1016/S1470-2045(18)30351-6] [PMID: 29875066]

[33]   Finn RS, Qin S, Ikeda M, *et al.* IMbrave150 Investigators. Atezolizumab plus bevacizumab in

unresectable hepatocellular carcinoma. N Engl J Med 2020; 382(20): 1894-905.
[http://dx.doi.org/10.1056/NEJMoa1915745] [PMID: 32402160]

[34] Alsaab HO, Sau S, Alzhrani R, Tatiparti K, Bhise K, Kashaw SK, *et al.* PD-1 and PD-L1 checkpoint signaling inhibition for cancer immunotherapy: mechanism, combinations, and clinical outcome. Vol. 8, Frontiers in Pharmacology. Frontiers Media S.A.; 2017.

[35] Dunn GP, Bruce AT, Ikeda H, Old LJ, Schreiber RD. Cancer immunoediting: from immunosurveillance to tumor escape. Nat Immunol 2002; 3(11): 991-8.
[http://dx.doi.org/10.1038/ni1102-991] [PMID: 12407406]

[36] Pardoll DM. The blockade of immune checkpoints in cancer immunotherapy. Nat Rev Cancer 2012; 12(4): 252-64.
[http://dx.doi.org/10.1038/nrc3239] [PMID: 22437870]

[37] Francisco LM, Salinas VH, Brown KE, *et al.* PD-L1 regulates the development, maintenance, and function of induced regulatory T cells. J Exp Med 2009; 206(13): 3015-29.
[http://dx.doi.org/10.1084/jem.20090847] [PMID: 20008522]

[38] Krummel MF, Allison JP. CD28 and CTLA-4 have opposing effects on the response of T cells to stimulation. J Exp Med 1995; 182(2): 459-65.
[http://dx.doi.org/10.1084/jem.182.2.459] [PMID: 7543139]

[39] Walunas TL, Bakker CY, Bluestone JA. CTLA-4 ligation blocks CD28-dependent T cell activation. J Exp Med 1996; 183(6): 2541-50.
[http://dx.doi.org/10.1084/jem.183.6.2541] [PMID: 8676075]

[40] Walunas TL, Lenschow DJ, Bakker CY, *et al.* CTLA-4 can function as a negative regulator of T cell activation. Immunity 1994; 1(5): 405-13.
[http://dx.doi.org/10.1016/1074-7613(94)90071-X] [PMID: 7882171]

[41] Harding FA, McArthur JG, Gross JA, Raulet DH, Allison JP. CD28-mediated signalling co-stimulates murine T cells and prevents induction of anergy in T-cell clones. Nature 1992; 356(6370): 607-9.
[http://dx.doi.org/10.1038/356607a0] [PMID: 1313950]

[42] Yasuda S, Sho M, Yamato I, *et al.* Simultaneous blockade of programmed death 1 and vascular endothelial growth factor receptor 2 (VEGFR2) induces synergistic anti-tumour effect *in vivo*. Clin Exp Immunol 2013; 172(3): 500-6.
[http://dx.doi.org/10.1111/cei.12069] [PMID: 23600839]

[43] Allen E, Jabouille A, Rivera LB, *et al.* Combined antiangiogenic and anti-PD-L1 therapy stimulates tumor immunity through HEV formation. Sci Transl Med 2017; 9(385): eaak9679.
[http://dx.doi.org/10.1126/scitranslmed.aak9679] [PMID: 28404866]

[44] Fu Y, Lin Q, Zhang Z, Zhang L. Therapeutic strategies for the costimulatory molecule OX40 in T-cel--mediated immunity. Vol. 10, Acta Pharmaceutica Sinica B. Chinese Academy of Medical Sciences; 2020. p. 414–33.

[45] Singh P, Toom S, Avula A, Kumar V, Rahma OE. The immune modulation effect of locoregional therapies and its potential synergy with immunotherapy in hepatocellular carcinoma. J Hepatocell Carcinoma 2020; 7: 11-7.
[http://dx.doi.org/10.2147/JHC.S187121] [PMID: 32104669]

[46] FDA grants accelerated approval to nivolumab for HCC previously treated with sorafenib | FDA [Internet]. [cited 2020 Dec 29]. Available from. https://www.fda.gov/drugs/resources-informatio--approved-drugs/fda-grants-accelerated-approval-nivolumab-hcc-previously-treated-sorafenib

[47] Yau T, Park JW, Finn RS, *et al.* CheckMate 459: A randomized, multi-center phase III study of nivolumab (NIVO) *vs* sorafenib (SOR) as first-line (1L) treatment in patients (pts) with advanced hepatocellular carcinoma (aHCC). Ann Oncol 2019; 30: v874-5.
[http://dx.doi.org/10.1093/annonc/mdz394.029]

[48] Sangro B, Park J, Finn R, *et al.* LBA-3 CheckMate 459: Long-term (minimum follow-up 33.6 months)

survival outcomes with nivolumab *versus* sorafenib as first-line treatment in patients with advanced hepatocellular carcinoma. Ann Oncol 2020; 31: S241-2.
[http://dx.doi.org/10.1016/j.annonc.2020.04.078]

[49]   Fessas P, Kaseb A, Wang Y, *et al.* Post-registration experience of nivolumab in advanced hepatocellular carcinoma: an international study. J Immunother Cancer 2020; 8(2): e001033.
[http://dx.doi.org/10.1136/jitc-2020-001033] [PMID: 32868393]

[50]   Choi W-M, Lee D, Shim JH, *et al.* Effectiveness and Safety of Nivolumab in Child-Pugh B Patients with Hepatocellular Carcinoma: A Real-World Cohort Study. Cancers (Basel) 2020; 12(7): 1968.
[http://dx.doi.org/10.3390/cancers12071968] [PMID: 32698355]

[51]   Finkelmeier F, Czauderna C, Perkhofer L, *et al.* Feasibility and safety of nivolumab in advanced hepatocellular carcinoma: real-life experience from three German centers. J Cancer Res Clin Oncol 2019; 145(1): 253-9.
[http://dx.doi.org/10.1007/s00432-018-2780-8] [PMID: 30374657]

[52]   Yu JI, Lee SJ, Lee J, *et al.* Clinical significance of radiotherapy before and/or during nivolumab treatment in hepatocellular carcinoma. Cancer Med 2019; 8(16): 6986-94.
[http://dx.doi.org/10.1002/cam4.2570] [PMID: 31588679]

[53]   Kudo M, Matilla A, Santoro A, Melero I, Gracian AC, Acosta-Rivera M, *et al.* Checkmate-040: Nivolumab (NIVO) in patients (pts) with advanced hepatocellular carcinoma (aHCC) and Child-Pugh B (CPB) status. J Clin Oncol 2019; 37(4_sppl): 327-7.

[54]   A Study of Nivolumab in Participants With Hepatocellular Carcinoma Who Are at High Risk of Recurrence After Curative Hepatic Resection or Ablation - Full Text View - ClinicalTrials.gov [Internet].   [cited   2021   Jan   14].   Available   from.
https://clinicaltrials.gov/ct2/show/NCT03383458?cond=nivolumab+hepatocellular+carcinoma&phase=2&draw=2&rank=3

[55]   Nivolumab in Combination With TACE/TAE for Patients With Intermediate Stage HCC - Full Text View   -   ClinicalTrials.gov   [Internet].   [cited   2021   Jan   14].   Available   from.
https://clinicaltrials.gov/ct2/show/NCT04268888?cond=nivolumab+hepatocellular+carcinoma&phase=2&draw=2&rank=5

[56]   Sorafenib and Nivolumab in Treating Participants With Unresectable, Locally Advanced or Metastatic Liver Cancer - Full Text View - ClinicalTrials.gov [Internet]. [cited 2021 Jan 14]. Available from.
https://clinicaltrials.gov/ct2/show/NCT03439891?cond=nivolumab+hepatocellular+carcinoma&phase=1&draw=2&rank=25

[57]   Regorafenib Followed by Nivolumab in Patients With Hepatocellular Carcinoma (GOING) - Full Text View   -   ClinicalTrials.gov   [Internet].   [cited   2021   Jan   14].   Available   from.
https://clinicaltrials.gov/ct2/show/NCT04170556?cond=nivolumab+hepatocellular+carcinoma&phase=1&draw=2&rank=11

[58]   Combination of Regorafenib and Nivolumab in Unresectable Hepatocellular Carcinoma - Full Text View   -   ClinicalTrials.gov   [Internet].   [cited   2021   Jan   14].   Available   from.
https://clinicaltrials.gov/ct2/show/NCT04310709?cond=nivolumab+hepatocellular+carcinoma&phase=1&draw=2&rank=1

[59]   Abemaciclib and Nivolumab for Subjects With Hepatocellular Carcinoma - Full Text View - ClinicalTrials.gov   [Internet].   [cited   2021   Jan   14].   Available   from.
https://clinicaltrials.gov/ct2/show/NCT03781960?cond=nivolumab+hepatocellular+carcinoma&phase=1&draw=2&rank=2

[60]   A Study of Relatlimab in Combination With Nivolumab in Participants With Advanced Liver Cancer Who Have Never Been Treated With Immuno-oncology Therapy After Prior Treatment With Tyrosine Kinase Inhibitors - Full Text View - ClinicalTrials.gov [Internet]. [cited 2021 Jan 14]. Available from.
https://clinicaltrials.gov/ct2/show/NCT04567615?cond=nivolumab+hepatocellular+carcinoma&phase=1&draw=2&rank=23

[61] A Trial to Evaluate the Safety and Efficacy of the Combination of the Oncolytic Immunotherapy Pexa-Vec With the PD-1 Receptor Blocking Antibody Nivolumab in the First-line Treatment of Advanced Hepatocellular Carcinoma (HCC) - Full Text View - ClinicalTrials.gov [Internet]. [cited 2021 Jan 14]. Available from. https://clinicaltrials.gov/ct2/show/NCT03071094?cond=nivolumab+hepatocellular+carcinoma&phase =1&draw=2&rank=16

[62] FDA grants accelerated approval to pembrolizumab for hepatocellular carcinoma | FDA [Internet]. [cited 2021 Jan 5]. Available from. https://www.fda.gov/drugs/fda-grants-accelerated-appro-al-pembrolizumab-hepatocellular-carcinoma

[63] Feun LG, Li YY, Wu C, *et al.* Phase 2 study of pembrolizumab and circulating biomarkers to predict anticancer response in advanced, unresectable hepatocellular carcinoma. Cancer 2019; 125(20): 3603-14.
[http://dx.doi.org/10.1002/cncr.32339] [PMID: 31251403]

[64] Finn RS, Ryoo BY, Merle P, *et al.* Pembrolizumab As Second-Line Therapy in Patients With Advanced Hepatocellular Carcinoma in KEYNOTE-240: A Randomized, Double-Blind, Phase III Trial. J Clin Oncol 2020; 38(3): 193-202.
[http://dx.doi.org/10.1200/JCO.19.01307] [PMID: 31790344]

[65] Study of Pembrolizumab (MK-3475) or Placebo Given With Best Supportive Care in Asian Participants With Previously Treated Advanced Hepatocellular Carcinoma (MK-347--394/KEYNOTE-394) - Full Text View - ClinicalTrials.gov [Internet]. [cited 2021 Jan 14]. Available from.
https://clinicaltrials.gov/ct2/show/NCT03062358?cond=hepatocellular+pembrolizumab&phase=2&dra w=2&rank=3

[66] Safety and Efficacy of Pembrolizumab (MK-3475) *versus* Placebo as Adjuvant Therapy in Participants With Hepatocellular Carcinoma (HCC) and Complete Radiological Response After Surgical Resection or Local Ablation (MK-3475-937 / KEYNOTE-937) - Full Text View - ClinicalTrials.gov [Internet]. [cited 2021 Jan 14]. Available from.
https://clinicaltrials.gov/ct2/show/NCT03867084?cond=hepatocellular+pembrolizumab&phase=2&dra w=2&rank=2

[67] Sorafenib Tosylate and Pembrolizumab in Treating Patients With Advanced or Metastatic Liver Cancer - Full Text View - ClinicalTrials.gov [Internet]. [cited 2021 Jan 14]. Available from. https://clinicaltrials.gov/ct2/show/NCT03211416?cond=hepatocellular+pembrolizumab&phase=1&dra w=3&rank=11

[68] Regorafenib Plus Tislelizumab as First-line Systemic Therapy for Patients With Advanced Hepatocellular Carcinoma - Full Text View - ClinicalTrials.gov [Internet]. [cited 2021 Jan 14]. Available from.
https://clinicaltrials.gov/ct2/show/NCT04183088?cond=tislelizumab+hepatocellular&draw=2&rank=3

[69] Pembrolizumab With or Without Elbasvir/Grazoprevir and Ribavirin in Treating Patients With Advanced Refractory Liver Cancer - Full Text View - ClinicalTrials.gov [Internet]. [cited 2021 Jan 14]. Available from.
https://clinicaltrials.gov/ct2/show/NCT02940496?cond=hepatocellular+pembrolizumab&phase=1&dra w=3&rank=13

[70] Study of Pembrolizumab Following TACE in Primary Liver Carcinoma - Full Text View - ClinicalTrials.gov [Internet]. [cited 2021 Jan 14]. Available from.
https://clinicaltrials.gov/ct2/show/NCT03397654?cond=hepatocellular+pembrolizumab&phase=1&dra w=3&rank=17

[71] IMMULAB - Immunotherapy With Pembrolizumab in Combination With Local Ablation in Hepatocellular Carcinoma (HCC) - Full Text View - ClinicalTrials.gov [Internet]. [cited 2021 Jan 14]. Available from.
https://clinicaltrials.gov/ct2/show/NCT03753659?cond=hepatocellular+pembrolizumab&phase=1&dra

w=3&rank=2

[72] Study of Pembrolizumab and Radiotherapy in Liver Cancer - Full Text View - ClinicalTrials.gov [Internet]. [cited 2021 Jan 14]. Available from. https://clinicaltrials.gov/ct2/show/NCT03316872?cond=hepatocellular+pembrolizumab&phase=1&dra w=3&rank=7

[73] GNOS-PV02 Personalized Neoantigen Vaccine, INO-9012 and Pembrolizumab in Subjects With Advanced HCC - Full Text View - ClinicalTrials.gov [Internet]. [cited 2021 Jan 14]. Available from. https://clinicaltrials.gov/ct2/show/NCT04251117?cond=hepatocellular+pembrolizumab&phase=1&dra w=3&rank=15

[74] Trial to Evaluate the Safety of Talimogene Laherparepvec Injected Into Tumors Alone and in Combination With Systemic Pembrolizumab MK-3475-611/Keynote-611 - Full Text View - ClinicalTrials.gov [Internet]. [cited 2021 Jan 14]. Available from. https://clinicaltrials.gov/ct2/show/NCT02509507?cond=hepatocellular+pembrolizumab&phase=1&dra w=3&rank=14

[75] Study of Y90-Radioembolization With Nivolumab in Asians With Hepatocellular Carcinoma - Full Text View - ClinicalTrials.gov [Internet]. [cited 2021 Jan 14]. Available from. https://clinicaltrials.gov/ct2/show/NCT03033446

[76] Hodi FS, Chesney J, Pavlick AC, *et al.* Combined nivolumab and ipilimumab *versus* ipilimumab alone in patients with advanced melanoma: 2-year overall survival outcomes in a multicentre, randomised, controlled, phase 2 trial. Lancet Oncol 2016; 17(11): 1558-68. [http://dx.doi.org/10.1016/S1470-2045(16)30366-7] [PMID: 27622997]

[77] Motzer RJ, Tannir NM, McDermott DF, *et al.* Nivolumab plus Ipilimumab *versus* Sunitinib in Advanced Renal-Cell Carcinoma. N Engl J Med 2018; 378(14): 1277-90. [http://dx.doi.org/10.1056/NEJMoa1712126] [PMID: 29562145]

[78] Overman MJ, Lonardi S, Wong KYM, *et al.* Durable clinical benefit with nivolumab plus ipilimumab in DNA mismatch repair-deficient/microsatellite instability-high metastatic colorectal cancer. J Clin Oncol 2018; 36(8): 773-9. [http://dx.doi.org/10.1200/JCO.2017.76.9901] [PMID: 29355075]

[79] Yau T, Kang Y-K, Kim T-Y, El-Khoueiry AB, Santoro A, Sangro B, *et al.* Nivolumab (NIVO) + ipilimumab (IPI) combination therapy in patients (pts) with advanced hepatocellular carcinoma (aHCC): Results from CheckMate 040. J Clin Oncol 2019; 37(15_suppl): 4012-2.

[80] FDA grants accelerated approval to nivolumab and ipilimumab combination for hepatocellular carcinoma | FDA [Internet]. [cited 2020 Dec 31]. Available from. https://www.fda.gov/drugs/ resources-information-approved-drugs/fda-grants-accelerated-approval-nivolumab-and-i-ilimumab-combination-hepatocellular-carcinoma

[81] A Study of Nivolumab in Combination With Ipilimumab in Participants With Advanced Hepatocellular Carcinoma - Full Text View - ClinicalTrials.gov [Internet]. [cited 2021 Jan 15]. Available from. https://clinicaltrials.gov/ct2/show/NCT04039607?cond=nivolumab+hepatocellular+carcinoma&phase =2&draw=2&rank=1

[82] A Study of Nivolumab and Ipilimumab in Combination With Transarterial ChemoEmbolization (TACE) in Participants With Intermediate Stage Liver Cancer - Full Text View - ClinicalTrials.gov [Internet]. [cited 2021 Jan 15]. Available from. https://clinicaltrials.gov/ct2/show/NCT04340193?cond=nivolumab+hepatocellular+carcinoma&phase =2&draw=2&rank=6

[83] Stereotactic Body Radiotherapy (SBRT) Followed by Immunotherapy in Liver Cancer - Full Text View - ClinicalTrials.gov [Internet]. [cited 2021 Jan 15]. Available from. https://clinicaltrials.gov/ct2/show/NCT03203304?cond=nivolumab+ipilimumab+hepatocellular&draw =2&rank=8

[84]   Cabozantinib Combined With Ipilimumab/Nivolumab and TACE in Patients With Hepatocellular Carcinoma - Full Text View - ClinicalTrials.gov [Internet]. [cited 2021 Jan 15]. Available from. https://clinicaltrials.gov/ct2/show/NCT04472767?cond=nivolumab+ipilimumab+hepatocellular&draw =2&rank=3

[85]   Safety and Bioactivity of Ipilimumab and Nivolumab Combination Prior to Liver Resection in Hepatocellular Carcinoma - Full Text View - ClinicalTrials.gov [Internet]. [cited 2021 Jan 15]. Available   from. https://clinicaltrials.gov/ct2/show/NCT03682276?cond=nivolumab+ipilimumab+hepatocellular&draw =2&rank=5

[86]   Reck M, Mok TSK, Nishio M, *et al.* Atezolizumab plus bevacizumab and chemotherapy in non-smal- -cell lung cancer (IMpower150): key subgroup analyses of patients with EGFR mutations or baseline liver metastases in a randomised, open-label phase 3 trial. Lancet Respir Med 2019; 7(5): 387-401. [http://dx.doi.org/10.1016/S2213-2600(19)30084-0] [PMID: 30922878]

[87]   Rini BI, Powles T, Atkins MB, *et al.* Atezolizumab plus bevacizumab *versus* sunitinib in patients with previously untreated metastatic renal cell carcinoma (IMmotion151): a multicentre, open-label, phase 3, randomised controlled trial. Lancet 2019; 393(10189): 2404-15. [http://dx.doi.org/10.1016/S0140-6736(19)30723-8] [PMID: 31079938]

[88]   Lee MS, Ryoo BY, Hsu CH, *et al.* Atezolizumab with or without bevacizumab in unresectable hepatocellular carcinoma (GO30140): an open-label, multicentre, phase 1b study. Lancet Oncol 2020; 21(6): 808-20. [http://dx.doi.org/10.1016/S1470-2045(20)30156-X] [PMID: 32502443]

[89]   Siegel AB, Cohen EI, Ocean A, *et al.* Phase II trial evaluating the clinical and biologic effects of bevacizumab in unresectable hepatocellular carcinoma. J Clin Oncol 2008; 26(18): 2992-8. [http://dx.doi.org/10.1200/JCO.2007.15.9947] [PMID: 18565886]

[90]   Boige V, Malka D, Bourredjem A, *et al.* Efficacy, safety, and biomarkers of single-agent bevacizumab therapy in patients with advanced hepatocellular carcinoma. Oncologist 2012; 17(8): 1063-72. [http://dx.doi.org/10.1634/theoncologist.2011-0465] [PMID: 22707516]

[91]   FDA approves lenvatinib for unresectable hepatocellular carcinoma | FDA [Internet]. [cited 2021 Jan 7]. Available from. https://www.fda.gov/drugs/resources-information-approved-drugs/fda-appr- ves-lenvatinib-unresectable-hepatocellular-carcinoma

[92]   FDA approves atezolizumab plus bevacizumab for unresectable hepatocellular carcinoma | FDA [Internet]. [cited 2021 Jan 7]. Available from. https://www.fda.gov/drugs/drug-approvals-a- d-databases/fda-approves-atezolizumab-plus-bevacizumab-unresectable-hepatocellular-carcinoma

[93]   Hack SP, Spahn J, Chen M, Cheng AL, Kaseb A, Kudo M, *et al.* IMbrave 050: A Phase III trial of atezolizumab plus bevacizumab in high-risk hepatocellular carcinoma after curative resection or ablation. Future Oncology. Future Medicine Ltd. 2020; Vol. 16: pp. 975-89.

[94]   A Study of Atezolizumab Plus Bevacizumab *versus* Active Surveillance as Adjuvant Therapy in Patients With Hepatocellular Carcinoma at High Risk of Recurrence After Surgical Resection or Ablation - Full Text View - ClinicalTrials.gov [Internet]. [cited 2021 Jan 15]. Available from. https://clinicaltrials.gov/ct2/show/NCT04102098?cond=atezolizumab+hepatocellular&draw=2&rank= 4

[95]   Study of Atezolizumab and Bevacizumab With Y-90 TARE in Patients With Unresectable Hepatocellular Carcinoma (HCC) - Full Text View - ClinicalTrials.gov [Internet]. [cited 2021 Jan 15]. Available   from. https://clinicaltrials.gov/ct2/show/NCT04541173?cond=atezolizumab+hepatocellular&draw=2&rank= 1

[96]   Atezolizumab/Bevacizumab Followed by On-demand TACE or Initial Synchronous Treatment With TACE and Atezolizumab/Bevacizumab - Full Text View - ClinicalTrialsgov [Internet] [cited 2021 Jan 15]   Available   from

https://clinicaltrials.gov/ct2/show/NCT04224636?cond=atezolizumab+hepatocellular&draw=2&rank=6

[97]   Desai J, Deva S, Lee JS, *et al.* Phase IA/IB study of single-agent tislelizumab, an investigational anti-PD-1 antibody, in solid tumors. J Immunother Cancer 2020; 8(1): e000453.
[http://dx.doi.org/10.1136/jitc-2019-000453] [PMID: 32540858]

[98]   Dahan R, Sega E, Engelhardt J, Selby M, Korman AJ, Ravetch JV. FcγRs Modulate the Anti-tumor Activity of Antibodies Targeting the PD-1/PD-L1 Axis. Cancer Cell 2015; 28(3): 285-95.
[http://dx.doi.org/10.1016/j.ccell.2015.08.004] [PMID: 26373277]

[99]   Feng Y, Hong Y, Sun H, *et al.* Abstract 2383: The molecular binding mechanism of tislelizumab, an investigational anti-PD-1 antibody, is differentiated from pembrolizumab and nivolumab. In: Cancer Research. American Association for Cancer Research (AACR); 2019. p. 2383–2383.

[100] Shen L, Guo J, Zhang Q, *et al.* Tislelizumab in Chinese patients with advanced solid tumors: an open-label, non-comparative, phase 1/2 study. J Immunother Cancer 2020; 8(1): e000437.
[http://dx.doi.org/10.1136/jitc-2019-000437] [PMID: 32561638]

[101] Phase 3 Study of Tislelizumab *versus* Sorafenib in Participants With Unresectable HCC - Full Text View - ClinicalTrials.gov [Internet]. [cited 2021 Jan 14]. Available from. https://clinicaltrials.gov/ct2/show/NCT03412773?cond=Tislelizumab+hepatocellular&draw=2&rank=8

[102] Qin S, Finn RS, Kudo M, *et al.* RATIONALE 301 study: tislelizumab *versus* sorafenib as first-line treatment for unresectable hepatocellular carcinoma. Future Oncol 2019; 15(16): 1811-22.
[http://dx.doi.org/10.2217/fon-2019-0097] [PMID: 30969136]

[103] A Study to Investigate Sitravatinib as Monotherapy and in Combination With Tislelizumab in Participants With Unresectable Locally Advanced or Metastatic Hepatocellular Carcinoma (HCC) or Gastric/Gastroesophageal Junction Cancer (GC/GEJC) - Full Text View - ClinicalTrials.gov [Internet]. [cited 2021 Jan 14]. Available from. https://clinicaltrials.gov/ct2/show/NCT03941873?cond=tislelizumab+hepatocellular&draw=2&rank=6

[104] Preliminary Antitumor Activity, Safety and Tolerability of Tislelizumab in Combination With Lenvatinib for Hepatocellular Carcinoma - Full Text View - ClinicalTrials.gov [Internet]. [cited 2021 Jan 14]. Available from. https://clinicaltrials.gov/ct2/show/NCT04401800?cond=tislelizumab+hepatocellular&draw=2&rank=5

[105] Tislelizumab in Combination With TACE in Advanced Hepatocellular Carcinoma - Full Text View - ClinicalTrials.gov [Internet]. [cited 2021 Jan 14]. Available from. https://clinicaltrials.gov/ct2/show/NCT04652492?cond=tislelizumab+hepatocellular&draw=2&rank=1

[106] TACE Combined With Sorafenib and Tislelizumab for Advanced HCC - Full Text View - ClinicalTrials.gov [Internet]. [cited 2021 Jan 14]. Available from. https://clinicaltrials.gov/ct2/show/NCT04599777?cond=tislelizumab+hepatocellular&draw=2&rank=7

[107] Tislelizumab Neo-adjuvant Treatment for Resectable RHCC - Full Text View - ClinicalTrials.gov [Internet]. [cited 2021 Jan 14]. Available from. https://clinicaltrials.gov/ct2/show/NCT04615143?cond=Tislelizumab+hepatocellular&draw=2&rank=4

[108] Markham A, Keam SJ. Camrelizumab: First Global Approval. Drugs 2019; 79(12): 1355-61.
[http://dx.doi.org/10.1007/s40265-019-01167-0] [PMID: 31313098]

[109] Qin S, Ren Z, Meng Z, *et al.* Camrelizumab in patients with previously treated advanced hepatocellular carcinoma: a multicentre, open-label, parallel-group, randomised, phase 2 trial. Lancet Oncol 2020; 21(4): 571-80.
[http://dx.doi.org/10.1016/S1470-2045(20)30011-5] [PMID: 32112738]

[110] Chen J, Hu X, Li Q, *et al.* Effectiveness and safety of toripalimab, camrelizumab, and sintilimab in a real-world cohort of hepatitis B virus associated hepatocellular carcinoma patients. Ann Transl Med

2020; 8(18): 1187-7.
[http://dx.doi.org/10.21037/atm-20-6063] [PMID: 33241036]

[111] A Trial of SHR-1210 (an Anti-PD-1 Inhibitor) in Combination With FOLFOX4 in Subjects With Advanced HCC Who Have Never Received Prior Systemic Treatment. - Full Text View - ClinicalTrials.gov [Internet]. [cited 2021 Jan 15]. Available from. https://clinicaltrials.gov/ct2/show/NCT03605706?cond=camrelizumab+hepatocellular&draw=2&rank=10

[112] Lenvatinib in Combination With Camrelizumab as First-Line Therapy in Patients With Advanced HCC - Full Text View - ClinicalTrials.gov [Internet]. [cited 2021 Jan 15]. Available from. https://clinicaltrials.gov/ct2/show/NCT04443309?cond=camrelizumab+hepatocellular&draw=2&rank=6

[113] Study of TACE Combined With Camrelizumab in the Treatment of HCC Patients - Full Text View - ClinicalTrials.gov [Internet]. [cited 2021 Jan 15]. Available from. https://clinicaltrials.gov/ct2/show/NCT04483284?cond=camrelizumab+hepatocellular&draw=2&rank=5

[114] Wainberg ZA, Segal NH, Jaeger D, Lee K-H, Marshall J, Antonia SJ, *et al.* Safety and clinical activity of durvalumab monotherapy in patients with hepatocellular carcinoma (HCC). J Clin Oncol 2017; 35(15_suppl): 4071-1.

[115] Sangro B, Gomez-Martin C, de la Mata M, *et al.* A clinical trial of CTLA-4 blockade with tremelimumab in patients with hepatocellular carcinoma and chronic hepatitis C. J Hepatol 2013; 59(1): 81-8.
[http://dx.doi.org/10.1016/j.jhep.2013.02.022] [PMID: 23466307]

[116] Safety and Efficacy of Lenvatinib (E7080/MK-7902) in Combination With Pembrolizumab (MK-3475) *versus* Lenvatinib as First-line Therapy in Participants With Advanced Hepatocellular Carcinoma (MK-7902-002/E7080-G000-311/LEAP-002) - Full Text View - ClinicalTrials.gov [Internet]. [cited 2021 Jan 14]. Available from. https://clinicaltrials.gov/ct2/show/NCT03713593?cond=lenvatinib+pembrolizumab+hepatocellular&draw=2&rank=3

[117] Safety and Efficacy of Lenvatinib (E7080/MK-7902) With Pembrolizumab (MK-3475) in Combination With Transarterial Chemoembolization (TACE) in Participants With Incurable/Non-metastatic Hepatocellular Carcinoma (MK-7902-012/E7080-G000-318/LEAP-012) - Full Text View - ClinicalTrials.gov [Internet]. [cited 2021 Jan 14]. Available from. https://clinicaltrials.gov/ct2/show/NCT04246177?cond=lenvatinib+pembrolizumab+hepatocellular&draw=2&rank=4

[118] FDA approves cabozantinib for hepatocellular carcinoma | FDA [Internet]. [cited 2021 Jan 14]. Available from. https://www.fda.gov/drugs/fda-approves-cabozantinib-hepatocellular-carcinoma

[119] Study of Cabozantinib in Combination With Atezolizumab to Subjects With Locally Advanced or Metastatic Solid Tumors - Full Text View - ClinicalTrials.gov [Internet]. [cited 2021 Jan 14]. Available from. https://clinicaltrials.gov/ct2/show/NCT03170960?cond=hepatocellular+atezolizumab&draw=3&rank=12

[120] Kelley RKW, W Oliver J, Hazra S, *et al.* Cabozantinib in combination with atezolizumab *versus* sorafenib in treatment-naive advanced hepatocellular carcinoma: COSMIC-312 Phase III study design. Future Oncol 2020; 16(21): 1525-36.
[http://dx.doi.org/10.2217/fon-2020-0283] [PMID: 32491932]

[121] Study of Cabozantinib in Combination With Atezolizumab *versus* Sorafenib in Subjects With Advanced HCC Who Have Not Received Previous Systemic Anticancer Therapy - Full Text View - ClinicalTrials.gov [Internet]. [cited 2021 Jan 14]. Available from. https://clinicaltrials.gov/ct2/show/NCT03755791?cond=hepatocellular+atezolizumab&draw=2&rank=5

[122] Escudier B, Gore M. Axitinib for the management of metastatic renal cell carcinoma. Drugs R D 2011; 11(2): 113-26.
[http://dx.doi.org/10.2165/11591240-000000000-00000] [PMID: 21679004]

[123] Motzer RJ, Penkov K, Haanen J, *et al.* Avelumab plus Axitinib *versus* Sunitinib for Advanced Renal-Cell Carcinoma. N Engl J Med 2019; 380(12): 1103-15.
[http://dx.doi.org/10.1056/NEJMoa1816047] [PMID: 30779531]

[124] FDA approves avelumab plus axitinib for renal cell carcinoma | FDA [Internet]. [cited 2021 Jan 14]. Available from. https://www.fda.gov/drugs/resources-information-approved-drugs/fda-appr-ves-avelumab-plus-axitinib-renal-cell-carcinoma

[125] Rajadurai P, Cheah PL, How SH, *et al.* Molecular testing for advanced non-small cell lung cancer in Malaysia: Consensus statement from the College of Pathologists, Academy of Medicine Malaysia, the Malaysian Thoracic Society, and the Malaysian Oncological Society. Lung Cancer 2019; 136: 65-73.
[http://dx.doi.org/10.1016/j.lungcan.2019.08.005] [PMID: 31446227]

[126] Xu J, Zhang Y, Jia R, *et al.* Anti-PD-1 antibody SHR-1210 combined with apatinib for advanced hepatocellular carcinoma, gastric, or esophagogastric junction cancer: An Open-label, Dose Escalation and Expansion Study. Clin Cancer Res 2019; 25(2): 515-23.
[http://dx.doi.org/10.1158/1078-0432.CCR-18-2484] [PMID: 30348638]

[127] Xu J, Shen J, Gu S, *et al.* Camrelizumab in combination with apatinib in patients with advanced hepatocellular carcinoma (RESCUE): a non-randomized, open-label, phase 2 trial. Clin Cancer Res 2020; 2571.

[128] Yuan G, Cheng X, Li Q, *et al.* Safety and efficacy of camrelizumab combined with apatinib for advanced hepatocellular carcinoma with portal vein tumor thrombus: A multicenter retrospective study. OncoTargets Ther 2020; 13: 12683-93.
[http://dx.doi.org/10.2147/OTT.S286169] [PMID: 33328740]

[129] Camrelizumab Combined With Apatinib for Perioperative Treatment of Resectable Primary Hepatocellular Carcinoma - Full Text View - ClinicalTrials.gov [Internet]. [cited 2021 Jan 14]. Available   from. https://clinicaltrials.gov/ct2/show/NCT04701060?cond=camrelizumab+apatinib+hepatocellular&draw=2&rank=2

[130] A Study to Evaluate Camrelizumab Plus Apatinib as Adjuvant Therapy in Patients With HCC at High Risk of Recurrence After Surgical Resection or Ablation - Full Text View - ClinicalTrials.gov [Internet].   [cited   2021   Jan   14].   Available   from. https://clinicaltrials.gov/ct2/show/NCT04639180?cond=camrelizumab+apatinib+hepatocellular&draw=2&rank=5

[131] Combination Camrelizumab (SHR-1210) and Apatinib for Downstaging/Bridging of HCC Before Liver Transplant - Full Text View - ClinicalTrials.gov [Internet]. [cited 2021 Jan 14]. Available from. https://clinicaltrials.gov/ct2/show/NCT04035876?cond=camrelizumab+apatinib+hepatocellular&draw=2&rank=3

[132] Evaluation Effectiveness and Safety of (cTACE or DEB-TACE + FOLFOX Regimen HAIC) Combined With Camrelizumab and Apatinib Mesylas in the Treatment of Advanced Hepatocellular Carcinoma - Full Text View - ClinicalTrials.gov [Internet]. [cited 2021 Jan 14]. Available from. https://clinicaltrials.gov/ct2/show/NCT04479527?cond=camrelizumab+apatinib+hepatocellular&draw=2&rank=4

[133] TACE Combined With Camrelizumab and Apatinib in Intermediate and Advanced Hepatocelluar Carcinoma - Full Text View - ClinicalTrials.gov [Internet]. [cited 2021 Jan 14]. Available from. https://clinicaltrials.gov/ct2/show/NCT04559607?cond=camrelizumab+apatinib+hepatocellular&draw=2&rank=6

[134] A Trial of Hepatic Arterial Infusion Combined With Apatinib and Camrelizumab for C-staged Hepatocellular Carcinoma in BCLC Classification - Full Text View - ClinicalTrials.gov [Internet].

[cited   2021   Jan   14].   Available   from.
https://clinicaltrials.gov/ct2/show/NCT04191889?cond=camrelizumab+apatinib+hepatocellular&draw
=2&rank=1

[135] Spratlin JL, Cohen RB, Eadens M, *et al.* Phase I pharmacologic and biologic study of ramucirumab
      (IMC-1121B), a fully human immunoglobulin G1 monoclonal antibody targeting the vascular
      endothelial growth factor receptor-2. J Clin Oncol 2010; 28(5): 780-7.
      [http://dx.doi.org/10.1200/JCO.2009.23.7537] [PMID: 20048182]

[136] Assess Efficacy and Safety of Durvalumab Alone or Combined With Bevacizumab in High Risk of
      Recurrence HCC Patients After Curative Treatment - Full Text View - ClinicalTrials.gov [Internet].
      [cited   2021   Jan   15].   Available   from.
      https://clinicaltrials.gov/ct2/show/NCT03847428?cond=durvalumab+bevacizumab+hepatocellular&dr
      aw=2&rank=3

[137] Kelley RK, Sangro B, Harris WP, Ikeda M, Okusaka T, Kang Y-K, *et al.* Efficacy, tolerability, and
      biologic activity of a novel regimen of tremelimumab (T) in combination with durvalumab (D) for
      patients (pts) with advanced hepatocellular carcinoma (aHCC). J Clin Oncol 2020; 38: 15_suppl-.:
      4508-8.

[138] Study of Durvalumab and Tremelimumab as First-line Treatment in Patients With Advanced
      Hepatocellular Carcinoma - Full Text View - ClinicalTrials.gov [Internet]. [cited 2021 Jan 11].
      Available from. https://clinicaltrials.gov/ct2/show/NCT03298451

[139] Duffy AG, Ulahannan SV, Makorova-Rusher O, *et al.* Tremelimumab in combination with ablation in
      patients with advanced hepatocellular carcinoma. J Hepatol 2017; 66(3): 545-51.
      [http://dx.doi.org/10.1016/j.jhep.2016.10.029] [PMID: 27816492]

[140] Durvalumab and Tremelimumab After Radioembolization for the Treatment of Unresectable, Locally
      Advanced Liver Cancer - Full Text View - ClinicalTrials.gov [Internet]. [cited 2021 Jan 15]. Available
      from.
      https://clinicaltrials.gov/ct2/show/NCT04605731?cond=tremelimumab+hepatocellular&draw=2&rank
      =7

[141] Durvalumab (MEDI4736) and Tremelimumab in Combination With Either Y-90 SIRT or TACE for
      Intermediate Stage HCC With Pick-the-winner Design - Full Text View - ClinicalTrials.gov [Internet].
      [cited   2021   Jan   15].   Available   from.
      https://clinicaltrials.gov/ct2/show/NCT04522544?cond=tremelimumab+hepatocellular&draw=2&rank
      =6

[142] Hypofractionated Radiotherapy Followed by Durvalumab With or Without Tremelimumab for the
      Treatment of Liver Cancer After Progression on Prior PD-1 Inhibition - Full Text View -
      ClinicalTrials.gov   [Internet].   [cited   2021   Jan   15].   Available   from.
      https://clinicaltrials.gov/ct2/show/NCT04430452?cond=tremelimumab+hepatocellular&draw=2&rank
      =8

[143] Ziogas IA, Evangeliou AP, Giannis D, Hayat MH, Mylonas KS, Tohme S, *et al.* The Role of
      Immunotherapy in Hepatocellular Carcinoma: A Systematic Review and Pooled Analysis of 2,402
      patients. Oncologist 2020.
      [PMID: 33314549]

[144] Nordness MF, Hamel S, Godfrey CM, *et al.* Fatal hepatic necrosis after nivolumab as a bridge to liver
      transplant for HCC: Are checkpoint inhibitors safe for the pretransplant patient? Am J Transplant
      2020; 20(3): 879-83.
      [http://dx.doi.org/10.1111/ajt.15617] [PMID: 31550417]

[145] Anugwom C, Leventhal T. Nivolumab-Induced Autoimmune-Like Cholestatic Hepatitis in a Liver
      Transplant Recipient. ACG Case Rep J 2020; 7(7): e00416.
      [http://dx.doi.org/10.14309/crj.0000000000000416] [PMID: 32766358]

[146] Pandey A, Cohen DJ. Ipilumumab for hepatocellular cancer in a liver transplant recipient, with durable

response, tolerance and without allograft rejection. Immunotherapy 2020; 12(5): 287-92.
[http://dx.doi.org/10.2217/imt-2020-0014] [PMID: 32248723]

[147] Amjad W, Kotiah S, Gupta A, Morris M, Liu L, Thuluvath PJ. Successful treatment of disseminated hepatocellular carcinoma after liver transplantation with nivolumab. J Clin Exp Hepatol 2020; 10(2): 185-7.
[http://dx.doi.org/10.1016/j.jceh.2019.11.009] [PMID: 32189935]

[148] DeLeon TT, Ahn DH, Bogenberger JM, *et al.* Novel targeted therapy strategies for biliary tract cancers and hepatocellular carcinoma. Future Oncol 2018; 14(6): 553-66.
[http://dx.doi.org/10.2217/fon-2017-0451] [PMID: 29460642]

[149] Gassmann D, Weiler S, Mertens JC, *et al.* Liver allograft failure after nivolumab treatment—A Case report with systematic literature research. Transplant Direct 2018; 4(8): e376.
[http://dx.doi.org/10.1097/TXD.0000000000000814] [PMID: 30255136]

[150] Rammohan A, Reddy MS, Farouk M, Vargese J, Rela M. Pembrolizumab for metastatic hepatocellular carcinoma following live donor liver transplantation: The silver bullet? Hepatology 2018; 67(3): 1166-8.
[http://dx.doi.org/10.1002/hep.29575] [PMID: 29023959]

[151] De Toni EN, Gerbes AL. Tapering of immunosuppression and sustained treatment with nivolumab in a liver transplant recipient. Gastroenterology 2017; 152(6): 1631-3.
[http://dx.doi.org/10.1053/j.gastro.2017.01.063] [PMID: 28384452]

[152] Friend BD, Venick RS, McDiarmid SV, *et al.* Fatal orthotopic liver transplant organ rejection induced by a checkpoint inhibitor in two patients with refractory, metastatic hepatocellular carcinoma. Pediatr Blood Cancer 2017; 64(12)
[http://dx.doi.org/10.1002/pbc.26682] [PMID: 28643391]

[153] Varkaris A, Lewis DW, Nugent FW. Preserved Liver Transplant After PD-1 Pathway Inhibitor for Hepatocellular Carcinoma. Am J Gastroenterol 2017; 112(12): 1895-6.
[http://dx.doi.org/10.1038/ajg.2017.387] [PMID: 29215617]

CHAPTER 5

Role of Biomarkers in Developing Therapies for Glioblastoma Multiforme

Vijeta Prakash[1] and **Reema Gabrani**[1,*]

[1] *Jaypee Institute of Information Technology, A-10, Sector-62, Noida, Uttar Pradesh 201309, India*

Abstract: Brain and nervous system cancer account for 28,142 new cases as of GLOBOCAN 2018. Glioblastoma multiforme (GBM) is a quite lethal and aggressive form of tumor which initiates from the cerebrum glial cells. Additionally, due to its aggressive nature of the infection, it is ranked as grade IV of astrocytoma by WHO and accounts for the most malignant cases of gliomas. The current standard of care includes surgical elimination of the tumor followed by radiotherapy and temozolomide (TMZ). The recent research focuses to identify its novel biomarkers as therapeutic targets. Currently, available drugs can be potentiated with adjuvant therapy. These include the inculcation of immunotherapy, phytochemicals, and chemotherapy. However, due to the tumor heterogeneity in GBM, there is a development of resistance majorly against the chemotherapeutic drugs. The most significant reason behind this is alteration and mutation in molecular pathways involved in functions like angiogenesis, migration, proliferation, and several other events. Therefore, moving towards personalized medicine, identification and characterization of biomarkers can promote prediction, diagnosis as well as treatment. Several biomarkers in molecular as well as metabolic pathways such as methylguanine-DNA methyltransferase (MGMT), receptor tyrosine kinase (RTK) pathways, TP53/MDM2/P14 and isocitrate dehydrogenase (IDH) for GBM have been identified. Apart from these, there are miRNA, GBM cancer stem cells (GSCs), and immune checkpoints, which can be used as biomarkers. This chapter reviews the research and progress of the biomarkers as an aid for GBM therapeutics.

Keywords: GBM cancer stem cells, Glial cells, Immunotherapy, miRNA, Molecular pathway.

INTRODUCTION

Glioblastoma multiforme (GBM) is one of the most aggressive tumors which develops in the central nervous system (CNS). There is an issue of poor prognosis in GBM since it shows 14.6 months of overall survival even after surgical and

** **Corresponding author Reema Gabrani:** Jaypee Institute of Information Technology, A-10, Sector-62, Noida, Uttar Pradesh 201309, India; Tel: 09717152115; E-mail: reema.gabrani@jiit.ac.in*

Atta-ur-Rahman & M. Iqbal Choudhary (Eds.)
All rights reserved-© 2021 Bentham Science Publishers

chemical interventions [1]. GBM is being treated with various methods, as shown in Fig. (1). Radiation therapy combined with chemotherapy (Temozolomide) is a standard care treatment, which is supported by different adjuvant methods. The advancements in genomics and proteomics have led to the introduction of the aspect of biomarkers in prognosis, as well as therapy. There are many important genes and proteins which have been studied as potential biomarkers. These biomarkers can be related to developmental pathways, immune checkpoints, micro RNAs (miRNAs) and GSCs since these are responsible for many important facets in tumor development [2].

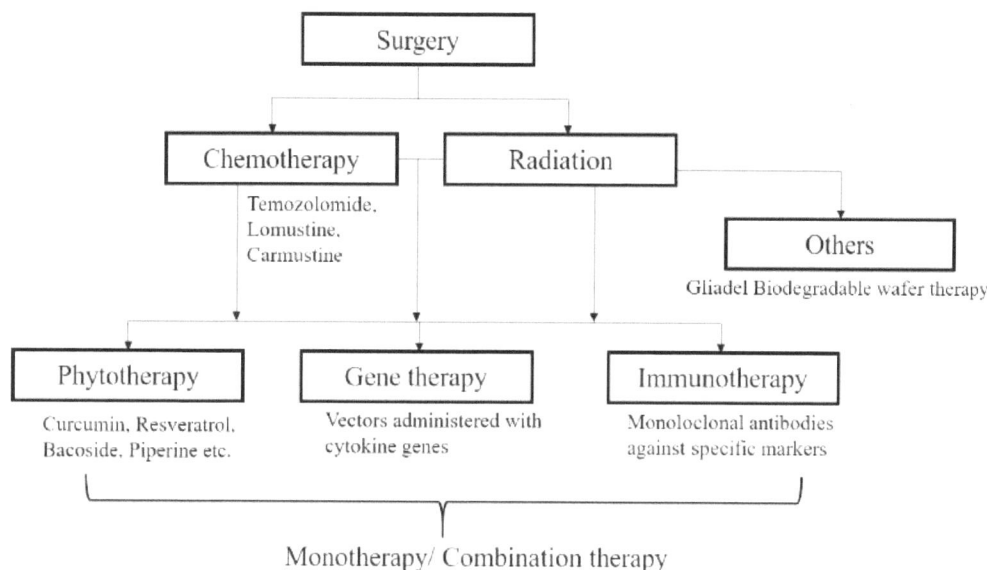

Fig. (1). The multipronged treatment for GBM is elicited in the flowchart. Patients can undergo surgical resection followed by radiation and chemotherapy as a single treatment or together. Subsequently, methods such as phytotherapy, gene therapy, and immunotherapy can be applied individually or in combination.

Biomarkers are of different types. Diagnostic biomarkers aid in better and accurate classification of the tumor based on the related features. Whereas prognostic biomarkers help understand the potential outcome such as overall survival and progression-free survival (PFS) [3]. Thus, exploring the avenues in this field can help in better patient management and can also lead to advancement in the treatment of GBM. Herein, we focus on the existing biomarkers and their development for the therapeutic and diagnostic regime.

BIOMARKERS IN MOLECULAR AND METABOLIC PATHWAYS

The progression and growth of GBM are dependent on different pathways linked to cell development and maturity. The pathways can activate certain growth factors/regulators, energy balance, cell survival and proliferation. There are several genes and proteins associated with these pathways, which readily aid the above processes.

Epidermal Growth Factor Receptor

Epidermal Growth Factor Receptor (EGFR) is one of the most significant proteins responsible for GBM progression. It is a transmembrane receptor, which upon activation, induces autophosphorylation and triggers a cascade of pathways, which leads to cell proliferation. However, certain alterations in the EGFR gene in glioma cells can lead to its overexpression, leading to the severity in tumors [4]. Isocitrate dehydrogenase (IDH) has been linked to the progression of glioma and has also been included in the new classification of gliomas by the World Health Organization. EGFR also happens to be coregulated with IDH, so its implication can be studied to bring out more effective markers or treatment. EGFR status in IDHwt GBM patients indicated that EGFR expression was negatively correlated to survival. It pointed towards shorter overall survival (OS), which is a major parameter employed in clinical research [5].

The most prominent alteration is the EGFRviii mutation, which arises from exon 2-7 deletion leading to activation of oncogenic response. This results in the gain of function and leads to excessive proliferation. The extracellular vesicles present in cerebrospinal fluid (CSF) showed the presence of wtEGFR as well as EGFRviii [6].

In a study done by Felsberg *et al.*, around 50% of the patients of GBM had EGFRviii mutation. EGFRviii mutation did not lead to a change in the overall survival. However, when studied along with O6-methylguanine DNA methyltransferase (MGMT), it was revealed that MGMT methylation, if co-occurred with EGFRviii, could lead to longer OS [7]. In another study, 38% of the patient samples were found to contain EGFRviii amplification after screening through PCR and sequencing [8]. Additionally, EGFR amplification affected certain cytokine levels. CD68$^+$ was more prevalent in the samples containing co-existing EGFR and EGFRviii along with other upregulated chemokines such as IL6, IL8, IL33, IL11 and CCL2 [9]. In addition, EGFR was also related to the mismatch repair protein (MMR) and it was observed that knockdown of EGFRviii led to its reduction. The MMR overexpression plays an important role in the development of resistance after treatment with temozolomide (TMZ) [10]. Hence, EGFRviii was observed to be linked with many factors, be it cytokines, developmental pathways, or repair mechanisms, so this could be utilized to develop EGFRviii as a diagnostic as well as therapeutic biomarker.

MGMT

MGMT being a mismatch repair protein, tends to inhibit apoptosis by readily alkylating O6 position of guanine at the DNA level. The efficacy of standard care treatment is observed to be affected by the expression of MGMT and therefore could be accounted as a prognostic, predictive and diagnostic biomarker. The methylation of the MGMT promoter can lead to its low expression and results in the improper repair of DNA [11]. Thus, the methylation of MGMT allows alkylating agents to inhibit DNA replication. Methylation of MGMT promoter is being recognized as a diagnostic biomarker since it helps in analyzing the status of progression of GBM tumor in patients. Additionally, it acts as a predictive biomarker [12] as it could envisage the treatment efficacy of alkylating agents in GBM. In addition, it can be considered as a prognostic biomarker [13] since it increased the overall survival of the patients.

In a xenograft study done by Shiv *et al.* in 2016, veliparib, a poly-ADP-ribose polymerase (PARP) inhibitor, was tested along with TMZ, which is an alkylating drug. It was observed that better survival was observed in MGMT promoter hypermethylated xenograft models compared to unmethylated groups. Additionally, these models were found to be extremely sensitive to TMZ. This proved that MGMT hypermethylation can be a great prognostic marker because of its correlation to survival [14]. This is supported by a study, which involved patients who experienced GBM recurrence post first surgery. MGMT methylation status remained significant even after the second surgery, which proved that MGMT promoter methylation can be considered as a diagnostic biomarker [15]. However, in an interesting twist to the significance of MGMT methylation in patient survival, it has been reported by Schiffgens *et al.* that methylated phenotype was associated only with the female group in a comparative study of 29 male patients and 24 female patients [16, 17].

The significance of MGMT expression was observed in GBM stem cells (GSCs) as well. In addition, MGMT was found to be correlated with markers of stemness like CD133$^+$. MGMT mRNA levels showed an increase in the presence of CD133$^+$ [18].

In a methylation study, it was observed that the median methylation level for MGMT was 64.65% in glioma patients. The level of methylation happened to be higher in high grade (71.75%) than low grade (56.55%) glioma patients. This study supported the fact that MGMT methylation could act as a good diagnostic biomarker [19]. Additionally, MGMT methylation led to an increase in PFS from 10 months to 19.2 months and OS from 21.7 months to 36.1 months, as reported by a study performed by Schaf *et al.* [17, 20].

Chen *et al.* reported the location of an enhancer in between promoter of Ki67 and MGMT gene. The activation of this enhancer led to TMZ resistant phenotype due to increased expression of MGMT. Deletion of the enhancer resulted in the loss of MGMT expression, and this could act as a potential GBM biomarker [21].

Tumor Protein p53

TP53 or tumor protein p53 encodes for tumor suppressor protein, which regulates the cell division, eventually stops the proliferation of tumor cells. These are usually mutated in the case of tumors like GBM, which directed the extensive proliferation. TP53 is found to be more prominently expressed in cancer tissues rather than normal brain tissue [22]. Dataset analysis has pointed toward the co-occurrence of alterations pertaining to several genes like TP53, loss of ATP-dependent helicase (ATRX) and IDH1 [23]. Due to the prominent presence and contribution toward GBM, TP53 can be a great candidate for a biomarker.

Additionally, TP53, along with MGMT, has been found to be associated with miR-125b, miR-21, and miR-34a with a negative correlation [24]. The mutations found in TP53 were mostly missense mutations in exon 8 of TP53. It has been reported that TP53 and MGMT methylation is correlated in 20.83% of the tumors. In addition, it has been observed that TP53 has OS of 3 months in the case of methylated phenotype, whereas 10 months in the case of unmethylated phenotype [25]. This indicates that TP53 can be considered as a prognostic biomarker candidate as it could be correlated with OS and PFS. Also, since it is related to several other checkpoints and has different implications, it can lead to an advanced and efficient prognosis.

Isocitrate Dehydrogenase

Isocitrate dehydrogenase (IDH) is responsible for oxidative carboxylation of isocitrate into α-ketoglutarate in the citric acid cycle [3, 26]. Mutations in IDH lead to the formation of 2-hydroxyglutarate (2-HG), which consumes NADPH instead of its production, during the catalysis process [27]. This results in hampering the defense against reactive oxygen species , hence leads to a tumorigenic phenotype [28]. Also, the importance of IDH mutation can be understood from the fact that WHO has classified glioblastoma based on the presence of IDH mutation. Glioblastoma falls in grade IV, which is further diverged into GBM IDH wild type, which has a poor prognosis and GBM IDH mutant, which has a better prognosis [29]. Due to the critical role of IDH, it can be a very significant marker for GBM as a diagnostic, prognostic and predictive marker [3, 30].

There is a prolonged survival associated with IDH mutation post-treatment, which is confirmed by a middle-east based study as well [31]. However, this prolonged survival of patients due to IDH mutation was observed to be linked to males more than females as per a study by Schiffgens *et al.* [16]. Though IDH holds a lot of importance as a biomarker, the prognostic value of IDH can be increased if it is studied along with other biomarkers such as 1p19q chromosome arm loss to distinguish the tumor characteristics. It has been observed that both biomarkers can be applied to grade II, III and IV gliomas [31]. Along with 1p19q deletion, many other genes could be clubbed to improve the prognosis of GBM, such as, a seven gene signature has been established which consists of ZNF419, FOXG1, STARD7, ZBTB16, CD180, SDK1, and CYP21A2 [32]. This can additionally help in stratifying GBM IDHwt tumors into low and high risk, thereby making the prognosis more effective [33].

Voltage-dependent Anion Channel

The voltage-dependent anion channel (VDAC) lies on the outer side of mitochondria and is often known as a porin. It is responsible for forming an interface between the cellular and mitochondrial mechanisms. It has been reported to be involved with various regulators of apoptosis, such as Bcl-2 [34].

The importance of VDAC was clearly depicted by Cierluk *et al.* whereupon administering cepharanthine, the dysregulation of VDAC resulted in a lack of ATP conductance between mitochondria and cytoplasm. VDAC was found responsible for cytoplasmic ROS generation [35]. VDAC associates with adenine nucleotide translocator (ANT), and both activate the mitochondrial apoptosis pathway. As a result of this pathway, many other molecules such as Smac/ Diablo, cytochrome c, and others get released, which have an apoptotic effect [36]. Apart from this, VDAC has also been observed to interact with hexokinase 2 and results in cytochrome c release [37].

Due to VDAC's ability to affect both pro-apoptotic and anti-apoptotic proteins, it becomes necessary to understand the mechanism and ensure it only potentiates apoptosis. As suggested by Shteinfer-Kuzmine *et al.*, VDAC1-based peptides can be recruited to selectively induce apoptotic cell death majorly through Ca^{2+} homeostasis and ROS generation [38]. In another research, it has been observed that si-VDAC1 could target cancer neurosphere formation [32]. Therefore, it is evident that VDAC can be an excellent target for GBM therapy and can serve as a biomarker since it targets certain cancer critical hallmarks.

MICRO RNA BIOMARKERS

Micro RNAs (miRNA) are single-stranded non-coding RNAs that majorly regulating gene expression and can be found circulating in CSF [39]. The miRNA profiling has been established to achieve a signature so as to predict GBM outcome in both high risk as well as low-risk patients [40]. Many miRNAs have a link with the cellular and metabolic development of GBM cells. As shown in Fig. (**2**), miRNA - biomarker network can assist in devising targeted therapies against GBM. One such miRNA signature included miR-9017, miR-15613, and miR-9625 [40]. Additionally, miRNAs are linked with various pathways and therefore, can be effective as prognostic as well as therapeutic biomarkers [41]. Some of the serum miRNAs have the potential to act as diagnostic markers as well [42, 43]. A prominent biomarker for GBM, miR-21, has been observed to be linked with cellular and molecular pathways through factors like insulin-like growth factor (IGF) binding protein-3 (IGFBP3), and osteoprotective proteins [44]. It has been observed that miR-300 gets downregulated in almost 75% of GBM cell line samples. The expression of miR-300 was shown to hamper the cell cycle, indicative of its role in cell development. It inhibited cell invasion and proliferation *in vitro*. The prime target of miR-300 was observed as ROCK1, rho associated serine-threonine kinase, involved in various cellular functions. The study also revealed the correlation of miR-300 with overall survival, which implied that lower miR-300 expression resulted in shorter OS [45]. Similarly, miR-1270 was associated with cancer regulation in various ways amongst different types of cancer. It was observed to be downregulated in GBM *in vitro* and *in vivo*. Additionally, miR-1270 differential expression in different tumor types can help in effective prognosis [46].

Another miRNA, miR-29b, was found to be downregulated in GBM. It was correlated with methylated MGMT as well as wild-type IDH and was found to be present in a higher amount as compared to other factors in blood serum samples. Also, postoperative levels for miR-29b were higher than those of preoperative, suggesting that it could be used as a therapeutic approach [47]. Additionally, miR 145 was downregulated, and its lower levels led to poor prognosis in GBM patients [48]. Many different miRNAs are being identified to be downregulated such as miR-3666 [49], miR-663 [50], miR-574 [51], miR-7, miR-23a, miR100 [52], miR-141 [53], miR-564, miR-1179 [54], miR-744 [55], whereas, miR-181 [56] and miR-365 [57] are upregulated in GBM. These are linked to critical gene expression, thus can be considered as good biomarkers (Table **1**).

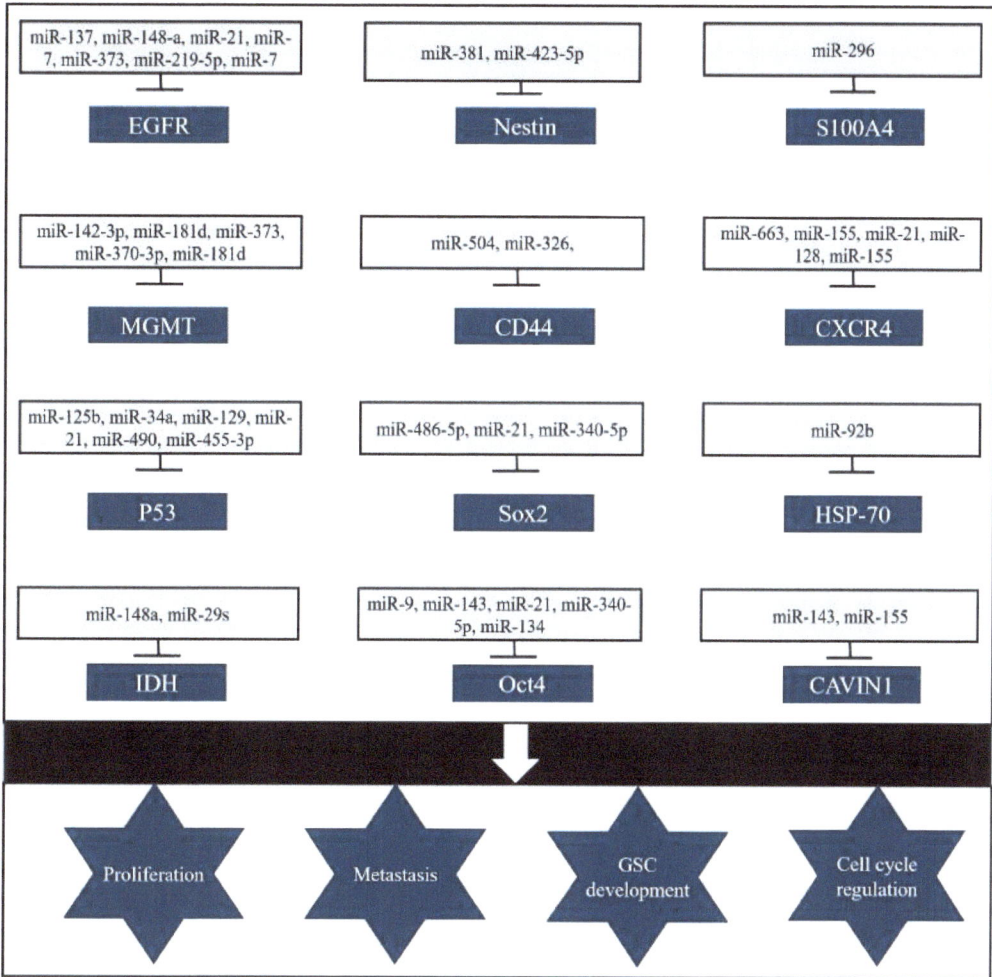

Fig. (2). The interaction of miRNAs with several oncogenic biomarkers is depicted. These biomarkers affect the endpoints proliferation, metastasis, GSC development, and cell cycle regulation.

Table 1. Role of several miRNA in GBM as biomarkers.

miRNA Type	Function Related to	Role as a Biomarker	References
Upregulated		-	-
miR-21	Apoptosis, migration, and invasiveness	Prognostic	[24]
miR-141	Inhibits proliferation	Prognostic	[52]
miR-1179	Inhibits proliferation and cell cycle progression	Prognostic	[54]
Downregulated		-	-
miR-300	Act on tumor suppressor gene through ROCK1	Prognostic	[45]

(Table 1) cont.....

miRNA Type	Function Related to	Role as a Biomarker	References
miR-1270	Tumor suppression through inverse regulating WT1 gene	Prognostic	[46]
miR-3666	Suppresses growth through KDM2A	Prognostic	[49]
miR-663	Inhibition of proliferation, migration and invasion	Prognostic	[50]
miR-574	Inhibition of cell proliferation and invasion	Prognostic and therapeutic	[51]
miR-7	Inhibition of viability, migration and invasion mainly through tyrosine kinase genes	Prognostic	[52]
miR-23a	Downregulation of tumor growth *in vivo* through Mdm2, TSC1	Prognostic	[52]
miR-100	Increase in radiosensitivity	Therapeutic	[52]
miR-744	Inhibits excessive cell proliferation through targeting NOB1	Therapeutic	[54]
miR-181	Inhibits cell growth through CCL8	Prognostic and therapeutic	[56]
miR-365	Suppression of cell proliferation and migration by PAX6	Prognostic	[57]

GBM CANCER STEM CELLS AS BIOMARKER BASED THERAPY

Stem cells have a critical role in managing the growth and development of all organisms. Most of the self-renewal and proliferative ability of GBM comes from glioblastoma stem cells (GSCs). These GSCs have been observed to show a characteristic neurosphere formation [58].

There are several antigens that happen to be associated with stem cells. One prominent marker, CD133, encoded by the PROM-1 gene, acts through its several isoforms and modulates tyrosine kinase phosphorylation [59]. High expression of CD133 is associated with poor overall survival and PFS [60]. The methylation pattern of CD133 was found to be associated with different grades of tumor, where higher promoter methylation was linked to low-grade GBM tumors. Additionally, its promoter methylation was positively correlated to PFS and OS [61]. Another marker of GSCs, CD90, also expressed differentially and was prominent in lower grade GBM. Interestingly, CD90 and CD133 happen to co-exist in GSCs [62]. Adding to the list is tetraspanin CD9, which is majorly related to invasion and apoptosis. CD9 is also related to GSCs in such a way that CD9 mRNA is overexpressed in GSCs as compared to normal astrocytes. Median survival happens to be inversely correlated with CD9 expression. Its silencing leads to loss of stemness and downregulates several cellular processes [63]. Thus, CD9 can be used as both a prognostic and therapeutic marker.

Another GSC marker, CD44, a ligand for ECM component hyaluronic acid, increases the invasiveness of GBM [64]. CD44 and Nestin have been observed to be co-localized in tumor cells membrane. CD44 additionally affected the migration capabilities of the cells in the case of GBM. The extracellular domain of CD44 was observed to interact with ECM and resulted in increased stemness of GSCs. The presence of CD44 has resulted in poor survival, making it a candidate for poor prognosis [65, 66]. CD 70 is another marker of GSCs, that is associated with a poor prognosis. It belongs to the tumor necrosis factor (TNF) receptor family. It leads to macrophage recruitment because of the production of chemokines such as IL-8 and CCL2 [67].

CD15 has been observed to be associated with hypoxia, which is linked to neurosphere formation. Sox-2, widely expressed in GBM cells, is also related to neurosphere formation and is responsible for GBM cells' plasticity. The knockdown of Sox-2 downregulated several other genes and biomarkers, namely PDGFRα, Krüppel-like factor 4(KLF4), aldehyde dehydrogenase 1 family member A1(ALDH1A1). Therefore, this can be a candidate for the GSC biomarker. ALDHs are crucial for cellular differentiation. It has been observed that its high expression leads to chemotherapeutic resistance. Knockout of ALDH1A3 increases the sensitivity of GBM cells *in vitro*. It can act as a predictive biomarker since it can predict metastasis. However, the proper role of ALDH1A3 as a biomarker has not been established yet [68]. Another stem cell-related biomarker is Nanog, which is reported to be overexpressed in cancerous cells and is specific to stem cells as it is downregulated upon onset of differentiation. Nanog is overexpressed in GBM, more than normal brain tissue, and due to its specificity to pluripotency, it is expressed only in poorly differentiated GSCs, hence can be a candidate for biomarkers [69].

There are other similar proteins, which can act as a marker of GSCs and can be a therapeutic candidate as well.

There are several different factors, which are related to GSCs and could be a potential biomarker. The gene S100A4, which encodes for a calcium-binding protein and interacts with p53, can upregulate GSCs self-renewal. Therefore, it can be a great candidate for prognostic biomarkers. Nestin is related to Notch signaling and regulates the stemness of GSCs [70]. Octamer-binding protein transcription factor 4 (OCT-4) is a biomarker found to be co-expressed by CD133 and Nestin. Oct-4 is additionally found to exist in a grade dependent manner and is associated with shorter survival. Therefore, it can be a good prognostic marker [71, 66]. The GSCs markers being related to GSCs molecular/cellular pathways can emerge as great candidates to be developed for prognosis and treatment.

IMAGING MODALITIES AS BIOMARKER

Apart from the presence or alterations of certain genes and various other factors, imaging has emerged as a potential biomarker for GBM. There are various ways in which imaging stands as a prognostic biomarker, such as measuring relative cerebral blood volume (rCBV), magnetic resonance (MR) perfusion studies, tumor enhancement and edema studies [26].

The standard treatment regime involves surgical resection followed by confirmation through an MRI scan. The patient is then provided with the standard of care treatment (TMZ + radiotherapy), which is followed up by subsequent MRI scans. In recent times, various other imaging options are being considered, such as positron emission tomography (PET), perfusion-weighted MRI (PWI), magnetic resonance spectroscopic imaging (MRSI) scans. This gives information about progression and necrosis induced by radiation [73].

The gliomas have several functional regions, contrast material–enhancing region (CER) and non-enhancing region (NER). NER does not include the CER and several other components. Though NER has biomarkers, which are of prognostic significance, they are not considered after the resection surgery. There is a need to identify other factors which can be imaging biomarkers. One such biomarker is the relative cerebral blood volume of NER (rCBVNER). In a study, GBM patients MR imaging analyses revealed that OS and PFS correlated with the rCBVNER. The study revealed that high rCBVNER can lead to poor survival. In addition, it was found that if NER crossed the midline of rCBV, then it can lead to poor survival of GBM patients [72].

MRI and PET scans can also help in the early prediction of GBM. MRI techniques can help in analyzing vascular density and tumor vasculature permeability, such as dynamic contrast-enhanced MRI (DCE-MRI), diffusion-weighted MRI (DWI) and PWI. Analysis of several biomarkers such as MGMT can be studied through features of MRI textures [73]. In 2018, a study by Małgorzata *et al.* considered 74 tumors and observed that DWI and PWI can aid in prognosis with some advancements [74].

Additionally, PET scans have also emerged as biomarkers for GBM since many imaging tracers can be utilized for prognosis, diagnosis as well as treatment of GBM [75]. Fluorodeoxyglucose (FDG-PET) is established as a biomarker for several cancer types, but it has a high baseline cerebral uptake making it difficult to be generally considered for GBM prognosis. Another issue with utilizing FDG-PET is that it hinders contrast enhancement, which is necessary for the process. But if used with other techniques like MR, it can come out as a great prognostic biomarker [76, 77]. Several other imaging markers can also prove to be prognostic such as 18F-FLT is associated with cellular proliferation and correlated to malignancy. Similarly, 18F-choline is related to membrane proliferation; 11c-methionine, 18F-FET and 18F-FDOPA are associated with amino acid metabolism. Additionally, 18F-RGD helps in analyzing angiogenesis and is a marker for integrin $\alpha V \beta 3$ [78].

Bosnyák *et al*. demonstrated that alpha[C-11]-L-methyl-tryptophan (AMT) PET scanning can help in determining tumor volume and some molecular markers such as EGFR and IDH. AMT imaging revealed that its higher uptake was correlated to OS. This makes AMT a great prognostic imaging biomarker for GBM patients [79].

Another way of incorporating imaging into the prognosis is through MR Dynamic susceptibility-weighted contrast-enhanced perfusion-weighted imaging (DSC-PWI). Here, labelling is done with the gadolinium-based agent to study the contrast. This technique helps to analyze the blood flow parameters. Several significant biomarkers such as mTOR and EGFR were significantly correlated with rCBV ratio of peri-enhancing tumor area (ratio of presence in area near tumor to internal control), making it a great candidate for prognosis [80]. Adding to this, arterial spin labeling perfusion-weighted imaging (ASL-PWI), can be utilized to get an understanding of molecular markers such as EGFR and IDH. This is a non- invasive technique as it uses magnetically labeled diffusible water for contrast imaging, making it safer than DSC-PWI [81].

It has been reported that branched-chain amino acid trasaminase1 (BCAT1), which converts α-ketoglutarate to glutamate, is associated with tumor growth. The level of this gene is more in patients harboring IDH wildtype glioma cells as investigated by MRSI. BCAT1was observed to be related to PFS in an inverse manner [82]. Therefore, this can be a good imaging candidate for prognosis since it will give an idea about the IDH status and correlate it for predicting the survival status. On similar lines, 2-hydroxyglutarate known as 2-HG, is a significant marker of glioblastoma since it is associated with IDH. Mutations in IDH lead to an imbalance in the level of 2-HG, eventually leading to increased survival of patients. 2-HG has been observed to be related to several genetic changes related to GBM [83]. The spectral characteristics of 2-HG can be studied via MRSI. Therefore, this correlation can be studied and incorporated into clinical practices for effective prognosis and better management of GBM [84]. The imaging biomarkers can be combined to improve prognosis.

IMMUNE CHECKPOINT AS BIOMARKER

Several factors and genes involved in eliciting the immune response have a great potential to be developed as biomarkers. Some of the immune checkpoint markers are discussed.

Programmed Cell Death Ligand

One of the important immune characteristics of GBM is the expression of immune checkpoint markers such as programmed cell death protein 1 (PD-1) and its ligand (PD-L1). PD-L1 present on the surface of antigen-presenting and tumor cells bind to PD1 expressed on T and pro-B cells. PDL-1 inactivates T cells and provides a conducive environment for tumor survival and growth [85]. PDL-1 expression was found to be inverse to the survival potential of patients [86]. Thus, PD-L1 can be considered as a good prognostic biomarker. Many studies have identified monoclonal antibodies effective against PD-1/PDL-1, which could be potentiated with anti-CD3 and/or anti-cytotoxic T-lymphocyte antigen 4 (CTLA-4) to mount enhanced immune response against GBM [87, 88].

CXCR4

Chemokines play an important role in the movement of motile cells based on chemical signals. One such chemokine is C-X-C motif chemokine receptor 4 (CXCR4), which is linked to activation of G protein and additionally phosphoinositide-3-kinase (PI3K)/Akt, associated with migration, invasion, apoptosis, and neo-vascularization. CXCR4 has been observed to be highly expressed in GBM and directs self-renewal of GSCs. This implies that CXCR4 is responsible for creating a microenvironment favorable for GBM development and its antagonist administration has shown anti-tumor effect [89]. The combination therapy of anti-CXCR4 and anti-PD-1 targeted tumor microenvironment improved ratios of $CD4^+/CD8^+$ and mediated better immune response [90]. Hence, it can be considered as a therapeutic marker.

ADAMTSL4

A disintegrin-like and metalloproteinase domain with thrombospondin type 1 motifs (ADAMTS) is involved mainly in angiogenesis and cell migration. From this family, ADAMTSL4 is highly expressed in GSCs and linked to immune checkpoints. Additionally, it was observed to be expressed differentially in different grades of the tumor, making it a great candidate for biomarker. ADAMTSL4 is also correlated to several important biomarkers such as unmethylated MGMT and wild type IDH1/2. ADAMTSL4 is strongly expressed in grade IV GBM and leads to shorter OS. Moreover, ADAMTSL4 was also related to other immune checkpoints such as PD-L1 and CTLA4. This strengthens it as a candidate for prognostic biomarker since it is significantly correlated with other immune checkpoints, GSCs and different type of GBM [91].

CAVIN1

Another protein related to immune checkpoints is caveolae-associated protein 1 (CAVIN1). This has been observed to be related to immunity regulation through the protection of human vascular endothelial cells from lysis. Upregulation of Cavin1 leads to poor survival of GBM cells. The levels of CAVIN1 were elevated in tumor cells as compared to the normal cells, making it a prognostic biomarker candidate. The higher expression of CAVIN1 was correlated with IDH and EGFR mutation. It was also observed that patients with low levels of CAVIN1 showed better treatment efficacy with radiation. So, employing proteins like ADAMTSL4 and CAVIN1 as biomarkers can aid in the prognosis of GBM [92].

Heat Shock Protein-70

The heat shock protein-70 (HSP-70) is another immune-related chaperone protein, which can aid in biomarker development. It is present in normal cells at extremely low levels, whereas, in tumor cells, its expression increases manifolds. The increase in expression of HSP-70 was found to be glioma grade dependent. The elevated HSP-70 was mainly related to anti-apoptotic effects by being associated with Bcl-2 related proteins. HSP70 corresponded to better PFS as compared to unmethylated phenotype [93, 94].

CONCLUSION

GBM is perceived to be an aggressive and complex kind of tumor, which has an issue of heterogeneity, and this poses challenges in the development of therapeutics. The heterogenic nature of GBM tumors and the development of resistance demands immediate attention.

Several biomarkers help in better identification and monitoring of the therapeutic effects. These include certain metabolic pathway genes, miRNAs, GBM stem cells, imaging modalities and immune checkpoint markers.

The genes and proteins pertaining to metabolic and molecular pathways have been in research for candidature as biomarkers for a long time. EGFRviii prevails to be the most common detectable biomarkers, and it can be utilized as a diagnostic and therapeutic type of biomarker. In addition to this, there are several other important genes such as MGMT, p53 and IDH, which hold an important part in GBM development and can be used as significant biomarkers as well. Apart from the pathway genes, there are miRNAs, which aid in biomarker research. There are many miRNAs involved in the diagnosis and therapeutic procedures. Hence, a miRNA signature can immensely help in differentiating risk factors in GBM patients and miRNAs such as miR-574, miR-100, miR-774 and others can be developed as therapeutic biomarkers.

GBM stem cells have emerged as a candidate for biomarker as there are many genes and antigens associated with GSCs, which can aid in the development of a therapeutic regime and detect the presence or development of GBM. Moreover, analyzing tumor contrast imaging with genomics variation and clinical factors can be a great way to analyse the progression of GBM. Therefore, many imaging modalities are being utilized for biomarker development. With the advancements such as ASL-PWI, DSC-PWI, FDG-PET and many others, several diagnostic parameters can be efficiently studied. Apart from these, immune checkpoint markers such as PD-L1, CXCR4, ADAMTSL4, CAVIN1 and HSP-70 are also emerging as significant biomarkers.

There is a significant development in therapeutic as well as diagnostic biomarkers for GBM. However, there is an urgent need to incorporate this in clinical practices to bring about a revolution, which can lead to better disease management.

ABBREVIATIONS

2-HG	2-hydroxyglutarate
ADAMTS	Thrombospondin Type 1 Motifs
ALDH1A1	Aldehyde Dehydrogenase 1 family, member A1
ALDHs	Aldehyde Dehydrogenases
AMT	alpha[C-11]-L-methyl-tryptophan
ANT	Adenine Nucleotide Translocator
ASL-PWI	Arterial Spin Labeling Perfusion-weighted Imaging
BCAT1	Branched-chain Amino Acid Trasaminase1
CAVIN1	Caveolae-associated Protein 1
CER	Contrast Material–enhancing Region
CNS	Central Nervous System
CSF	Cerebrospinal Fluid
CTLA-4	Cytotoxic T-lymphocyte Antigen 4
CXCR4	C-X-C Motif Chemokine Receptor 4
DCE-MRI	Dynamic Contrast-enhanced MRI

DSC-PWI	MR Dynamic susceptibility-weighted Contrast-enhanced Perfusion Weighted Imaging
EGFR	Epidermal Growth Factor Receptor
FDG	Fluorodeoxyglucose
GBM	Glioblastoma Multiforme
HSP-70	heat Shock Protein-70
IDH	Isocitrate Dehydrogenase
IGF	Insulin-like Growth Factor
IGFBP3	Insulin-like Growth Factor Binding Protein-3
KLF4	Krüppel-like factor 4
MGMT	O6-methylguanine DNA methyltransferase
miRNA	micro RNAs
MMR	Mismatch Repair Protein
MRSI	Magnetic Resonance Spectroscopic Imaging
NER	non-enhancing region
OS	Overall Survival
PD-1	Programmed Cell Death Protein 1
PET	positron Emission Tomography
PFS	Progression Free Survival
PWI	Perfusion-weighted MRI
rCBV	Relative Cerebral Blood Volume
rCBVNER	Relative Cerebral Blood Volume of NER
TMZ	Temozolomide
TNF	Tumor Necrosis Factor
TP53	Tumor Protein p53
VDAC	Voltage-dependent Anion Channel

CONSENT FOR PUBLICATION

Not applicable.

CONFLICT OF INTEREST

The author declares no conflict of interest, financial or otherwise.

ACKNOWLEDGEMENTS

The authors acknowledge Jaypee Institute of Information Technology, Noida, for all the support provided.

REFERENCES

[1]   Tamimi AF, Juweid M. Epidemiology and outcome of glioblastoma. Exon Publ 2017; pp. 143-53.
        [http://dx.doi.org/10.15586/codon.glioblastoma.2017.ch8]

[2]   Hassn Mesrati M, Behrooz AB, Y Abuhamad A, Syahir A. Understanding Glioblastoma Biomarkers:
        Knocking a Mountain with a Hammer. Cells 2020; 9(5): 1236.
        [http://dx.doi.org/10.3390/cells9051236] [PMID: 32429463]

[3]   Szopa W, Burley TA, Kramer-Marek G, Kaspera W. Diagnostic and therapeutic biomarkers in
        glioblastoma: current status and future perspectives. Biomed Res Int 2017; 2017: 8013575.
        [http://dx.doi.org/10.1155/2017/8013575]

[4]   Saadeh FS, Mahfouz R, Assi HI. EGFR as a clinical marker in glioblastomas and other gliomas. Int J
        Biol Markers 2018; 33(1): 22-32.
        [http://dx.doi.org/10.5301/ijbm.5000301] [PMID: 28885661]

[5]   Armocida D, Pesce A, Frati A, Santoro A, Salvati M. EGFR amplification is a real independent
        prognostic impact factor between young adults and adults over 45yo with wild-type glioblastoma? J
        Neurooncol 2020; 146(2): 275-84.
        [http://dx.doi.org/10.1007/s11060-019-03364-z] [PMID: 31889239]

[6]   Figueroa JM, Skog J, Akers J, *et al.* Detection of wild-type EGFR amplification and EGFRvIII
        mutation in CSF-derived extracellular vesicles of glioblastoma patients. Neuro-oncol 2017; 19(11):
        1494-502.
        [http://dx.doi.org/10.1093/neuonc/nox085] [PMID: 28453784]

[7]   Felsberg J, Hentschel B, Kaulich K, *et al.* Epidermal growth factor receptor variant III (EGFRvIII)
        positivity in EGFR-amplified glioblastomas: prognostic role and comparison between primary and
        recurrent tumors. Clin Cancer Res 2017; 23(22): 6846-55.
        [http://dx.doi.org/10.1158/1078-0432.CCR-17-0890] [PMID: 28855349]

[8]   Koga T, Li B, Figueroa JM, *et al.* Mapping of genomic EGFRvIII deletions in glioblastoma: insight
        into rearrangement mechanisms and biomarker development. Neuro-oncol 2018; 20(10): 1310-20.
        [http://dx.doi.org/10.1093/neuonc/noy058] [PMID: 29660021]

[9]   An Z, Knobbe-Thomsen CB, Wan X, Fan QW, Reifenberger G, Weiss WA. EGFR cooperates with
        EGFRvIII to recruit macrophages in glioblastoma. Cancer Res 2018; 78(24): 6785-94.
        [http://dx.doi.org/10.1158/0008-5472.CAN-17-3551] [PMID: 30401716]

[10]   Struve N, Binder ZA, Stead LF, *et al.* EGFRvIII upregulates DNA mismatch repair resulting in
        increased temozolomide sensitivity of MGMT promoter methylated glioblastoma. Oncogene 2020;
        39(15): 3041-55.
        [http://dx.doi.org/10.1038/s41388-020-1208-5] [PMID: 32066879]

[11]   Metro G, Pierini T, La Starza R. MGMT promoter methylation in glioma: esmo biomarker factsheet

[12]   Brandes AA, Franceschi E, Tosoni A, *et al.* MGMT promoter methylation status can predict the
        incidence and outcome of pseudoprogression after concomitant radiochemotherapy in newly
        diagnosed glioblastoma patients. J Clin Oncol 2008; 26(13): 2192-7.
        [http://dx.doi.org/10.1200/JCO.2007.14.8163] [PMID: 18445844]

[13]   Chen Y, Hu F, Zhou Y, Chen W, Shao H, Zhang Y. MGMT promoter methylation and glioblastoma
        prognosis: a systematic review and meta-analysis. Arch Med Res 2013; 44(4): 281-90.
        [http://dx.doi.org/10.1016/j.arcmed.2013.04.004] [PMID: 23608672]

[14]   Gupta SK, Kizilbash SH, Carlson BL, *et al.* Delineation of MGMT hypermethylation as a biomarker
        for veliparib-mediated temozolomide-sensitizing therapy of glioblastoma. JNCI. J Natl Cancer Inst
        2015; 108(5): djv369.
        [http://dx.doi.org/10.1093/jnci/djv369] [PMID: 26615020]

[15]   Brandes AA, Franceschi E, Paccapelo A, *et al.* Role of MGMT methylation status at time of diagnosis
        and recurrence for patients with glioblastoma: clinical implications. Oncologist 2017; 22(4): 432-7.

[http://dx.doi.org/10.1634/theoncologist.2016-0254] [PMID: 28275120]

[16] Schiffgens S, Wilkens L, Brandes AA, *et al.* Sex-specific clinicopathological significance of novel (Frizzled-7) and established (MGMT, IDH1) biomarkers in glioblastoma. Oncotarget 2016; 7(34): 55169-80.
[http://dx.doi.org/10.18632/oncotarget.10465] [PMID: 27409829]

[17] Zhao H, Wang S, Song C, Zha Y, Li L. The prognostic value of MGMT promoter status by pyrosequencing assay for glioblastoma patients' survival: a meta-analysis. World J Surg Oncol 2016; 14(1): 261.
[http://dx.doi.org/10.1186/s12957-016-1012-4] [PMID: 27733166]

[18] Happold C, Stojcheva N, Silginer M, *et al.* Transcriptional control of O^6 -methylguanine DNA methyltransferase expression and temozolomide resistance in glioblastoma. J Neurochem 2018; 144(6): 780-90.
[http://dx.doi.org/10.1111/jnc.14326] [PMID: 29480969]

[19] Gong M, Shi W, Qi J, *et al.* Alu hypomethylation and MGMT hypermethylation in serum as biomarkers of glioma. Oncotarget 2017; 8(44): 76797-806.
[http://dx.doi.org/10.18632/oncotarget.20012] [PMID: 29100349]

[20] Schaff LR, Yan D, Thyparambil S, *et al.* Characterization of MGMT and EGFR protein expression in glioblastoma and association with survival. J Neurooncol 2020; 146(1): 163-70.
[http://dx.doi.org/10.1007/s11060-019-03358-x] [PMID: 31823165]

[21] Chen X, Zhang M, Gan H, *et al.* A novel enhancer regulates MGMT expression and promotes temozolomide resistance in glioblastoma. Nat Commun 2018; 9(1): 2949.
[http://dx.doi.org/10.1038/s41467-018-05373-4] [PMID: 30054476]

[22] Geng R-X, Li N, Xu Y, *et al.* Identification of core biomarkers associated with outcome in glioma: evidence from bioinformatics analysis 2018.
[http://dx.doi.org/10.1155/2018/3215958]

[23] Ghasimi S, Wibom C, Dahlin AM, *et al.* Genetic risk variants in the CDKN2A/B, RTEL1 and EGFR genes are associated with somatic biomarkers in glioma. J Neurooncol 2016; 127(3): 483-92.
[http://dx.doi.org/10.1007/s11060-016-2066-4] [PMID: 26839018]

[24] Jesionek-Kupnicka D, Braun M, Trąbska-Kluch B, *et al.* MiR-21, miR-34a, miR-125b, miR-181d and miR-648 levels inversely correlate with MGMT and TP53 expression in primary glioblastoma patients. Arch Med Sci 2019; 15(2): 504-12.
[http://dx.doi.org/10.5114/aoms.2017.69374] [PMID: 30899304]

[25] Manuel J-M, Ghosh D, Narasinga Rao K, Sibin M, Venkatesh H. Role of concurrent methylation pattern of MGMT, TP53 and CDKN2A genes in the prognosis of high grade glioma. J Carcinog Mutagen 2016; 7(1): 2.
[http://dx.doi.org/10.4172/2157-2518.1000250]

[26] McNamara MG, Sahebjam S, Mason WP. Emerging biomarkers in glioblastoma. Cancers (Basel) 2013; 5(3): 1103-19.
[http://dx.doi.org/10.3390/cancers5031103] [PMID: 24202336]

[27] Dang L, White DW, Gross S, *et al.* Cancer-associated IDH1 mutations produce 2-hydroxyglutarate. Nature 2009; 462(7274): 739-44.
[http://dx.doi.org/10.1038/nature08617] [PMID: 19935646]

[28] Reiter-Brennan C, Semmler L, Klein A. The effects of 2-hydroxyglutarate on the tumorigenesis of gliomas. Contemp Oncol (Pozn) 2018; 22(4): 215-22.
[http://dx.doi.org/10.5114/wo.2018.82642] [PMID: 30783384]

[29] Johnson DR, Guerin JB, Giannini C, Morris JM, Eckel LJ, Kaufmann TJ. 2016 updates to the WHO brain tumor classification system: what the radiologist needs to know. Radiographics 2017; 37(7): 2164-80.

[http://dx.doi.org/10.1148/rg.2017170037] [PMID: 29028423]

[30]　Chen J-R, Yao Y, Xu H-Z, Qin Z-Y. Isocitrate dehydrogenase (IDH) 1/2 mutations as prognostic markers in patients with glioblastomas. Medicine (Baltimore) 2016; 95(9): e2583.
[http://dx.doi.org/10.1097/MD.0000000000002583] [PMID: 26945349]

[31]　Ayoub Z, Geara F, Najjar M, *et al.* Prognostic significance of O6-methylguanine-D-A-methyltransferase (MGMT) promoter methylation and isocitrate dehydrogenase-1 (IDH-1) mutation in glioblastoma multiforme patients: A single-center experience in the Middle East region. Clin Neurol Neurosurg 2019; 182: 92-7.
[http://dx.doi.org/10.1016/j.clineuro.2019.04.008] [PMID: 31108342]

[32]　Liu YQ, Wu F, Li J-J, *et al.* Gene Expression Profiling Stratifies IDH-Wildtype Glioblastoma With Distinct Prognoses. Front Oncol 2019; 9: 1433.
[http://dx.doi.org/10.3389/fonc.2019.01433] [PMID: 31921684]

[33]　Deluche E, Bessette B, Durand S, *et al.* CHI3L1, NTRK2, 1p/19q and IDH status dependent anion channel 1 in tumor cells. Biochimica et Biophysica Acta (BBA)-. Biomembranes 2015; 1848(10): 2547-75.

[34]　Cierluk K, Szlasa W, Rossowska J, *et al.* Cepharanthine induces ROS stress in glioma and neuronal cells via modulation of VDAC permeability. Saudi Pharm J 2020; 28(11): 1364-73.
[http://dx.doi.org/10.1016/j.jsps.2020.08.026] [PMID: 33250643]

[35]　Veenman L, Shandalov Y, Gavish M. VDAC activation by the 18 kDa translocator protein (TSPO), implications for apoptosis. J Bioenerg Biomembr 2008; 40(3): 199-205.
[http://dx.doi.org/10.1007/s10863-008-9142-1] [PMID: 18670869]

[36]　Wolf A, Agnihotri S, Micallef J, *et al.* Hexokinase 2 is a key mediator of aerobic glycolysis and promotes tumor growth in human glioblastoma multiforme. J Exp Med 2011; 208(2): 313-26.
[http://dx.doi.org/10.1084/jem.20101470] [PMID: 21242296]

[37]　Shteinfer-Kuzmine A, Amsalem Z, Arif T, Zooravlov A, Shoshan-Barmatz V. Selective induction of cancer cell death by VDAC1-based peptides and their potential use in cancer therapy. Mol Oncol 2018; 12(7): 1077-103.
[http://dx.doi.org/10.1002/1878-0261.12313] [PMID: 29698587]

[38]　Arif T, Krelin Y, Nakdimon I, *et al.* VDAC1 is a molecular target in glioblastoma, with its depletion leading to reprogrammed metabolism and reversed oncogenic properties. Neuro-oncol 2017; 19(7): 951-64.
[http://dx.doi.org/10.1093/neuonc/now297] [PMID: 28339833]

[39]　Shoshan-Barmatz V, Ben-Hail D, Admoni L, Krelin Y, Tripathi SS. The mitochondrial voltage-dependent anion channel 1 in tumor cells. Biochim Biophys Acta 2015; 1848(10 Pt B): 2547-75.
[http://dx.doi.org/10.1016/j.bbamem.2014.10.040] [PMID: 25448878]

[40]　Kopkova A, Sana J, Machackova T, *et al.* Cerebrospinal fluid microRNA signatures as diagnostic biomarkers in brain tumors. Cancers (Basel) 2019; 11(10): 1546.
[http://dx.doi.org/10.3390/cancers11101546] [PMID: 31614872]

[41]　Yuan Y, Zhang H, Liu X, *et al.* MicroRNA signatures predict prognosis of patients with glioblastoma multiforme through the Cancer Genome Atlas. Oncotarget 2017; 8(35): 58386-93.
[http://dx.doi.org/10.18632/oncotarget.16878] [PMID: 28938564]

[42]　Saadatpour L, Fadaee E, Fadaei S, *et al.* Glioblastoma: exosome and microRNA as novel diagnosis biomarkers. Cancer Gene Ther 2016; 23(12): 415-8.
[http://dx.doi.org/10.1038/cgt.2016.48] [PMID: 27834360]

[43]　Ebrahimkhani S, Vafaee F, Hallal S, *et al.* Deep sequencing of circulating exosomal microRNA allows non-invasive glioblastoma diagnosis. NPJ Precis Oncol 2018; 2(1): 28.
[http://dx.doi.org/10.1038/s41698-018-0071-0] [PMID: 30564636]

[44]　Akers JC, Hua W, Li H, *et al.* A cerebrospinal fluid microRNA signature as biomarker for

glioblastoma. Oncotarget 2017; 8(40): 68769-79.
[http://dx.doi.org/10.18632/oncotarget.18332] [PMID: 28978155]

[45]   Masoudi MS, Mehrabian E, Mirzaei H. MiR-21: A key player in glioblastoma pathogenesis. J Cell Biochem 2018; 119(2): 1285-90.
[http://dx.doi.org/10.1002/jcb.26300] [PMID: 28727188]

[46]   Zhou F, Li Y, Hao Z, *et al.* MicroRNA-300 inhibited glioblastoma progression through ROCK1. Oncotarget 2016; 7(24): 36529-38.
[http://dx.doi.org/10.18632/oncotarget.9068] [PMID: 27145462]

[47]   Wei L, Li P, Zhao C, Wang N, Wei N. Upregulation of microRNA-1270 suppressed human glioblastoma cancer cell proliferation migration and tumorigenesis by acting through WT1. OncoTargets Ther 2019; 12: 4839-48.
[http://dx.doi.org/10.2147/OTT.S192521] [PMID: 31417281]

[48]   Zhong F, Huang T, Leng J. Serum miR-29b as a novel biomarker for glioblastoma diagnosis and prognosis. Int J Clin Exp Pathol 2019; 12(11): 4106-12.
[PMID: 31933806]

[49]   Shi L, Wang B, Gu X, Zhang S, Li X, Zhu H. miR-145 is a potential biomarker for predicting clinical outcome in glioblastomas. J Cell Biochem 2018; 120(5): 8016-20.
[http://dx.doi.org/10.1002/jcb.28079] [PMID: 30485503]

[50]   Shou T, Yang H, Lv J, Liu D, Sun X. MicroRNA□3666 suppresses the growth and migration of glioblastoma cells by targeting KDM2A. Mol Med Rep 2019; 19(2): 1049-55.
[PMID: 30483744]

[51]   Li Q, Cheng Q, Chen Z, *et al.* MicroRNA-663 inhibits the proliferation, migration and invasion of glioblastoma cells via targeting TGF-β1. Oncol Rep 2016; 35(2): 1125-34.
[http://dx.doi.org/10.3892/or.2015.4432] [PMID: 26717894]

[52]   Mao Y, Wei F, Wei C, Wei C. microRNA-574 inhibits cell proliferation and invasion in glioblastoma multiforme by directly targeting zinc finger E-box-binding homeobox 1. Mol Med Rep 2018; 18(2): 1826-34.
[http://dx.doi.org/10.3892/mmr.2018.9106] [PMID: 29901177]

[53]   Zhang Y, Cruickshanks N, Pahuski M, *et al.* Noncoding RNAs in glioblastoma. Exon Publications 2017; pp. 95-130.
[http://dx.doi.org/10.15586/codon.glioblastoma.2017.ch6]

[54]   Xiong X, Deng J, Zeng C, Jiang Y, Tang S, Sun X. MicroRNA-141 is a tumor regulator and prognostic biomarker in human glioblastoma. Oncol Lett 2017; 14(4): 4455-60.
[http://dx.doi.org/10.3892/ol.2017.6735] [PMID: 28943957]

[55]   Xu X, Cai N, Zhi T, *et al.* MicroRNA-1179 inhibits glioblastoma cell proliferation and cell cycle progression via directly targeting E2F transcription factor 5. Am J Cancer Res 2017; 7(8): 1680-92.
[PMID: 28861324]

[56]   Deng Y, Li Y, Fang Q, Luo H, Zhu G. microRNA-744 is downregulated in glioblastoma and inhibits the aggressive behaviors by directly targeting NOB1. Am J Cancer Res 2018; 8(11): 2238-53.
[PMID: 30555741]

[57]   Zhai F, Chen X, He Q, *et al.* MicroRNA-181 inhibits glioblastoma cell growth by directly targeting CCL8. Oncol Lett 2019; 18(2): 1922-30.
[http://dx.doi.org/10.3892/ol.2019.10480] [PMID: 31423262]

[58]   Yuan F, Liu J, Pang H, *et al.* MicroRNA-365 suppressed cell proliferation and migration via targeting PAX6 in glioblastoma. Am J Transl Res 2019; 11(1): 361-9.
[PMID: 30787993]

[59]   Jhanwar-Uniyal M, Labagnara M, Friedman M, Kwasnicki A, Murali R. Glioblastoma: molecular pathways, stem cells and therapeutic targets. Cancers (Basel) 2015; 7(2): 538-55.

[http://dx.doi.org/10.3390/cancers7020538] [PMID: 25815458]

[60] Grosse-Gehling P, Fargeas CA, Dittfeld C, *et al.* CD133 as a biomarker for putative cancer stem cells in solid tumours: limitations, problems and challenges. J Pathol 2013; 229(3): 355-78.
[http://dx.doi.org/10.1002/path.4086] [PMID: 22899341]

[61] Zhang W, Chen H, Lv S, Yang H. High CD133 expression is associated with worse prognosis in patients with glioblastoma. Mol Neurobiol 2016; 53(4): 2354-60.
[http://dx.doi.org/10.1007/s12035-015-9187-1] [PMID: 25983032]

[62] Wu X, Wu F, Xu D, Zhang T. Prognostic significance of stem cell marker CD133 determined by promoter methylation but not by immunohistochemical expression in malignant gliomas. J Neurooncol 2016; 127(2): 221-32.
[http://dx.doi.org/10.1007/s11060-015-2039-z] [PMID: 26757925]

[63] He J, Liu Y, Zhu T, *et al.* CD90 is identified as a candidate marker for cancer stem cells in primary high-grade gliomas using tissue microarrays. Mol Cell Proteomics 2012; 11(6): 010744.
[http://dx.doi.org/10.1074/mcp.M111.010744] [PMID: 22203689]

[64] Podergajs N, Motaln H, Rajčević U, *et al.* Transmembrane protein CD9 is glioblastoma biomarker, relevant for maintenance of glioblastoma stem cells. Oncotarget 2016; 7(1): 593-609.
[http://dx.doi.org/10.18632/oncotarget.5477] [PMID: 26573230]

[65] Wang P, Wan WW, Xiong SL, Feng H, Wu N. Cancer stem-like cells can be induced through dedifferentiation under hypoxic conditions in glioma, hepatoma and lung cancer. Cell Death Discov 2017; 3(1): 16105.
[http://dx.doi.org/10.1038/cddiscovery.2016.105] [PMID: 28179999]

[66] Krogh Petersen J, Jensen P, Dahl Sørensen M, Winther Kristensen B. Expression and prognostic value of Oct-4 in astrocytic brain tumors. PLoS One 2016; 11(12): e0169129.
[http://dx.doi.org/10.1371/journal.pone.0169129] [PMID: 28030635]

[67] Berezovsky AD, Poisson LM, Cherba D, *et al.* Sox2 promotes malignancy in glioblastoma by regulating plasticity and astrocytic differentiation. Neoplasia 2014; 16(3): 193-206, 206.e19-206.e25.
[http://dx.doi.org/10.1016/j.neo.2014.03.006] [PMID: 24726753]

[68] Wu W, Schecker J, Würstle S, Schneider F, Schönfelder M, Schlegel J. Aldehyde dehydrogenase 1A3 (ALDH1A3) is regulated by autophagy in human glioblastoma cells. Cancer Lett 2018; 417: 112-23.
[http://dx.doi.org/10.1016/j.canlet.2017.12.036] [PMID: 29306018]

[69] Zhang W, Yan W, You G, *et al.* Genome-wide DNA methylation profiling identifies ALDH1A3 promoter methylation as a prognostic predictor in G-CIMP- primary glioblastoma. Cancer Lett 2013; 328(1): 120-5.
[http://dx.doi.org/10.1016/j.canlet.2012.08.033] [PMID: 22960273]

[70] Soni P, Qayoom S, Husain N, *et al.* CD24 and nanog expression in stem cells in glioblastoma: correlation with response to chemoradiation and overall survival. Asian Pacific journal of cancer prevention. Asian Pac J Cancer Prev 2017; 18(8): 2215-9.
[PMID: 28843258]

[71] Jin X, Jin X, Jung J-E, Beck S, Kim H. Cell surface Nestin is a biomarker for glioma stem cells. Biochem Biophys Res Commun 2013; 433(4): 496-501.
[http://dx.doi.org/10.1016/j.bbrc.2013.03.021] [PMID: 23524267]

[72] Fuster-Garcia E, García-Gómez JM, De Angelis E, Sraum A, Molnar A, Van Huffel S, *et al.* Use case II: imaging biomarkers and new trends for integrated glioblastoma management Imaging Biomarkers. Springer 2017; pp. 181-94.

[73] Jain R, Poisson LM, Gutman D, *et al.* Outcome prediction in patients with glioblastoma by using imaging, clinical, and genomic biomarkers: focus on the nonenhancing component of the tumor. Radiology 2014; 272(2): 484-93.
[http://dx.doi.org/10.1148/radiol.14131691] [PMID: 24646147]

[74]   Korfiatis P, Kline TL, Coufalova L, *et al.* MRI texture features as biomarkers to predict MGMT methylation status in glioblastomas. Med Phys 2016; 43(6): 2835-44.
         [http://dx.doi.org/10.1118/1.4948668] [PMID: 27277032]

[75]   Neska-Matuszewska M, Bladowska J, Sąsiadek M, Zimny A. Differentiation of glioblastoma multiforme, metastases and primary central nervous system lymphomas using multiparametric perfusion and diffusion MR imaging of a tumor core and a peritumoral zone-Searching for a practical approach. PLoS One 2018; 13(1): e0191341.
         [http://dx.doi.org/10.1371/journal.pone.0191341] [PMID: 29342201]

[76]   Verger A, Langen K-J. PET Imaging in glioblastoma: Use in clinical practice. Exon Publications 2017; pp. 155-74.
         [http://dx.doi.org/10.15586/codon.glioblastoma.2017.ch9]

[77]   Hassanzadeh C, Rao YJ, Chundury A, *et al.* Multiparametric MRI and [18F] fluorodeoxyglucose positron emission tomography imaging is a potential prognostic imaging biomarker in recurrent glioblastoma. Front Oncol 2017; 7: 178.
         [http://dx.doi.org/10.3389/fonc.2017.00178] [PMID: 28868256]

[78]   O'Halloran PJ, Viel T, Murray DW, *et al.* Mechanistic interrogation of combination bevacizumab/dual PI3K/mTOR inhibitor response in glioblastoma implementing novel MR and PET imaging biomarkers. Eur J Nucl Med Mol Imaging 2016; 43(9): 1673-83.
         [http://dx.doi.org/10.1007/s00259-016-3343-3] [PMID: 26975402]

[79]   Sinigaglia M, Assi T, Besson FL, *et al.* Imaging-guided precision medicine in glioblastoma patients treated with immune checkpoint modulators: research trend and future directions in the field of imaging biomarkers and artificial intelligence. EJNMMI Res 2019; 9(1): 78.
         [http://dx.doi.org/10.1186/s13550-019-0542-5] [PMID: 31432278]

[80]   Bosnyák E, Michelhaugh SK, Klinger NV, *et al.* Prognostic molecular and imaging biomarkers in primary glioblastoma. Clin Nucl Med 2017; 42(5): 341-7.
         [http://dx.doi.org/10.1097/RLU.0000000000001577] [PMID: 28195901]

[81]   Liu X, Mangla R, Tian W, *et al.* The preliminary radiogenomics association between MR perfusion imaging parameters and genomic biomarkers, and their predictive performance of overall survival in patients with glioblastoma. J Neurooncol 2017; 135(3): 553-60.
         [http://dx.doi.org/10.1007/s11060-017-2602-x] [PMID: 28889246]

[82]   Yoo R-E, Yun TJ, Hwang I, *et al.* Arterial spin labeling perfusion-weighted imaging aids in prediction of molecular biomarkers and survival in glioblastomas. Eur Radiol 2020; 30(2): 1202-11.
         [http://dx.doi.org/10.1007/s00330-019-06379-2] [PMID: 31468161]

[83]   Cho HR, Jeon H, Park C-K, Park S-H, Kang KM, Choi SH. BCAT1 is a new MR imaging-related biomarker for prognosis prediction in IDH1-wildtype glioblastoma patients. Sci Rep 2017; 7(1): 17740.
         [http://dx.doi.org/10.1038/s41598-017-17062-1] [PMID: 29255149]

[84]   Leather T, Jenkinson MD, Das K, Poptani H. Magnetic resonance spectroscopy for detection of 2-hydroxyglutarate as a biomarker for IDH mutation in gliomas. Metabolites 2017; 7(2): 29.
         [http://dx.doi.org/10.3390/metabo7020029] [PMID: 28629182]

[85]   Choi C, Raisanen JM, Ganji SK, *et al.* Prospective longitudinal analysis of 2-hydroxyglutarate magnetic resonance spectroscopy identifies broad clinical utility for the management of patients with IDH-mutant glioma. J Clin Oncol 2016; 34(33): 4030-9.
         [http://dx.doi.org/10.1200/JCO.2016.67.1222] [PMID: 28248126]

[86]   Ricklefs FL, Alayo Q, Krenzlin H, *et al.* Immune evasion mediated by PD-L1 on glioblastoma-derived extracellular vesicles. Sci Adv 2018; 4(3): eaar2766.
         [http://dx.doi.org/10.1126/sciadv.aar2766] [PMID: 29532035]

[87]   Chen RQ, Liu F, Qiu XY, Chen XQ. The prognostic and therapeutic value of PD-L1 in glioma. Front

Pharmacol 2019; 9: 1503.
[http://dx.doi.org/10.3389/fphar.2018.01503] [PMID: 30687086]

[88]   Litak J, Mazurek M, Grochowski C, Kamieniak P, Roliński J. PD-L1/PD-1 Axis in Glioblastoma Multiforme. Int J Mol Sci 2019; 20(21): 5347.
[http://dx.doi.org/10.3390/ijms20215347] [PMID: 31661771]

[89]   Park J, Kwon M, Kim KH, *et al.* Immune checkpoint inhibitor-induced reinvigoration of tumor-infiltrating CD8+ T cells is determined by their differentiation status in glioblastoma. Clin Cancer Res 2019; 25(8): 2549-59.
[http://dx.doi.org/10.1158/1078-0432.CCR-18-2564] [PMID: 30659023]

[90]   Gravina GL, Mancini A, Marampon F, *et al.* The brain-penetrating CXCR4 antagonist, PRX177561, increases the antitumor effects of bevacizumab and sunitinib in preclinical models of human glioblastoma. J Hematol Oncol 2017; 10(1): 5.
[http://dx.doi.org/10.1186/s13045-016-0377-8] [PMID: 28057017]

[91]   Wu A, Maxwell R, Xia Y, *et al.* Combination anti-CXCR4 and anti-PD-1 immunotherapy provides survival benefit in glioblastoma through immune cell modulation of tumor microenvironment. J Neurooncol 2019; 143(2): 241-9.
[http://dx.doi.org/10.1007/s11060-019-03172-5] [PMID: 31025274]

[92]   Zhao Z, Zhang K-N, Chai R-C, *et al.* ADAMTSL4, a secreted glycoprotein, is a novel immune-related biomarker for primary glioblastoma multiforme 2019.
[http://dx.doi.org/10.1155/2019/1802620]

[93]   Guo Q, Guan GF, Cheng W, *et al.* Integrated profiling identifies caveolae-associated protein 1 as a prognostic biomarker of malignancy in glioblastoma patients. CNS Neurosci Ther 2019; 25(3): 343-54.
[http://dx.doi.org/10.1111/cns.13072] [PMID: 30311408]

[94]   Lämmer F, Delbridge C, Würstle S, *et al.* Cytosolic Hsp70 as a biomarker to predict clinical outcome in patients with glioblastoma. PLoS One 2019; 14(8): e0221502.
[http://dx.doi.org/10.1371/journal.pone.0221502] [PMID: 31430337]

CHAPTER 6

Poly (ADP-Ribose) Polymerases as New Drug Targets in Cancer Treatment

Fatih Tok[1,*] and **Bedia Koçyiğit-Kaymakçıoğlu**[1]

[1] Department of Pharmaceutical Chemistry, Faculty of Pharmacy, Marmara University, Istanbul, 34854, Turkey

Abstract: Cancer is the second leading cause of death worldwide, remains one of the most major health problems worldwide. Chemotherapeutic agents play an important role in cancer therapy. However, many anticancer drugs have potential disadvantages, such as non-selective toxicity, few drug targets, higher medical costs. Furthermore, since rapid resistance to chemotherapeutics, medicinal chemists aim to develop new anticancer drugs with better properties. The development of new anticancer drugs is one of the most vital areas of research in chemical science. Poly (ADP-ribose) polymerase (PARP) is an important nuclear enzyme responsible for the genomic repair, telomerase regulation, transcription, and regulation of cell death. Poli (ADP-ribose) polymerase inhibitors have recently been approved for cancer treatment, especially breast and ovarian cancer. In this study, we explained the roles of PARP inhibitors in cancer treatment and their mechanisms of action with their structure-activity relationship. Therefore, this article will provide readers with a new perspective on cancer diseases and its treatment with PARP inhibitors.

Keywords: Benzamide, BRCA, Breast cancer, Cancer treatment, DNA damage, DNA repair, Dual inhibitors, Nicotinamide, Olaparib, Poly (ADP-ribose) polymerase, PARP inhibitors, Veliparib.

INTRODUCTION

Cancer, a great global health concern, is the leading cause of every one in six deaths in the world. It was estimated that 18.1 million cancer cases and 9.6 million deaths from cancer occur in 2018. By 2040, these numbers will increase significantly, cancer incidence and cancer mortality will reach 29.5 million and 16.3 million burdens worldwide, respectively [1].

[*] **Corresponding author Fatih Tok**: Department of Pharmaceutical Chemistry, Faculty of Pharmacy, Marmara University, Istanbul, Turkey; Tel: +9021 6775 5200/5338; E-mail: fatih.tok@marmara.edu.tr

Atta-ur-Rahman & M. Iqbal Choudhary (Eds.)
All rights reserved-© 2021 Bentham Science Publishers

Lung cancer (11.6% of all cases) and breast cancer (11.6% of all cases) are the most diagnosed types of cancer in the world. Although there are many treatment methods, such as chemotherapy, radiotherapy, immunotherapy, endocrine therapy and surgery; cancer management is complicated and more complex than other diseases. Cancer affected not only patients but also their families and countries' health system negatively. These families experience difficult psychological and financial distress. Cancer control leads to great economic loss for countries each year [2].

Breast cancer is the most common type of cancer in women. It is predicted that breast cancer is diagnosed more than 30% new cancer cases in women and constitutes 15% of female cancer deaths globally in 2020. Ovarian cancer cases are reported as the second most common gynecological cancer, approximately 2.5% of female cancer patients, and the fifth leading cause of cancer-related deaths in women, approximately %5 of female cancer deaths. The reason for the high mortality rate is late-stage diagnosis [3, 4]. Older age, being female, family story (cancer susceptibility genes, BRCA mutations), high-dose radiation are the strongest risk factors for ovarian and breast cancer [5].

Surgery is an option depends on the cancer stage with radiation therapy. However, if cancer has spread through the body, surgery may be restricted to patients. Radiotherapy is another option for cancer treatment, but radiotherapy is limited because of its high toxicity and localized therapy [6]. Therefore, chemo therapeutics play a critical role in cancer treatment. Many chemotherapeutics have some risk factors such as poor bioavailability, toxic side effects, drug-resistance, non-specific target, higher medical cost. Thereby, scientific advances in the area of cancer drug design and discovery are extremely important for the future of humans.

Mechanisms of DNA Damage and Repair

The human genome, DNA, must maintain its integrity and stability to ensure cell survival. Exogenous factors, such as ultraviolet light, reactive oxygen species, chemical agents, cause many DNA lesions. Not only exogenous factors but also endogenous factors create some DNA lesions during the replication process. These problems induce genetic instability and threaten cell viability and homeostasis [7]. However, DNA can face up difficulties because of its unique repair mechanisms. These DNA repair pathways refer to as single-strand break repair (SSR), base excision repair (BER), nucleotide excision repair (NER), homologous recombination (HR) and non-homologous end-joining (NHEJ), mismatch repair (MMR). When repair mechanisms are insufficient, apoptosis or necrosis activates, and cell death occurs [8].

The MMR system is responsible for recognizing and correcting mismatched bases after the replication process and repair of insertion/deletion single-strand DNA loops. This repair mechanism carries genetic information accurately. A system fault may cause at the beginning of the oncogenesis process. MMR pathway constitutes three steps: (i) mismatch recognition, (ii) recruitment of the excision machinery, (iii) re-synthesis, and ligation [9]. The NER system is responsible for recognizing helix-distorting DNA lesions created by ultraviolet (UV) radiation. Firstly, this repair system opens the DNA duplex and cuts the damaged DNA strand. Then it provides the resynthesis and ligation of the DNA strand [10]. The BER system plays a critical role in repairing small base lesions induced by endogenous oxidation, alkylation. BER pathway constitutes three steps: (i) small base excision, (ii) DNA backbone incision, (iii) DNA end processing and repair [11].

The NHEJ system ensures the repair of double-strand DNA breaks during the G1 phases of the cell cycle. Several proteins, such as Ku, DNA-PKcs and Artemis are required for repair. NHEJ can not repair according to original DNA sequences. NHEJ plays roles throughout the cell cycle as different from HR [12]. The HR system provides repair of single and double-strand DNA breaks accurately during the S and G2 phases [8]. The HR system is a higher fidelity mechanism, according to NHEJ. However, the HR repair mechanism is limited only the S and G2 phases of the cell cycle [13, 14].

The BER mechanism plays a critical role in the repair of single-strand DNA breaks. However, the PARP enzyme is essential in the stimulation of DNA glycosylase and endonuclease enzymes [15]. RAD51 and BRCA1/2 proteins are critical roles in the BER mechanism. Different repair mechanisms and proteins are used in the repair of double-strand DNA breaks. Homologous recombination (HR) is the most important mechanism to repair the double-strand DNA breaks with high fidelity. HR restores DNA integrity. However, the result mechanisms such as NHEJ and MMEJ may show error-prone. The PARP-1 enzyme prevents the binding of Ku proteins to DNA, and so inhibits NHEJ, which is associated with error-prone [16]. NHEJ components such as Ku70, Ku80 and Artemis may not be sufficient to repair double-strand DNA breaks [17] (Fig. **1**).

PARP Inhibitors and Their Mechanisms of Action

Poli (ADP-ribose) polymerase (PARP) is a nuclear enzyme that plays an important role in DNA repair. The PARP family enzyme consists of 18 members in mammalian cells [18]. The most important member of the family is PARP-1 and PARP-2 [19].

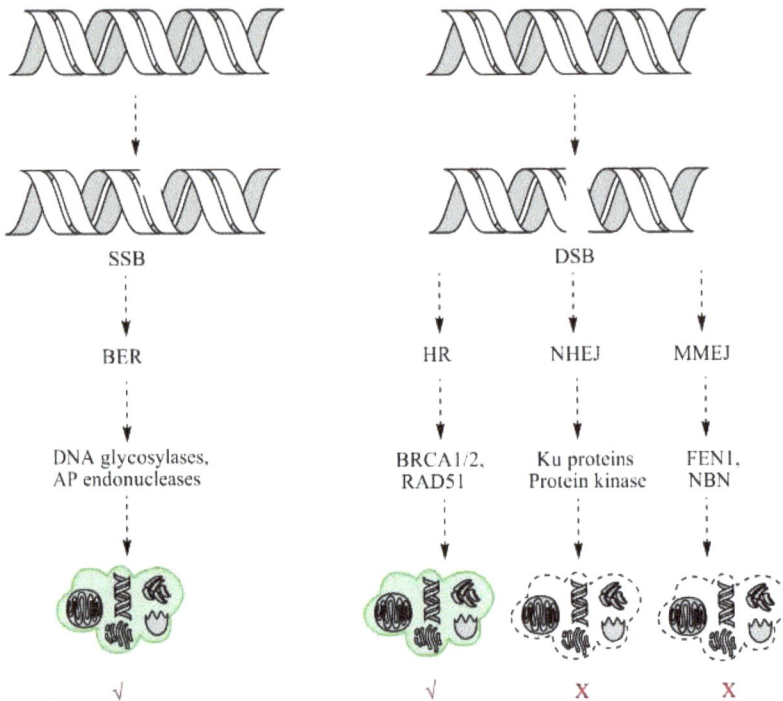

Fig. (1). Single and double-strand DNA breaks and repair mechanisms. *Figures were drawn by using ChemBioDraw Ultra 11.0 Programs.

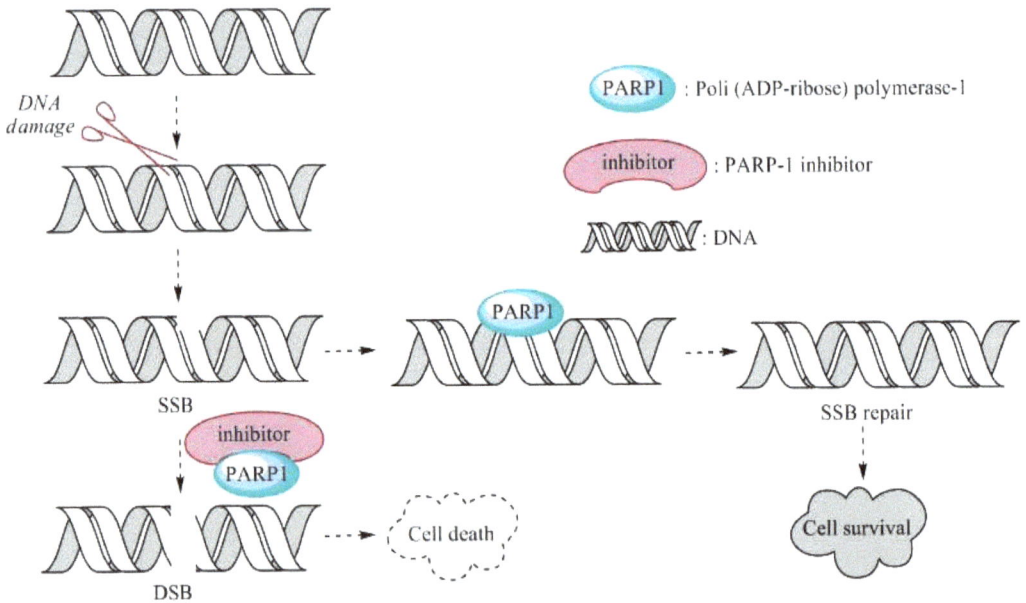

Fig. (2). Mechanism of action of poly (ADP-ribose) polymerase-1 and its inhibitor.

PARP-1 is responsible for the repair of single-strand DNA breaks (SSB). If it prevents, double-strand DNA breaks (DSB) can form and this could lead to cell death as depicted in Fig. (**2**) [20].

PARP-1 consists of three major domains: (i) Zinc-finger domain, (ii) catalytic domain, (iii) automodification domain [21]. When PARP-1 is free, it has a disordered structure and acts as "beads on a long chain".

   i. The zinc-finger domain recognizes and binds to damaged DNA regions with high selectivity. These disordered structures gather around the same damaged region and form PARP-1 and DNA complex easily [22].

   ii. The catalytic domain comprises an ADP-ribosyltransferase (ART) catalytic domain. PARylation process initiates *via* an active ART catalytic domain. PARP enzyme cofactor, NAD^+, binds on ART catalytic domain and PARP-1 substrates. Then, the transfer of ADP-ribose subunits is catalyzed from nicotinamide adenine dinucleotide (NAD^+) to target proteins [23]. Thus the DNA repair process completes *via* modifying the chromatin structure and DNA repair effectors [24].

   iii. The automodification domain is responsible for binding NAD^+ to the ART catalytic domain according to DNA lesions. When there are not any DNA lesions, this automodification domain prevents the binding of NAD^+ and acts auto-inhibitory domain [22, 25].

Apart from DNA repair, the second most important role of PARP-1: the regulation of transcription by coupling with many transcription factors such as NF-kB [26]. NF-kB is a central module and responsible for the inflammation process during "ischemia" [27]. PARP-1 also regulates hypoxia-inducible factors that mediate many hypoxia-regulated mechanisms such as glucose transport, glycolysis, erythropoiesis or angiogenesis [28].

BRCA1 and BRCA2 genes are tumor suppressor genes that protect the integrity of the genome [29]. These genes produce some proteins which are used in homologs recombination repair. If a mutation develops in BRCA1/2 genes, HR can not protect the genome stability with high fidelity and the risk of ovarian and breast cancer increases. Notably, PARP-1 inhibitors contribute some benefits in the treatment of ovarian and breast cancer in BRCA1/2 deficient cells [30, 31]. Therefore, olaparib was the first PARP-1 inhibitor that has been approved for the treatment of patients with BRCA-mutated breast cancer in 2004 by the Food and Drug Administration (FDA) [32]. After all, reports showing successful treatment, olaparib has also been approved for the treatment of recurrent epithelial ovarian, fallopian tube, or primary peritoneal cancer in 2017 [33]. Also, PARP inhibitors combined with other chemotherapeutic agents can be used for the treatment of other cancer diseases such as gastric, prostate, lung and pancreatic cancer [34 - 37].

Development and Clinical Trials of PARP Inhibitors in Cancer Treatment

PARP-1 inhibitors were designed to have the ability of competition with NAD^+ to the catalytic site of the enzyme [38]. The earliest studies showed that the structures of 3-aminobenzamide and nicotinamide interacted and inhibited the PARP-1 enzyme easily [39].

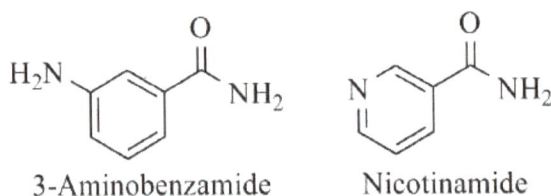

3-Aminobenzamide   Nicotinamide

Three basic structural features are very important for designing new PARP-1 inhibitors: (i) Aromatic ring, (ii) carboxamide moiety, (iii) a side chain extending into the deep pocket located in the automodification domain of PARP-1 (Fig. **3**). The carboxamide group can be implemented into a ring system or it can stay separately [40].

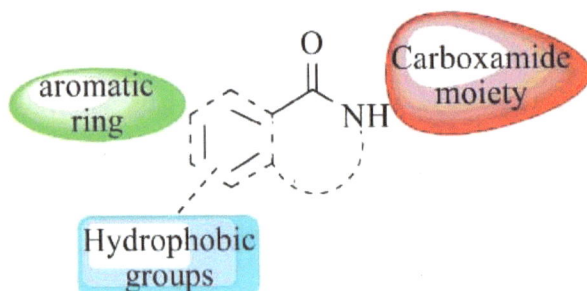

Fig. (3). Pharmacophore structure of PARP-1 inhibitors.

3-Aminobenzamide is a known first-generation PARP-1 inhibitor. Nicotinamide, isostere of benzamide, is obtained as a result of the replacement of carbon and nitrogen atom. PARP inhibitors carrying the structure of nicotinamide and 3-aminobenzamide compete against NAD^+ for binding PARP enzyme [41, 42]. However, these compounds exhibit low efficacy and selectivity [43]. In the view of points, new molecules having more effective-selective and good pharmacokinetic profiles have been investigated by medicinal chemists.

Therefore, the second generation of PARP inhibitors bearing quinazoline analogs was discovered in the 1990s (Fig. **4**). Molecules in this group were more effective than 3-aminobenzamide analogs. For instance; while 8-hydroxy-2-methyl quinazolin-4-[3H]-one (NU1025) inhibited the PARP-1 enzyme ($IC_{50} = 400$ nM), PJ34 also inhibited with the value of $IC_{50} = 20$ nM. Compounds PJ34 were investigated their effect on vascular dysfunction, stroke and nephropathy with *in vitro* and *in vivo* models. Compounds PJ34 are selective PARP-1 inhibitors and their clinical studies are continuing as new drug candidates [44]. Carboxamide functional groups in these molecules formed hydrogen bonds with serine and glycine amino acids in the catalytic domain of PARP-1. The aromatic ring also exhibited π-π interactions with the tyrosine amino acid of PARP-1 easily. Therefore, benzamide core played an important role in showing significant activity [45].

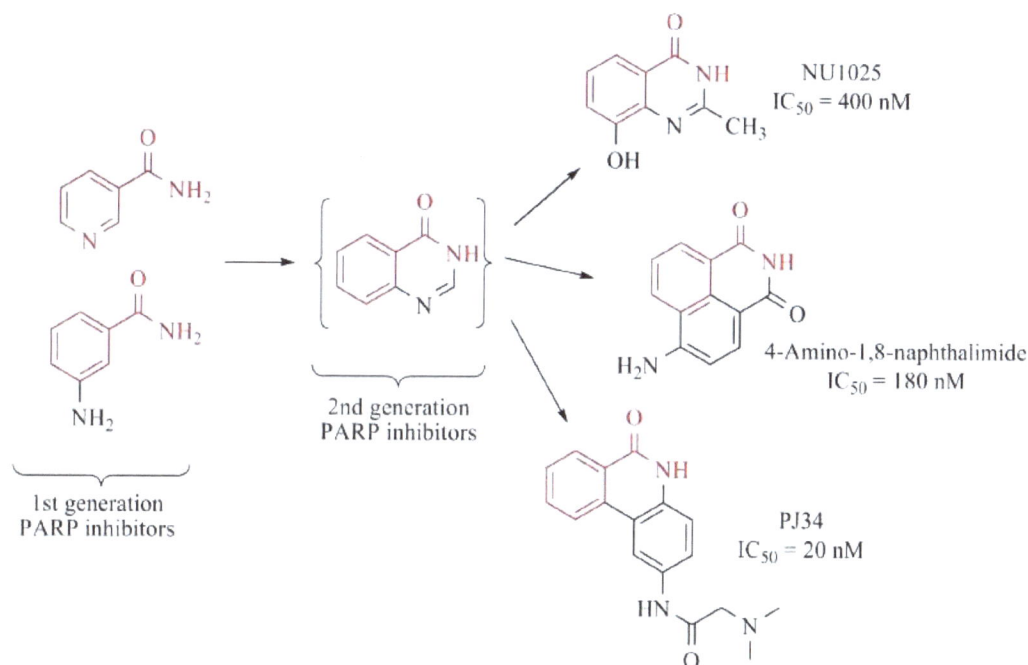

Fig. (4). The structure of 1st and 2nd generation PARP inhibitors.

Compounds PJ34 is a selective PARP-1 inhibitor and its clinical studies continue as a new drug candidate. PJ34 resisted the mitochondrial structure and cell survival. PJ34 also induced in accumulation of DNA breaks and reactivation of the tumor suppressor gen p53 transcriptional functions. The effects of PJ34 and temozolomide or cisplatin with combined therapy were investigated on the B16F10 *in vitro* melanoma model. It was reported that PJ34 increased the cytotoxic effects of antineoplastic drugs as alkylating agents in combined therapy [46, 47].

Most of the PARP-1 inhibitor molecules have a benzamide structure as a pharmacophore group. In view of this point, the third generation of PARP inhibitors was developed. It was reported that these molecules carried benzimidazole in their structure generally. Molecules in this group are more potent and selective. Several drug molecules in the third generation are currently available in the market or currently undergoing clinical trials [45].

Many studies carried out about the second generation of PARP inhibitors. Quinazolin-4(3H)-one core was an important structure to design new PARP-1 inhibitors. Especially 2- and 8-position at the quinazolin-4(3H)-one derivatives were chosen to be able to optimize the activity [48]. For example, Maksimainen *et al.* designed and synthesized thieno[2,3-c]isoquinolin-5(4H)-one derivatives as a PARP-1 inhibitor. It was reported that the molecule whose structure was given below, had a potential anti-ischemic effect [49]. Giannini *et al.* discovered more potent PARP-1 inhibitory activity than olaparib and veliparib (IC_{50} = 9.8 nM for the structure of molecule was given below, IC_{50} = 10 nM for olaparib, IC_{50} = 10 nM for veliparib). Differences between the existing quinazolinone derivatives and this article contained a propanoyl side chain. Structure-activity relationships showed that the propanoyl side-chain provided additional hydrogen bonds with the binding site of the enzyme [50]. McPherson *et al.* reported a new PARP-1 inhibitor, which provided a successful strategy for the treatment of colorectal cancer. Sensitivity to the PARP-1 inhibitors in cancer cells increased when the combination of this molecule with DNA damaging chemotherapeutic agents such as cisplatin or oxaliplatin [51]. An example of the third generation of PARP inhibitors was given the synthesis of 2-substituted benzo[d]imidazole--carboxamide derivatives by Zhong *et al.* The following lead compound demonstrated the same inhibitory activity with olaparib (both of them IC_{50} values = 25 nM) [52] (Fig. **5**).

Table 1. Some adverse effects in patients using olaparib.

Adverse Effect (AE)	Olaparib (N=136)	Placebo (N=128)
Patients with any AE	132	119
Fatigue	71	50
Nausea	96	46
Vomiting	46	18

(Table 1) cont.....

Adverse Effect (AE)	Olaparib (N=136)	Placebo (N=128)
Abdominal pain	34	34
Diarrhea	37	31
Headache	28	16
Constipation	28	14
Poor appetite	28	17
Anemia	29	7

Olaparib (Lynparza, AstraZeneca), the best-known PARP inhibitor, was the first approved in PARP inhibitors for the treatment of ovarian cancer with BRCA1 and BRCA2 mutations [53, 54].

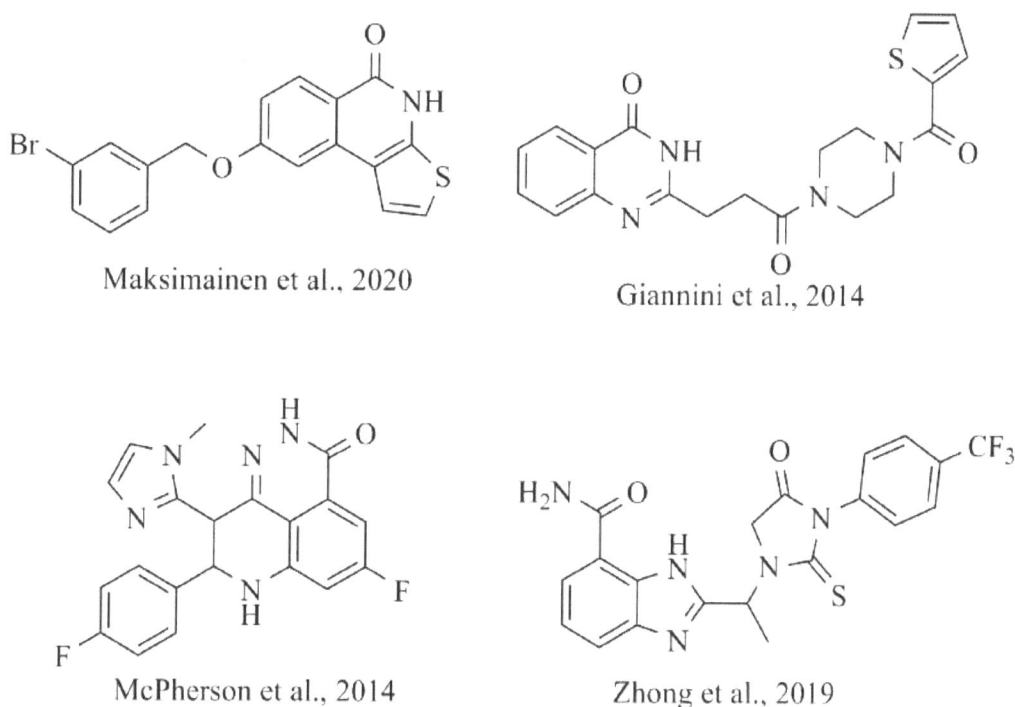

Maksimainen et al., 2020

Giannini et al., 2014

McPherson et al., 2014

Zhong et al., 2019

Fig. (5). The structure of some 2nd and 3rd generation PARP-1 inhibitors.

It was investigated what kind of adverse effects occurred when the use of olaparib in patients with an ovarian cancer diagnosis. When the drug was given to 136 patients and placebo to 128 patients, the incidence of adverse effects in the table was obtained as below (Table **1**). While olaparib was determined well tolerated with BRCA mutated patients, some gastrointestinal adverse effects were reported. Other PARP inhibitors had similar adverse effects. Furthermore, it was indicated that thrombocytopenia could be formed in treatment with niraparib. In addition, liver enzymes (alanine aminotransferase (ALT)/aspartate aminotransferase (AST)) must be monitored at the treatment with rucaparib [55].

Rucaparib (Rubraca, Clovis Oncology) was approved for the treatment of some gynecologic disorders such as both platinum-sensitive and platinum-resistant epithelial ovarian, primary peritoneal and fallopian tube cancers with germline and somatic BRCA mutations. Rucaparib was administered orally like olaparib [56]. Rucaparib was the second PARP inhibitor which was approved in December 2016 by FDA [57].

Niraparib, (Zejula, Tesaro) was approved by the FDA and EMA for the treatment of recurrent epithelial ovarian and fallopian tube cancer which is platinum-sensitive. However, patients treated with niraparib showed long term benefits in progression-free survival with recurrent germline BRCA mutated [56, 58].

Veliparib (ABT888, Abbvie), was reported some benefits on breast, ovarian and lung cancer, but it has not been approved any agency, yet. Because some adverse effects such as significant myelosuppression were reported when combined with other chemotherapeutics (cyclophosphamide, topotecan, and doxorubicin) [53, 56].

Talazoparib (BMN673, Medivation) provided significantly radio-sensitization effects in stem cells so it potentiated the effects of radiation and chemotherapy. When Talazoparib compared to other PARP inhibitors as olaparib, Talazoparib was almost 100 fold more efficient in PARP enzyme binding [59, 60]. Talazoparib had excellent pharmacokinetic properties after oral administration [61]. Chemical structures of PARP inhibitors carrying benzamide structure as a pharmacophore group were given below (Fig. **6**). Furthermore, the approval histories, targets, BRCA status, indications, relative PARP trapping potencies of PARP inhibitors were compared and can be found in Table **2** [56, 62 - 63].

Recent Advances with PARP Inhibitor Research

The first PARP enzyme was discovered by scientists in France and Japan in the 1960s. PARP-1 is a commonly abundant form among the PARP enzymes and localize in the nucleus [64]. PARP-1, PARP-2 and PARP-3 are important roles in the repair of DNA lesions. PARP-1 repairs both single and double-strand DNA breaks and performs with many repair pathways such as HR, BER, NHEJ and NER [65]. PARP-2 is largely similar to PARP-1. PARP-2 is responsible for only single-strand DNA breaks and helps DNA repair in regions where PARP-1 is not available. However, the DNA binding region in PARP-2 is different from PARP-1 and there is no central automodification domain in PARP-2. On the other hand, PARP-3 helps the repair of double-strand DNA breaks [66]. Furthermore, PARP-2 is especially involved in the development of T-cells, spermatogenesis, adipogenesis and chronic anemia. While selective PARP-1 inhibitors can be used as anticancer drugs, selective PARP-2 inhibitors can function more broadly in many areas such as inflammation, tumor invasion, angiogenesis and cellular metabolism. Therefore, selective inhibition of PARP-2 can attempt on tumor cells more widely [67].

Table 2. The differences of currently available PARP inhibitors.

PARP Inhibitors	Approval	Company	Target	BRCA Status	Indications	PARP Trapping Potency (Relative to Olaparib)	IC_{50} in DT40 Cells, nM)
Olaparib	2014 FDA, 2014 EMA	Astra Zeneca	PARP1 PARP2 PARP3	Germline and somatic	Treatment of BRCA-mutated ovarian cancer, metastatic breast and pancreatic cancers	1	6
Rucaparib	2016 FDA, 2018 EMA	Clovis	PARP1 PARP2 PARP3	Germline and somatic	Treatment of BRCA-mutated ovarian cancer, platinum-sensitive recurrent epithelial ovarian and peritoneal cancers	1	21
Niraparib	2017 FDA, 2017 EMA	Tesaro	PARP1 PARP2	Not required	Treatment of platinum-sensitive ovarian cancer, HR deficiency advanced ovarian and peritoneal cancers	2	60
Veliparib	-	Abbvie	PARP1 PARP2	Germline	Not yet approved by any agency. But its efficacy in lung cancer, breast cancer, ovarian cancer was determined.	<0.2	30
Talazoparib	2018 FDA, 2019 EMA	Pfizer	PARP1 PARP2	Germline	Treatment of BRCA-mutated metastatic breast cancers	~100	4

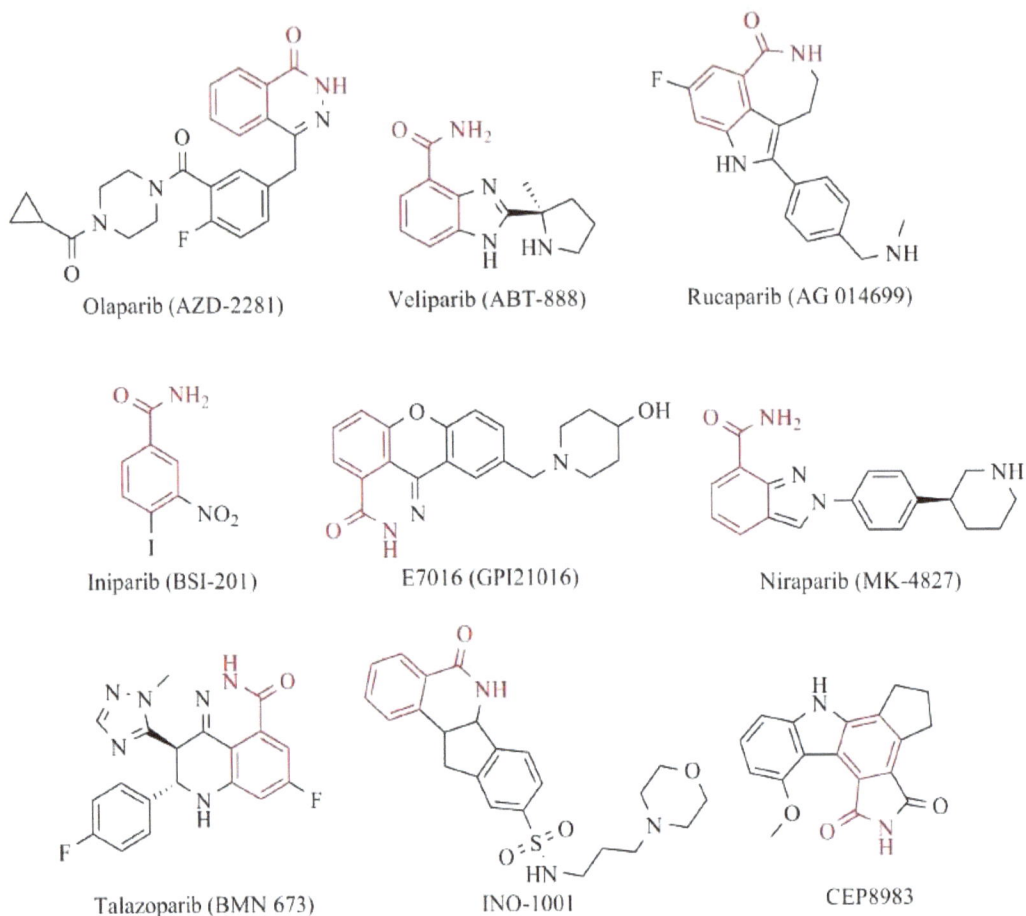

Fig. (6). The structure of PARP-1 inhibitors that have been approved or undergoing clinical trials.

The benefits of using PARP inhibitors in HR-deficient ovarian cancer and breast cancer are known. However, Ji *et al.* reported that consumption of the homologous recombination genes BRCA1 and BRCA2 in non-small cell lung cancer and these HR-deficient cancer cells were very hypersensitive to some PARP inhibitors. Therefore using PARP inhibitors in HR-deficient lung cancer was a new useful option and the effectiveness of PARP inhibitors was showed clearly [68]. The enhancement of PARP levels was reported to some cancers in melanoma, breast, ovarian and lung cancer. Almahli *et al.* designed and synthesized new PARP-1 inhibitors and investigated their cytotoxicity on A549 lung adenocarcinoma cells. They reported that PARP-1 inhibitors induced apoptosis *via* attenuation of AKT phosphorylation, so cell proliferation in lung adenocarcinoma inhibited [60].

There are three critical bonds in the interaction of PARP inhibitors with the enzyme. Two important amino acid residues such as Gly863 and Ser904 in the PARP enzyme's active site and the carboxamide moiety in inhibitors can form three hydrogen bonds between carboxamide NH to Gly C=O, carboxamide C=O to Gly NH and carboxamide C=O to Ser OH. Additionally, π-π stacking interaction was observed between the phenyl moiety of Tyr907 and the nicotinamide of NAD⁺. Attempts to increase the binding affinity of PARP inhibitors were focused on freely rotatable or enclosing the carboxamide group into a bicyclic system [69].

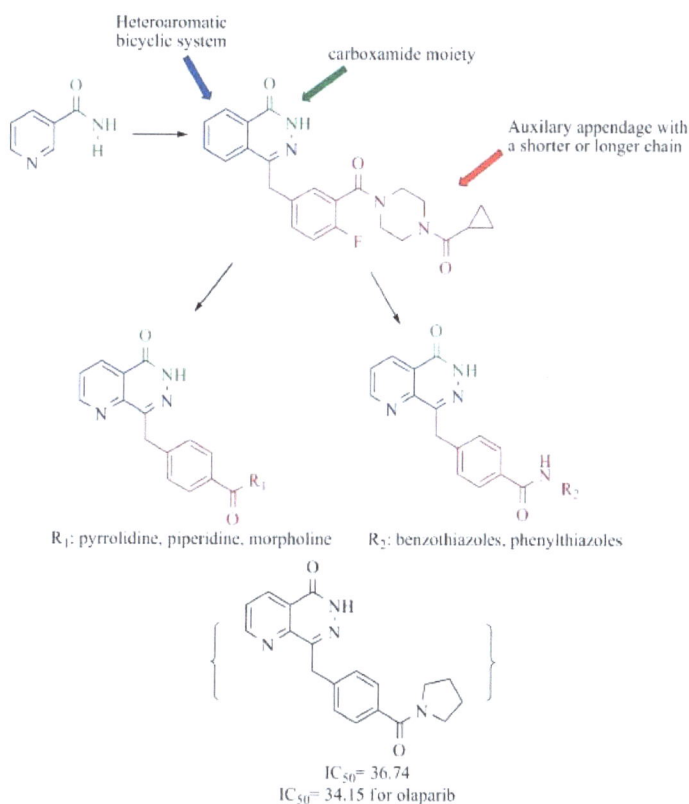

Fig. (7). Designed molecules from nicotinamide based PARP-1 inhibitors.

The structures of PARP-1 inhibitors in the literature are usually carrying phthalazinones, quinazolinones or isoquinolinones, none of them feature the nicotinamide moiety (pyridine ring and carboxamide at 3 positions). Pyridopyridazinone scaffold obtains an isosteric replacement of the phthalazinone nucleus. In addition, these pyridopyridazinones have lower central nervous system's side effects because of lower lipid solubility and blood-brain barrier permeability. To extend the half-life of a molecule, the benzyl group at position 4 of the pyridopyridazinone scaffold was attached through a lactam moiety. In Fig. 7, the inhibitory potencies of these designed molecules are comparable to olaparib [69].

The majority of PARP-1 inhibitors comprise the nicotinamide pharmacophore group and describe as NAD competitors [70]. However, these classical NAD competitors may affect other NAD-dependent pathways. They may prevent some enzyme's functions which are used in nucleotides as cofactors such as kinase enzymes because of their structural similarities to nucleotides [71]. Due to these limitations, new structures that inhibited PARP-1 enzyme but NAD non-dependent molecules were investigated. Two important additional routes were depicted in Fig. (**8**), and were reported for the inhibition of PARP-1 enzyme: it was aimed to prevent PARP-1 from binding with DNA and to disrupt the interaction of histone H4 and PARP-1 [72, 73]. In particular, the second route was very specific to PARP-1. The H4-dependent route was found stronger and better than DNA-dependent activation. Thus these H4-dependent PARP-1 inhibitors were greater activity than olaparib which was currently an approved NAD competitor drug in many cancer cells [74]. Moreover, PARP-1 activation with NAD-dependent led to many toxic effects, as NAD was an important metabolic currency. PARP inhibitors non-analog NAD exhibited minimum toxic effects [74].

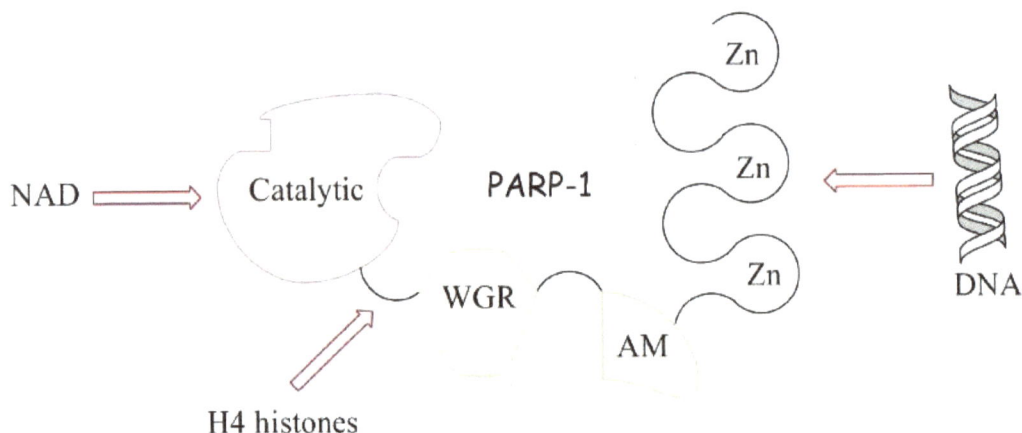

Fig. (8).   Three ways of PARP-1 activation. 1) NAD-dependent pathways, 2) specific H4 histone-dependent pathways, and 3) DNA-dependent pathways.

The benzimidazole ring in the veliparib is extremely sensitive to oxidation, which reduces the bioavailability of the molecule. Therefore, Wang *et al.* designed a molecule with better pharmacokinetic and physicochemical properties by introducing a fluorine atom to the benzimidazole ring. As a result of the structure-activity relationship, a strong PARP-1 inhibitor was found whose structure was given below (Fig. **9**). Molecular docking studies showed that the carbonyl oxygen formed three hydrogen bonds with the amino acids of the enzyme serine, glycine and histidine. Besides, it was determined that the fluorine atom at the 5-position of the benzimidazole ring strengthened the interaction of the PARP-1 active site by a binding extra hydrogen bond with the hydroxyl group of the serine amino acid [75].

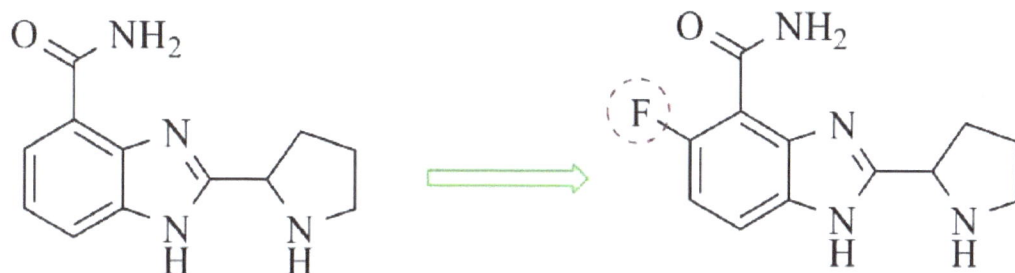

Fig. (9). The structure of a new PARP-1 inhibitor having better pharmacokinetic and physicochemical properties than veliparib.

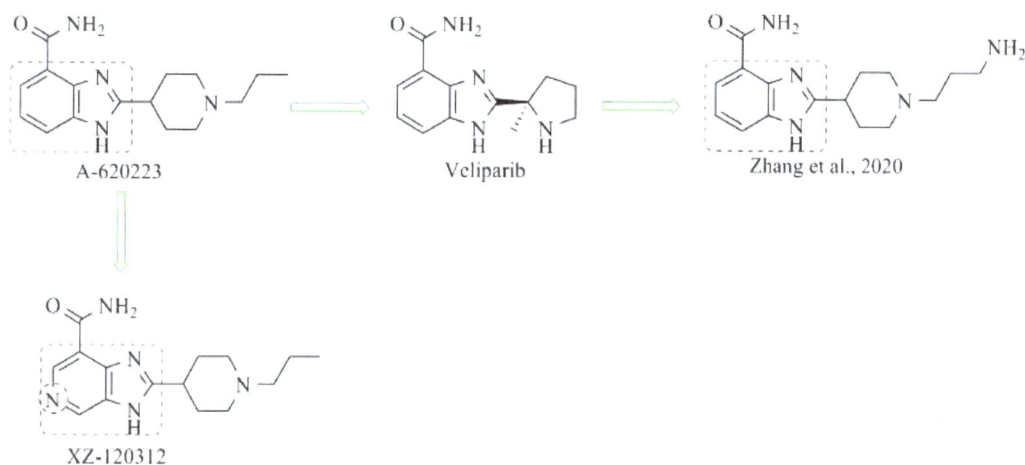

Fig. (10). Structures of benzimidazole-4-carboxamide and imidazo[4,5-c]pyridine derivatives as PARP-1 inhibitors.

The group lead by Golding and Griffin described a series of benzimidazole- 4-carboxamide, which were exhibited PARP-1 inhibitory activity in the mid-1990s. It was reported that the structure of benzimidazole-4-carboxamide was essential for inhibitory activity, the modification could be made at the 2nd position of the benzimidazole ring. Many studies showed that veliparib bearing pyrrolidine substitution with a quaternary carbon was better activity than A-620223 bearing piperidyl skeleton. However, Zhang *et al.* designed a new series of piperidyl-benzimidazole skeleton, which exhibited more significant PARP-1 inhibitory activity than veliparib [76]. Zhu *et al.* also reported a new series of cyclic amine-substituted imidazo[4,5-c]pyridine analogs as a similar PARP-1 inhibitor's study (Fig. **10**). For example, compound XZ-120312 exhibited significant PARP-1 inhibitory activity with the IC_{50} of 8.6 nM [77].

Scientists carry out some studies on the application of PARP inhibitors together with chemotherapy, radiotherapy and immunotherapy. In preclinical studies, it was reported that combined therapy with PARP inhibitors increased the sensitivity of chemotherapy and radiotherapy because of their synergistic activities. Studies on the combined olaparib and veliparib with chemotherapeutics such as topotecan and paclitaxel reduced the side effects of chemotherapy and tolerated better [78].

PARP inhibitors can block DNA repair and provide tumor cells more sensitive to cytotoxic agents [79]. Similarly, PARP inhibitors can act as radiosensitizing and chemosensitizing agents in combination therapies [80]. Combining PARP inhibitors with cytotoxic agents can increase the efficacy of PARP inhibitors and the administered doses of drugs may be decreased [81]. Combination therapy, using drugs that work by different mechanisms, plays a critical role in cancer-fighting. Both PARP-1 and topoisomerases are very important for genome stability. Topoisomerase inhibitors are another effective way for cancer treatment [82]. Therefore, new dual inhibitors against both PARP-1 and topoisomerase enzyme were developed as depicted in Fig. (**11**). 4-Amidobenzimidazole acridine derivatives were designed from acridine analogs having topoisomerase inhibitors and benzimidazole-4-carboxamide moiety whose skeleton of veliparib [83]. In another study, similar dual inhibitors were designed from olaparib and acridine analogs [84]. These two studies showed significant synergistic antitumor effects.

An example of dual inhibitors can also be given PARP-1 and histone deacetylases (HDAC) acting as synergistic antitumor agents. HDAC regulates some biological effects such as neurodegeneration, inflammation, metabolic disorders. To overcome the sensitization of tumor cells to antineoplastic agents in combination therapy was used both PARPi and HDACi. Therefore, target compounds P1 and P2 were designed and synthesized based on olaparib and panobinostat (HDAC inhibitor) by molecular hybridization (Fig. **12**). Compound P1 demonstrated more antiproliferative activities against MDA-MB-231, HCC1937 and, Raji cancer cells than olaparib and 4.1-fold less cytotoxicity to normal cells MCF-10A [85].

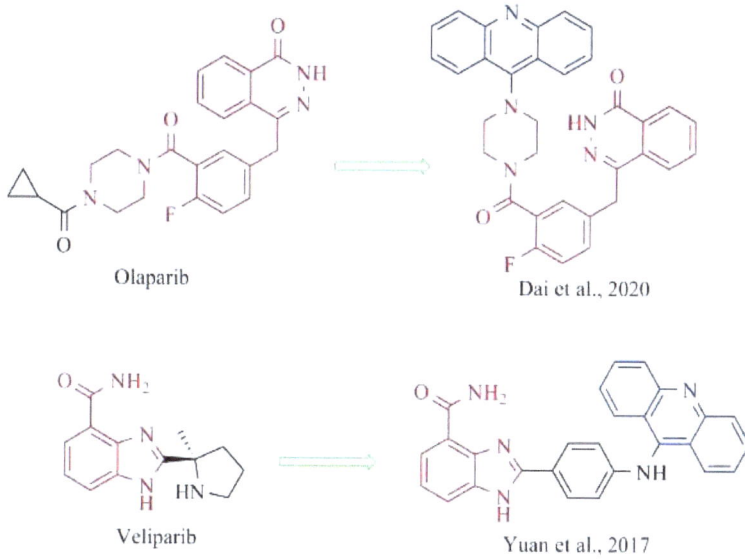

Fig. (11). New dual inhibitors developed from olaparib and veliparib.

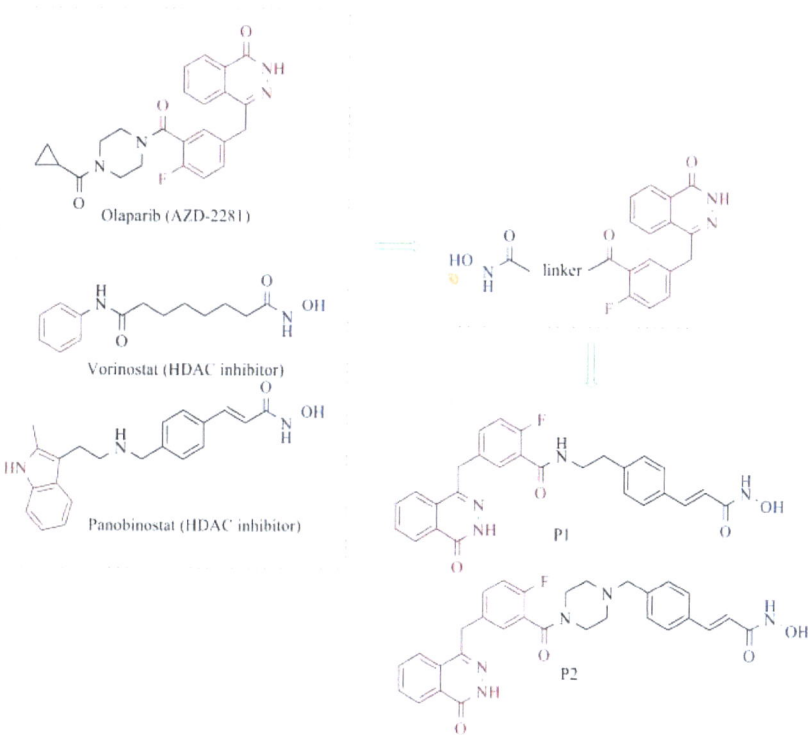

Fig. (12). New dual inhibitors acting as synergistic antitumor effects.

PARP inhibition alone can not be sufficient in the treatment of cancer because DNA damage caused by PARP inhibitors is tried to be repaired by other DNA repair mechanisms. Therefore, many clinical kinds of research on using PARP inhibitors in combination with other chemotherapeutic agents remain under investigation. Olaparib demonstrated barely bioactivity in the treatment of tumor cells if homologous recombination repair mechanisms are proficient. HSP90 protects protein stability and stabilizes BRCA protein. HSP90 confers resistance to PARP inhibitors because of its less susceptibility to enzymatic breakdown. Lin *et al.* designed new dual inhibitors based on PARP-1 inhibitor olaparib with HSP90 inhibitor C0817 by molecular hybridization (Fig. **13**). For example, compound 1 showed better inhibitory activity in MDA-MB-231, MCF-7 and SKBR3 cancer cells compared to olaparib [86]. One more example of such combined inhibitors is veliparib with ganetespib. Ganetespib is a second-generation HSP90 inhibitor, destabilizes the protein expression of BRCA1, BRCA2, and RAD51. Ganetespib and veliparib in combined therapy were observed synergistic anti-tumor effects and they didn't exhibit any systemic toxicity *in vivo* mouse model [87].

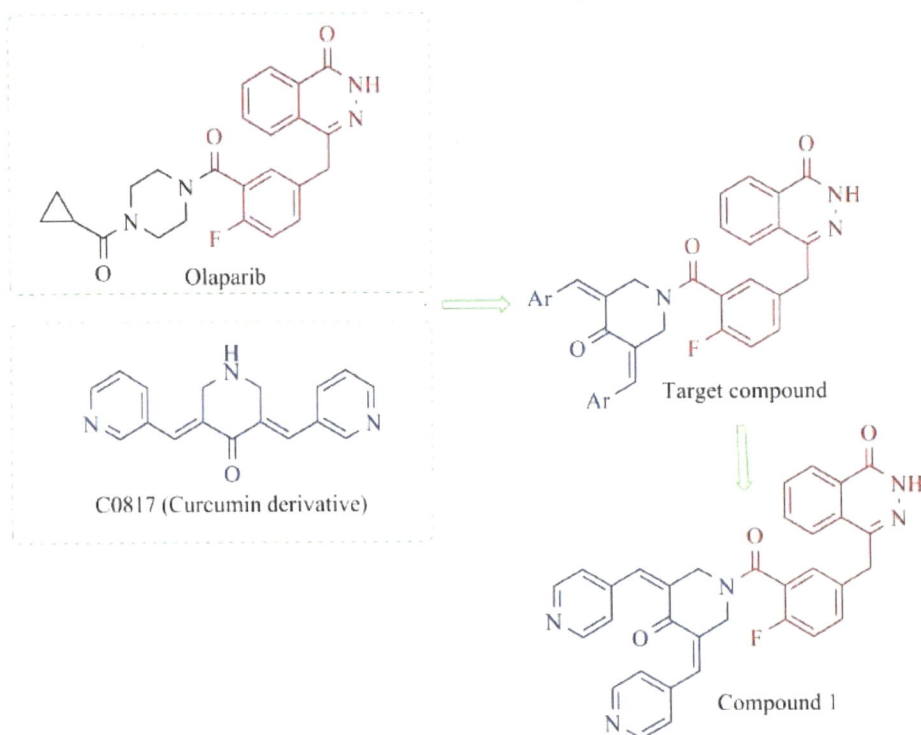

Fig. (13). Design route of novel dual-target inhibitors of PARP-1 and HSP90.

Many anticancer studies on homoerythrina alkaloid derivatives were reported in the literature. Li *et al.* discovered the PARP-1 inhibitory activity of erythrina. Compound B-10n isolated from erythrina alkaloid bearing a 1,2,3-triazole moiety was the most promising one. Nitrogen heterocyclic compounds such as 1,2,3-triazole skeleton were observed in many structures of effective anticancer drugs [88]. Classic PARP-1 inhibitors are generally containing amide fractions to be able to bind enzymes. Although compound B-10n does not bear an amide group, it can be a new non-amide-based PARP-1 inhibitors. The target compound whose structure was depicted in Fig. (**14**), discovered from erythrina. MTT assay results showed significant antiproliferative activity against A549 and the selectivity index of the target compound was higher than rucaparib. PARP-1 inhibitory activity of the target compound also was better than rucaparib [89].

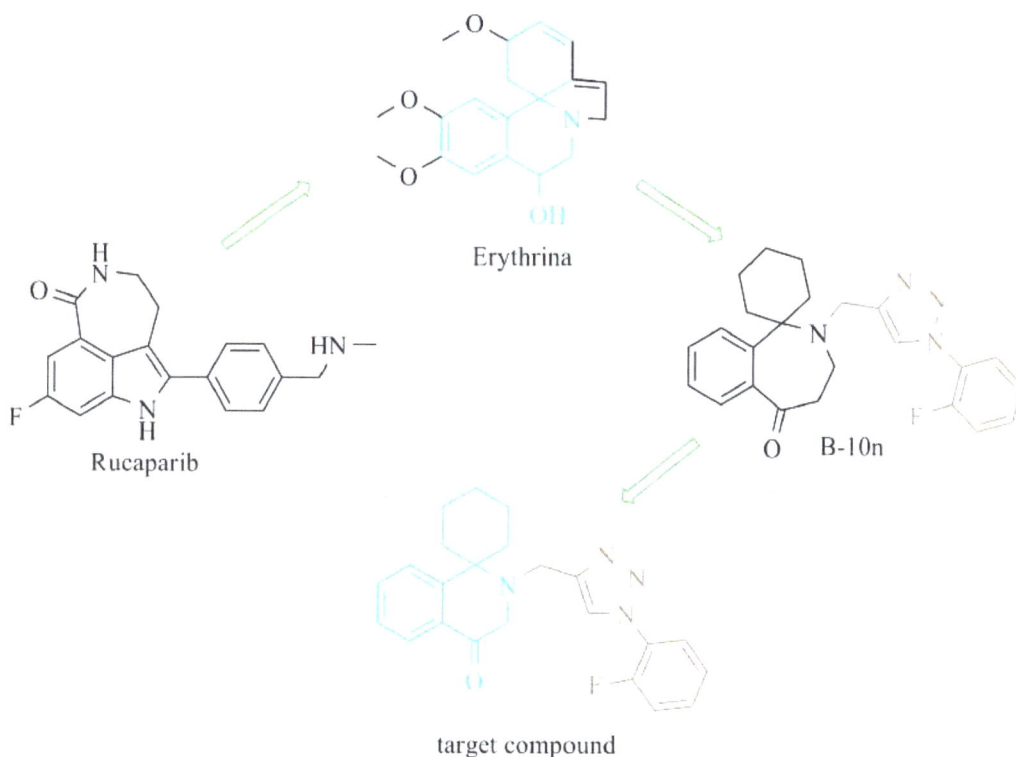

Fig. (14). Design route of target compound from rucaparib and erythrina alkaloid derivatives.

Xie *et al.* designed and synthesized a new 2,3-dihydro-1H- [1, 2]diazepino [4,5,6-*cd*]indole-1,4(6H)-dion structure based on a PARP-1 inhibitor rucaparib. Substituted aromatic rings were attached to the 6th position of the indole ring and the effectiveness of these molecules against the PARP-1 enzyme and BRCA1 mutated MDA-MB-436 and MCF-7 cells were evaluated [90]. Designed molecules form hydrogen bonds with glycine and serine, π-π stacking interaction with the aryl ring of tyrosine amino acids of the PARP enzyme (Fig. **15**). Different size basic groups on the aromatic ring determined the strength of the activity.

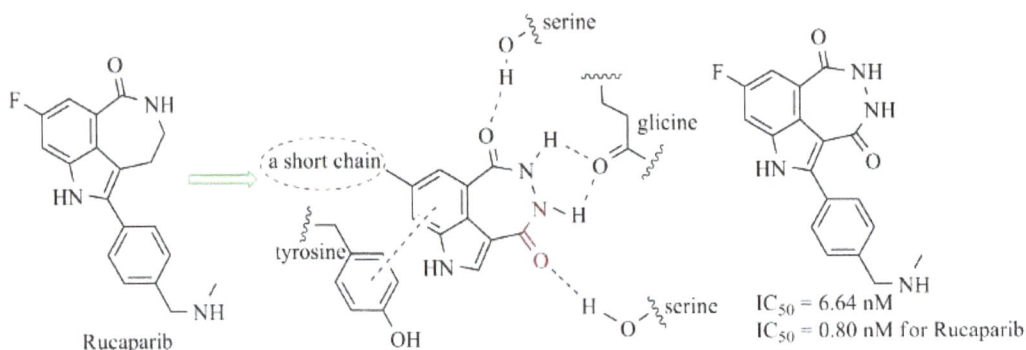

Fig. (15). The model of novel core-binding to PARP -1 enzyme.

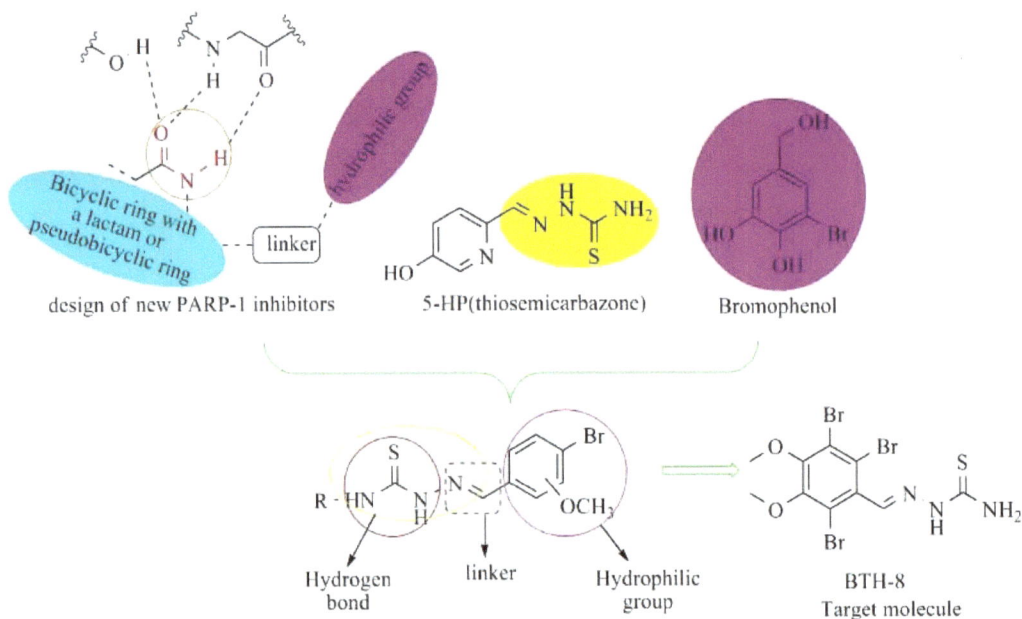

Fig. (16). Design of multifunctional hybrids bearing bromophenol–thiosemicarbazone and common structure of PARP-1 inhibitors.

It is extremely important to discover effective molecules in cancer treatment. Thiosemicarbazone derivatives and bromophenols were developed in clinical trials as anticancer agents, many years ago. To accomplish more effective molecules in cancer treatment were designed a hybrid molecule bearing multiple pharmacophore groups such as bromophenol, thiosemicarbazone and also common structure of PARP-1 inhibitors [91] (Fig. **16**). As a result, target molecule BTH-8 was discovered, and it exhibited significant antitumor activity against BRCA deficient cells such as HCC-1937 and Capan-1 by inducing cell apoptosis. It was reported that BTH-8 could be a lead molecule to treat breast cancer [92].

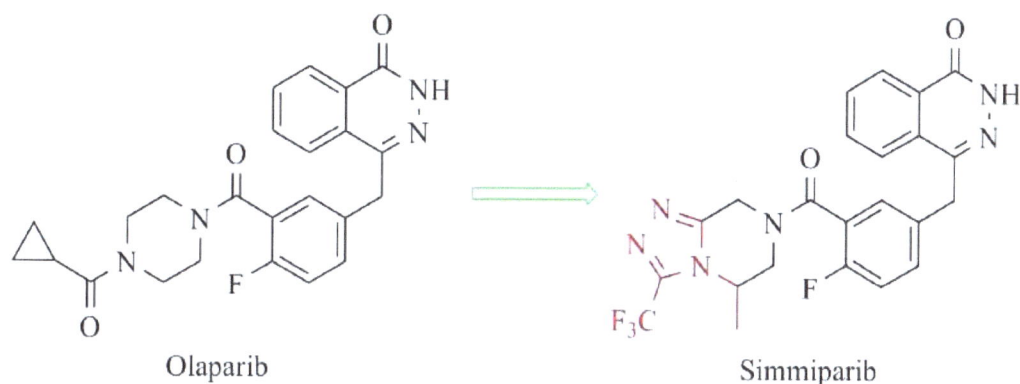

Olaparib   Simmiparib

Fig. (17). The structure of simmiparib as a new PARP-1 inhibitor molecule.

Yuan *et al.* discovered a new PARP enzyme inhibitor drug, simmiparib, from olaparib (Fig. **17**). It was determined that the antiproliferative effect of this new molecule had a much higher than olaparib. Simmiparib also inhibited the PARP-1 enzyme more selectively. *In vitro* and *in vivo* studies showed that simmiparib had good pharmacokinetic properties. Clinical trials of this molecule continue in China. All these features support it's a new PARP-1 inhibitor drug [93].

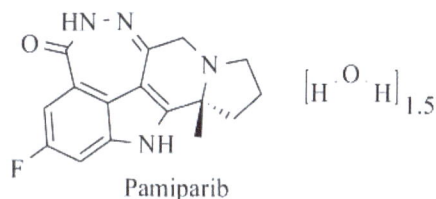

Pamiparib

Xiong *et al.* discovered pamiparib, is a strong and selective PARP-1/2 inhibitor. It was reported that pamiparib was 16-fold more potent than olaparib and it could be used in combined therapy with DNA alkylating agents such as temozolomide. Pamiparib showed strong antitumor activity against brain tumors in mice models because of its good penetration across the blood-brain barrier. Clinical development of pamiparib against brain tumors is currently underway [94].

Photoactivatable prodrugs strategy presents temporal and spatial control for the release of active molecules by UV irradiation. These prodrugs are designed by blocking the pharmacophore group with a photoactivatable protecting group. Especially photoactivatable prodrugs are an important approach for cancer treatment. When a photoactivatable protecting group as o-nitrobenzyl derivative binded to the lactam pharmacophore of talazoparib as depicted in Fig. (**18**), the inhibitory effect of the prodrug of talazoparib was significantly reduced. Therefore talazoparib's systemic side effects were prevented and its activity was observed only in the cancer tissues [95].

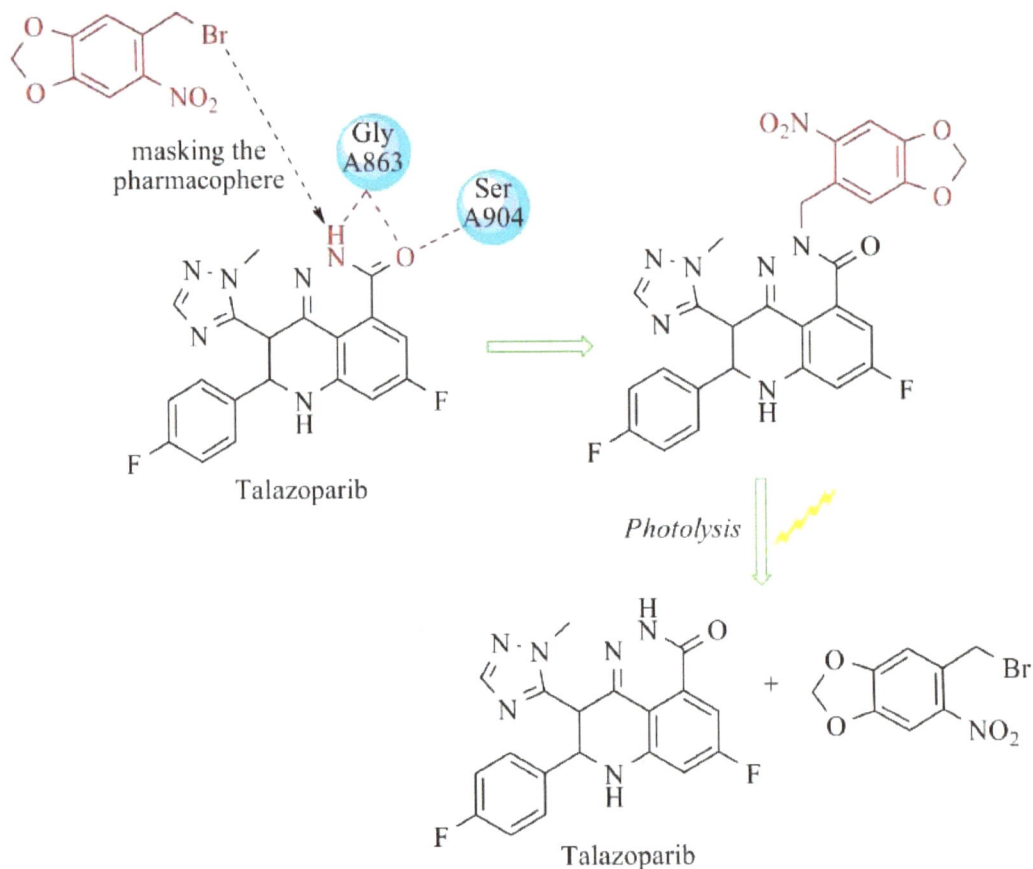

Fig. (18). The design of photoactivatable prodrugs with talazoparib.

While olaparib inhibits the PARP-1 enzyme significantly, the resistance to PARP inhibitors can occur easily because of acting as substrates of the p-glycoprotein efflux pump. As a result, Baptista *et al.* identified and considered as new candidate molecules for PARP-1 inhibitor. These compounds interacted not only with the nicotinamide binding region (glycine, tyrosine) of the PARP enzyme but also with some donor sites (methionine). This situation showed higher PARP-1 inhibition values [96] (Fig. **19**).

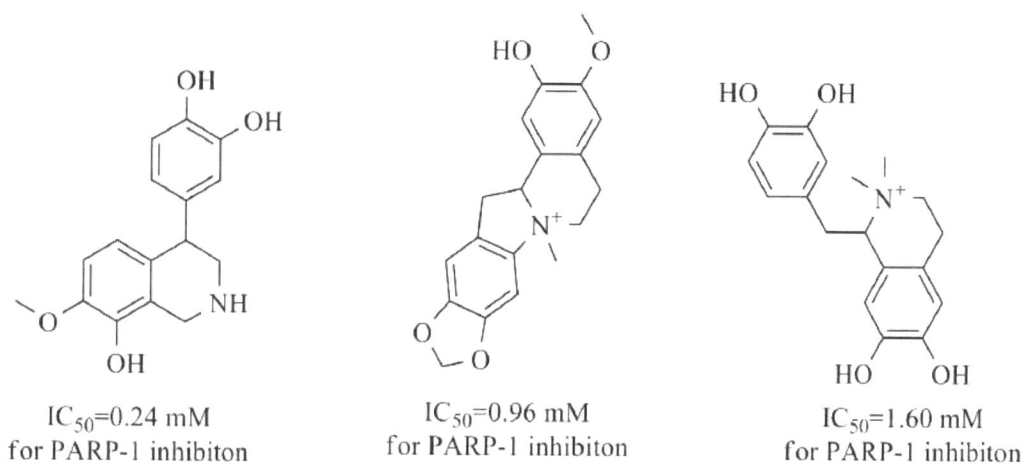

IC_{50}=0.24 mM	IC_{50}=0.96 mM	IC_{50}=1.60 mM
for PARP-1 inhibiton	for PARP-1 inhibiton	for PARP-1 inhibiton

Fig. (19). The structure with higher PARP-1 trapping activity.

PARP enzymes play a critical role not only in cancer but also in neuroinflammatory and neurodegenerative disorders [97]. However, there are limited brain-uptake of molecules due to P-glycoprotein (P-gb) [98]. For example, olaparib is a good P-gp substrate so it can excrete from the brain by the drug-efflux pump. Therefore, compound AZD2461 was discovered as a weak P-gp substrate by AstraZeneca. Then, veliparib and BGB-290 were reported as weak P-gp substrates [99] (Fig. **20**). These weak P-gp substrates can be lead compounds for the treatment of neurodegenerative disorders.

PARP overactivation may cause depletion of ATP, macrophage activation and inflammation. Its overactivation leads to many pathologies such as cardiac dysfunction, myocardial infarction [100]. PARP enzymes also regulate autophagy, the biology of lymphocyte and other immune cells [101, 102]. Nowadays, many scientists try to fight against the coronavirus disease 2019 (COVID-19), which turned into a pandemic disease in 2020. A cytokine storm, macrophage overactivation and increased reactive oxygen species were observed in this viral infection. PARP inhibitors may benefit the treatment of viral infection. PARP inhibitors have some evidence to reduce reactive species and inflammation. Furthermore, PARP inhibitors have a protective feature of lung cells. Because these drugs can decrease lung fibrosis and inflammation which a common symptom of COVID-19. Also, it was reported that PARP inhibitors such as olaparib and INO-1001 could reduce serum interleukin levels (IL-1, IL6) in the lung [103]. SARS-CoV-2 positive patients showed an increased risk of intravascular coagulation, coagulopathy and thrombosis. However, the anti-thrombotic effect of PARP-1 inhibitors was reported in the literature [104]. Because of all these reasons, PARP inhibitors should regard as a possible option in the treatment of COVID-19.

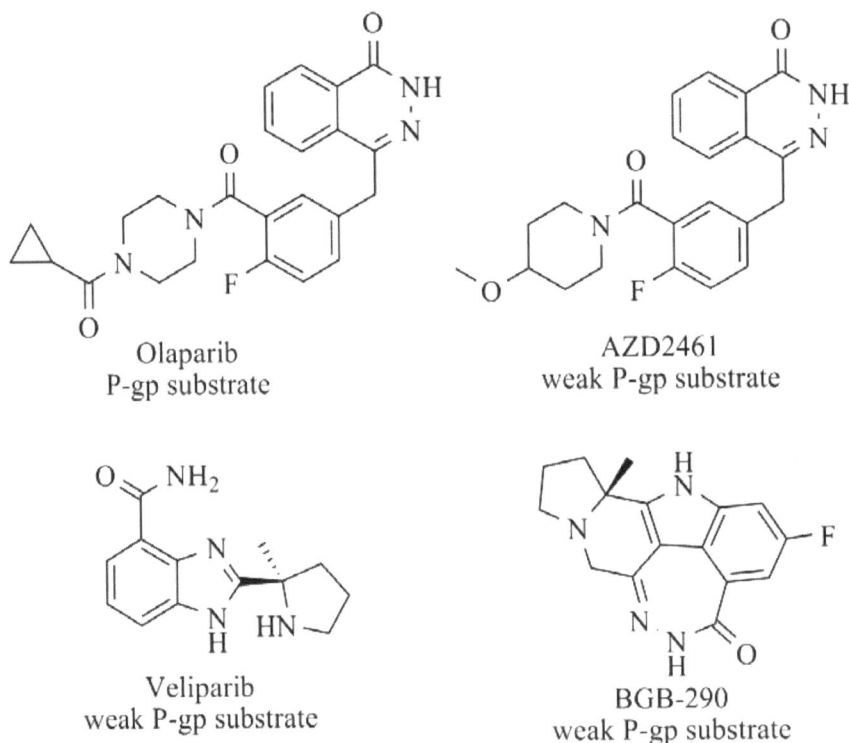

Olaparib
P-gp substrate

AZD2461
weak P-gp substrate

Veliparib
weak P-gp substrate

BGB-290
weak P-gp substrate

Fig. (20). The structures of PARP-1 inhibitors having high or weak P-gp substrate.

CONCLUSION

Poli (ADP-ribose) polymerase is a nuclear enzyme that regulates DNA repair, transcription, cell-cycle progression and genome integrity. PARP enzyme catalyzes the repair of single-strand DNA breaks. PARP inhibition causes the accumulation of DNA lesions and cell deaths by the mechanism of synthetic lethality.

The design and investigation of new PARP inhibitors, which started with 3-aminobenzamide and nicotinamide core continued with the discovery of more potent quinazoline, phthalazinone and benzimidazole derivatives. PARP inhibitors were approved for the treatment of breast and ovarian cancer with BRCA mutations by FDA. Nowadays, many PARP inhibitors are undergoing clinical trials. Many studies suggest that PARP inhibitors have some advantages to fight not only cancer but also other diseases such as inflammation, viral infection, ischemia.

Although there are also clinical benefits in using PARP inhibitors with monotherapy, the combination of PARP inhibitors with chemotherapeutic agents enhances PARP catalytic activity and chemotherapy cytotoxicity. Therefore, PARP inhibitors with chemotherapy, immunotherapy and radiotherapy combinations are widely used in cancer patients.

CONSENT FOR PUBLICATION

Not applicable.

CONFLICT OF INTEREST

The author declares no conflict of interest, financial or otherwise.

ACKNOWLEDGEMENTS

Declared none.

REFERENCES

[1]   Ferlay J, Colombet M, Soerjomataram I, *et al.* Estimating the global cancer incidence and mortality in 2018: GLOBOCAN sources and methods. Int J Cancer 2019; 144(8): 1941-53.
        [http://dx.doi.org/10.1002/ijc.31937] [PMID: 30350310]

[2]   WHO report on cancer: setting priorities, investing wisely and providing care for all. Geneva: World Health Organization; Licence: CC BY-NC-SA 3.0 IGO. 2020.

[3]   Torre LA, Trabert B, DeSantis CE, *et al.* Ovarian cancer statistics, 2018. CA Cancer J Clin 2018; 68(4): 284-96.
        [http://dx.doi.org/10.3322/caac.21456] [PMID: 29809280]

[4]   Bi Y, Verginadis II, Dey S, *et al.* Radiosensitization by the PARP inhibitor olaparib in BRCA1-proficient and deficient high-grade serous ovarian carcinomas. Gynecol Oncol 2018; 150(3): 534-44.
        [http://dx.doi.org/10.1016/j.ygyno.2018.07.002] [PMID: 30025822]

[5]   American Cancer Society. Cancer Facts & Fig 2020 Atlanta: American Cancer Society. 2020.

[6]   Tiong SS, Dickie C, Haas RL, O'Sullivan B. The role of radiotherapy in the management of localized soft tissue sarcomas. Cancer Biol Med 2016; 13(3): 373-83.
        [http://dx.doi.org/10.20892/j.issn.2095-3941.2016.0028] [PMID: 27807504]

[7]   Souliotis VL, Vlachogiannis NI, Pappa M, Argyriou A, Ntouros PA, Sfikakis PP. DNA damage response and oxidative stress in systemic autoimmunity. Int J Mol Sci 2019; 21(1): 1-24.
        [http://dx.doi.org/10.3390/ijms21010055] [PMID: 31861764]

[8]   Mota MBS, Carvalho MA, Monteiro ANA, Mesquita RD. DNA damage response and repair in perspective: *Aedes aegypti, Drosophila melanogaster* and *Homo sapiens.* Parasit Vectors 2019; 12(1): 533.
        [http://dx.doi.org/10.1186/s13071-019-3792-1] [PMID: 31711518]

[9]   Bak ST, Sakellariou D, Pena-Diaz J. The dual nature of mismatch repair as antimutator and mutator: for better or for worse. Front Genet 2014; 5(287): 287.
[http://dx.doi.org/10.3389/fgene.2014.00287] [PMID: 25191341]

[10]   Gavande NS, VanderVere-Carozza PS, Hinshaw HD, *et al.* DNA repair targeted therapy: The past or future of cancer treatment? Pharmacol Ther 2016; 160: 65-83.
[http://dx.doi.org/10.1016/j.pharmthera.2016.02.003] [PMID: 26896565]

[11]   Stratigopoulou M, van Dam TP, Guikema JEJ. Base excision repair in the immune system: small dna lesions with big consequences. Front Immunol 2020; 11(1084): 1084.
[http://dx.doi.org/10.3389/fimmu.2020.01084] [PMID: 32547565]

[12]   Zhao B, Watanabe G, Lieber MR. Polymerase μ in non-homologous DNA end joining: importance of the order of arrival at a double-strand break in a purified system. Nucleic Acids Res 2020; 48(7): 3605-18.
[http://dx.doi.org/10.1093/nar/gkaa094] [PMID: 32052035]

[13]   O'Dea R, Santocanale C. Non-canonical regulation of homologous recombination DNA repair by the USP9X deubiquitylase. J Cell Sci 2020; 133(3): 1-40.
[http://dx.doi.org/10.1242/jcs.233437] [PMID: 31964704]

[14]   Oing C, Tennstedt P, Simon R, *et al.* BCL2-overexpressing prostate cancer cells rely on PARP1-dependent end-joining and are sensitive to combined PARP inhibitor and radiation therapy. Cancer Lett 2018; 423: 60-70.
[http://dx.doi.org/10.1016/j.canlet.2018.03.007] [PMID: 29526801]

[15]   Prasad R, Horton JK, Dai DP, Wilson SH. Repair pathway for parp-1 dna-protein crosslinks. DNA Repair (Amst) 2019; 73: 71-7.
[http://dx.doi.org/10.1016/j.dnarep.2018.11.004] [PMID: 30466837]

[16]   Konecny GE, Kristeleit RS. Parp inhibitors for BRCA1/2-mutated and sporadic ovarian cancer: current practice and future directions. Br J Cancer 2016; 115(10): 1157-73.
[http://dx.doi.org/10.1038/bjc.2016.311] [PMID: 27736844]

[17]   Hurley RM, Wahner Hendrickson AE, Visscher DW, *et al.* 53BP1 as a potential predictor of response in PARP inhibitor-treated homologous recombination-deficient ovarian cancer. Gynecol Oncol 2019; 153(1): 127-34.
[http://dx.doi.org/10.1016/j.ygyno.2019.01.015] [PMID: 30686551]

[18]   Abdullah I, Chee CF, Lee YK, *et al.* Benzimidazole derivatives as potential dual inhibitors for PARP-1 and DHODH. Bioorg Med Chem 2015; 23(15): 4669-80.
[http://dx.doi.org/10.1016/j.bmc.2015.05.051] [PMID: 26088338]

[19]   Ray Chaudhuri A, Nussenzweig A. The multifaceted roles of PARP1 in DNA repair and chromatin remodelling. Nat Rev Mol Cell Biol 2017; 18(10): 610-21.
[http://dx.doi.org/10.1038/nrm.2017.53] [PMID: 28676700]

[20]   Stoepker C, Faramarz A, Rooimans MA, *et al.* DNA helicases FANCM and DDX11 are determinants of PARP inhibitor sensitivity. DNA Repair (Amst) 2015; 26: 54-64.
[http://dx.doi.org/10.1016/j.dnarep.2014.12.003] [PMID: 25583207]

[21]   Alemasova EE, Lavrik OI. Poly(ADP-ribosyl)ation by PARP1: reaction mechanism and regulatory proteins. Nucleic Acids Res 2019; 47(8): 3811-27.
[http://dx.doi.org/10.1093/nar/gkz120] [PMID: 30799503]

[22]   Lord CJ, Ashworth A. Parp inhibitors: the first synthetic lethal targeted therapy. Europe PMC Funders Group 2017; 355(630): 1152-8.
[PMID: 28302823]

[23]   Tok F, Koçyiğit-Kaymakçıoğlu B, İlhan R, Yılmaz S, Ballar-Kırmızıbayrak P, Taşkın-Tok T. Design, synthesis, biological evaluation and molecular docking of novel molecules to PARP-1 enzyme. Turk J Chem 2019; 43: 1290-305.

[http://dx.doi.org/10.3906/kim-1905-15]

[24]   Mateo J, Lord CJ, Serra V, *et al.* A decade of clinical development of PARP inhibitors in perspective. Ann Oncol 2019; 30(9): 1437-47.
[http://dx.doi.org/10.1093/annonc/mdz192] [PMID: 31218365]

[25]   Dawicki-McKenna JM, Langelier MF, DeNizio JE, *et al.* PARP-1 activation requires local unfolding of an autoinhibitory domain. Mol Cell 2015; 60(5): 755-68.
[http://dx.doi.org/10.1016/j.molcel.2015.10.013] [PMID: 26626480]

[26]   Raineri A, Prodomini S, Fasoli S, Gotte G, Menegazzi M. Influence of onconase in the therapeutic potential of PARP inhibitors in A375 malignant melanoma cells. Biochem Pharmacol 2019; 167: 173-81.
[http://dx.doi.org/10.1016/j.bcp.2019.06.006] [PMID: 31185226]

[27]   Castri P, Lee YJ, Ponzio T, *et al.* Poly(ADP-ribose) polymerase-1 and its cleavage products differentially modulate cellular protection through NF-kappaB-dependent signaling. Biochim Biophys Acta 2014; 1843(3): 640-51.
[http://dx.doi.org/10.1016/j.bbamcr.2013.12.005] [PMID: 24333653]

[28]   Gonzalez-Flores A, Aguilar-Quesada R, Siles E, *et al.* Interaction between PARP-1 and HIF-2α in the hypoxic response. Oncogene 2014; 33(7): 891-8.
[http://dx.doi.org/10.1038/onc.2013.9] [PMID: 23455322]

[29]   Gorodetska I, Kozeretska I, Dubrovska A. *BRCA* genes: the role in genome stability, cancer stemness and therapy resistance. J Cancer 2019; 10(9): 2109-27.
[http://dx.doi.org/10.7150/jca.30410] [PMID: 31205572]

[30]   Karakashev S, Zhu H, Yokoyama Y, *et al.* BET bromodomain inhibition synergizes with parp inhibitor in epithelial ovarian cancer. Cell Rep 2017; 21(12): 3398-405.
[http://dx.doi.org/10.1016/j.celrep.2017.11.095] [PMID: 29262321]

[31]   Rodriguez-Freixinos V, Fariñas-Madrid L, Gil-Martin M, *et al.* Chemotherapy and parp inhibitors in heavily pretreated brca1/2 mutation ovarian cancer (bmoc) patients. Gynecol Oncol 2019; 152(2): 270-7.
[http://dx.doi.org/10.1016/j.ygyno.2018.11.036] [PMID: 30551885]

[32]   Deben C, Lardon F, Wouters A, *et al.* APR-246 (PRIMA-1(MET)) strongly synergizes with AZD2281 (olaparib) induced PARP inhibition to induce apoptosis in non-small cell lung cancer cell lines. Cancer Lett 2016; 375(2): 313-22.
[http://dx.doi.org/10.1016/j.canlet.2016.03.017] [PMID: 26975633]

[33]   Sulai NH, Tan AR. Development of poly(ADP-ribose) polymerase inhibitors in the treatment of BRCA-mutated breast cancer. Clin Adv Hematol Oncol 2018; 16(7): 491-501.
[PMID: 30067621]

[34]   Gu L, Du N, Jin Q, *et al.* Magnitude of benefit of the addition of poly ADP-ribose polymerase (PARP) inhibitors to therapy for malignant tumor: A meta-analysis. Crit Rev Oncol Hematol 2020; 147: 102888.
[http://dx.doi.org/10.1016/j.critrevonc.2020.102888] [PMID: 32018126]

[35]   Marshall CH, Antonarakis ES. Emerging treatments for metastatic castration-resistant prostate cancer: Immunotherapy, PARP inhibitors, and PSMA-targeted approaches. Cancer Treat Res Commun 2020; 23: 100164.
[http://dx.doi.org/10.1016/j.ctarc.2020.100164] [PMID: 31978677]

[36]   Zhu H, Wei M, Xu J, *et al.* PARP inhibitors in pancreatic cancer: molecular mechanisms and clinical applications. Mol Cancer 2020; 19(1): 49.
[http://dx.doi.org/10.1186/s12943-020-01167-9] [PMID: 32122376]

[37]   Wu W, Zhu H, Liang Y, *et al.* Expression of PARP-1 and its active polymer PAR in prostate cancer and benign prostatic hyperplasia in Chinese patients. Int Urol Nephrol 2014; 46(7): 1345-9.

[http://dx.doi.org/10.1007/s11255-014-0642-0] [PMID: 24436031]

[38]   Karpova Y, Wu C, Divan A, *et al.* Non-NAD-like PARP-1 inhibitors in prostate cancer treatment. Biochem Pharmacol 2019; 167: 149-62.
[http://dx.doi.org/10.1016/j.bcp.2019.03.021] [PMID: 30880062]

[39]   Pavlović M, Tadić A, Gligorijević N, *et al.* Synthesis, chemical characterization, PARP inhibition, DNA binding and cellular uptake of novel ruthenium(II)-arene complexes bearing benzamide derivatives in human breast cancer cells. J Inorg Biochem 2020; 210: 111155.
[http://dx.doi.org/10.1016/j.jinorgbio.2020.111155] [PMID: 32768729]

[40]   Boraei ATA, Singh PK, Sechi M, Satta S. Discovery of novel functionalized 1,2,4-triazoles as PARP-1 inhibitors in breast cancer: Design, synthesis and antitumor activity evaluation. Eur J Med Chem 2019; 182: 111621.
[http://dx.doi.org/10.1016/j.ejmech.2019.111621] [PMID: 31442685]

[41]   Goodfellow E, Senhaji Mouhri Z, Williams C, Jean-Claude BJ. Design, synthesis and biological activity of novel molecules designed to target PARP and DNA. Bioorg Med Chem Lett 2017; 27(3): 688-94.
[http://dx.doi.org/10.1016/j.bmcl.2016.09.054] [PMID: 28003142]

[42]   Papeo G, Posteri H, Borghi D, *et al.* Discovery of 2-[1-(4,4-difluorocyclohexyl)piperidin-4-yl]-6-fluoro-3-oxo-2,3-dihydro-1H-isoindole-4-carboxamide (NMS-P118): a potent, orally available, and highly selective PARP-1 inhibitor for cancer therapy. J Med Chem 2015; 58(17): 6875-98.
[http://dx.doi.org/10.1021/acs.jmedchem.5b00680] [PMID: 26222319]

[43]   Siavashpour A, Khalvati B, Azarpira N, Mohammadi H, Niknahad H, Heidari R. Poly (ADP-Ribose) polymerase-1 (PARP-1) overactivity plays a pathogenic role in bile acids-induced nephrotoxicity in cholestatic rats. Toxicol Lett 2020; 330: 144-58.
[http://dx.doi.org/10.1016/j.toxlet.2020.05.012] [PMID: 32422328]

[44]   Passeri D, Camaioni E, Liscio P, *et al.* Concepts and molecular aspects in the polypharmacology of parp-1 inhibitors. ChemMedChem 2016; 11(12): 1219-26.
[http://dx.doi.org/10.1002/cmdc.201500391] [PMID: 26424664]

[45]   Malyuchenko NV, Kotova EY, Kulaeva OI, Kirpichnikov MP, Studitskiy VM. PARP1 Inhibitors: antitumor drug design. Acta Naturae 2015; 7(3): 27-37.
[http://dx.doi.org/10.32607/20758251-2015-7-3-27-37] [PMID: 26483957]

[46]   Cseh AM, Fabian Z, Quintana-Cabrera R, *et al.* PARP Inhibitor PJ34 protects mitochondria and induces DNA-damage mediated apoptosis in combination with Cisplatin or Temozolomide in B16F10 melanoma cells. Front Physiol 2019; 10(538): 538.
[http://dx.doi.org/10.3389/fphys.2019.00538] [PMID: 31133874]

[47]   Bai XT, Moles R, Chaib-Mezrag H, Nicot C. Small PARP inhibitor PJ-34 induces cell cycle arrest and apoptosis of adult T-cell leukemia cells. J Hematol Oncol 2015; 8(117): 117.
[http://dx.doi.org/10.1186/s13045-015-0217-2] [PMID: 26497583]

[48]   Nathubhai A, Haikarainen T, Hayward PC, *et al.* Structure-activity relationships of 2-arylquinazolin-4-ones as highly selective and potent inhibitors of the tankyrases. Eur J Med Chem 2016; 118: 316-27.
[http://dx.doi.org/10.1016/j.ejmech.2016.04.041] [PMID: 27163581]

[49]   Maksimainen MM, Nurmesjärvi A, Terho RA, Threadgill MD, Lehtiö L, Heiskanen JP. Derivatives of a PARP Inhibitor TIQ-A through the Synthesis of 8-Alkoxythieno[2,3-*c*]isoquinolin-5(4*H*)-ones. ACS Omega 2020; 5(22): 13447-53.
[http://dx.doi.org/10.1021/acsomega.0c01879] [PMID: 32548533]

[50]   Giannini G, Battistuzzi G, Vesci L, *et al.* Novel PARP-1 inhibitors based on a 2-propanoyl--H-quinazolin-4-one scaffold. Bioorg Med Chem Lett 2014; 24(2): 462-6.
[http://dx.doi.org/10.1016/j.bmcl.2013.12.048] [PMID: 24388690]

[51]   McPherson LA, Shen Y, Ford JM. Poly (ADP-ribose) polymerase inhibitor LT-626: Sensitivity

correlates with MRE11 mutations and synergizes with platinums and irinotecan in colorectal cancer cells. Cancer Lett 2014; 343(2): 217-23.
[http://dx.doi.org/10.1016/j.canlet.2013.10.034] [PMID: 24215868]

[52] Zhong Y, Meng Y, Xu X, *et al.* Design, synthesis and evaluation of phthalazinone thiohydantoin-based derivative as potent PARP-1 inhibitors. Bioorg Chem 2019; 91: 103181.
[http://dx.doi.org/10.1016/j.bioorg.2019.103181] [PMID: 31404795]

[53] Chen Y, Du H. The promising PARP inhibitors in ovarian cancer therapy: From Olaparib to others. Biomed Pharmacother 2018; 99: 552-60.
[http://dx.doi.org/10.1016/j.biopha.2018.01.094] [PMID: 29895102]

[54] Franzese E, Centonze S, Diana A, *et al.* PARP inhibitors in ovarian cancer. Cancer Treat Rev 2019; 73: 1-9.
[http://dx.doi.org/10.1016/j.ctrv.2018.12.002] [PMID: 30543930]

[55] Ledermann JA, El-Khouly F. PARP inhibitors in ovarian cancer: Clinical evidence for informed treatment decisions. Br J Cancer 2015; 113 (Suppl. 1): S10-6.
[http://dx.doi.org/10.1038/bjc.2015.395] [PMID: 26669450]

[56] Zheng F, Zhang Y, Chen S, Weng X, Rao Y, Fang H. Mechanism and current progress of Poly ADP-ribose polymerase (PARP) inhibitors in the treatment of ovarian cancer. Biomed Pharmacother 2020; 123: 109661.
[http://dx.doi.org/10.1016/j.biopha.2019.109661] [PMID: 31931287]

[57] Mirza MR, Pignata S, Ledermann JA. Latest clinical evidence and further development of PARP inhibitors in ovarian cancer. Ann Oncol 2018; 29(6): 1366-76.
[http://dx.doi.org/10.1093/annonc/mdy174] [PMID: 29750420]

[58] Matulonis UA, Herrstedt J, Tinker A, *et al.* Long-term benefit of niraparib treatment of recurrent ovarian cancer (OC). J Clin Oncol 2017; 35: 5534.
[http://dx.doi.org/10.1200/JCO.2017.35.15_suppl.5534]

[59] Lakomy DS, Urbauer DL, Westin SN, Lin LL. Phase I study of the PARP inhibitor talazoparib with radiation therapy for locally recurrent gynecologic cancers. Clin Transl Radiat Oncol 2019; 21: 56-61.
[http://dx.doi.org/10.1016/j.ctro.2019.12.005] [PMID: 31993510]

[60] Almahli H, Hadchity E, Jaballah MY, *et al.* Development of novel synthesized phthalazinone-based PARP-1 inhibitors with apoptosis inducing mechanism in lung cancer. Bioorg Chem 2018; 77: 443-56.
[http://dx.doi.org/10.1016/j.bioorg.2018.01.034] [PMID: 29453076]

[61] Wang B, Chu D, Feng Y, Shen Y, Aoyagi-Scharber M, Post LE. Discovery and Characterization of (8S,9R)-5-Fluoro-8-(4-fluorophenyl)-9-(1-methyl-1H-1,2,4-triazol-5-yl)-2,7,8-9-tetrahydro-3H-pyrido[4,3,2-de]phthalazin-3-one (BMN 673, Talazoparib), a Novel, Highly Potent, and Orally Efficacious Poly(ADP-ribose) Polymerase-1/2 Inhibitor, as an Anticancer Agent. J Med Chem 2016; 59(1): 335-57.
[http://dx.doi.org/10.1021/acs.jmedchem.5b01498] [PMID: 26652717]

[62] Min A, Im SA. Parp inhibitors as therapeutics: beyond modulation of parylation. Cancers (Basel) 2020; 12(2): 1-16.
[http://dx.doi.org/10.3390/cancers12020394] [PMID: 32046300]

[63] Lim JSJ, Tan DSP. Understanding resistance mechanisms and expanding the therapeutic utility of parp inhibitors. Cancers (Basel) 2017; 9(8): 1-14.
[http://dx.doi.org/10.3390/cancers9080109] [PMID: 28829366]

[64] Plummer R. Poly(ADP-ribose)polymerase (PARP) inhibitors: from bench to bedside. Clin Oncol (R Coll Radiol) 2014; 26(5): 250-6.
[http://dx.doi.org/10.1016/j.clon.2014.02.007] [PMID: 24602564]

[65] Césaire M, Ghosh U, Austry JB, *et al.* Sensitization of chondrosarcoma cells with PARP inhibitor and high-LET radiation. J Bone Oncol 2019; 17: 100246.

[http://dx.doi.org/10.1016/j.jbo.2019.100246] [PMID: 31312595]

[66] Langelier MF, Riccio AA, Pascal JM. PARP-2 and PARP-3 are selectively activated by 5′ phosphorylated DNA breaks through an allosteric regulatory mechanism shared with PARP-1. Nucleic Acids Res 2014; 42(12): 7762-75.
[http://dx.doi.org/10.1093/nar/gku474] [PMID: 24928857]

[67] Zhao H, Ji M, Cui G, *et al.* Discovery of novel quinazoline-2,4(1H,3H)-dione derivatives as potent PARP-2 selective inhibitors. Bioorg Med Chem 2017; 25(15): 4045-54.
[http://dx.doi.org/10.1016/j.bmc.2017.05.052] [PMID: 28622906]

[68] Ji W, Weng X, Xu D, Cai S, Lou H, Ding L. Non-small cell lung cancer cells with deficiencies in homologous recombination genes are sensitive to PARP inhibitors. Biochem Biophys Res Commun 2020; 522(1): 121-6.
[http://dx.doi.org/10.1016/j.bbrc.2019.11.050] [PMID: 31753490]

[69] Elmasry GF, Aly EE, Awadallah FM, El-Moghazy SM. Design and synthesis of novel PARP-1 inhibitors based on pyridopyridazinone scaffold. Bioorg Chem 2019; 87: 655-66.
[http://dx.doi.org/10.1016/j.bioorg.2019.03.068] [PMID: 30952061]

[70] Wigle TJ, Blackwell DJ, Schenkel LB, *et al. In Vitro* and cellular probes to study PARP enzyme target engagement. Cell Chem Biol 2020; 27(7): 877-887.e14.
[http://dx.doi.org/10.1016/j.chembiol.2020.06.009] [PMID: 32679093]

[71] Antolín AA, Mestres J. Linking off-target kinase pharmacology to the differential cellular effects observed among PARP inhibitors. Oncotarget 2014; 5(10): 3023-8.
[http://dx.doi.org/10.18632/oncotarget.1814] [PMID: 24632590]

[72] Kirsanov KI, Kotova E, Makhov P, *et al.* Minor grove binding ligands disrupt PARP-1 activation pathways. Oncotarget 2014; 5(2): 428-37.
[http://dx.doi.org/10.18632/oncotarget.1742] [PMID: 24504413]

[73] Makhov P, Uzzo RG, Tulin AV, Kolenko VM. Histone-dependent PARP-1 inhibitors: A novel therapeutic modality for the treatment of prostate and renal cancers. Urol Oncol Semin Ori 2020; S1078-1439(20): 30145-9.

[74] Thomas C, Ji Y, Lodhi N, *et al.* Non-NAD-Like poly(ADP-Ribose) Polymerase-1 Inhibitors effectively eliminate cancer *in vivo.* EBioMedicine 2016; 13: 90-8.
[http://dx.doi.org/10.1016/j.ebiom.2016.10.001] [PMID: 27727003]

[75] Wang J, Wang X, Li H, *et al.* Design, synthesis and biological evaluation of novel 5-fluoro--H-benzimidazole-4-carboxamide derivatives as potent PARP-1 inhibitors. Bioorg Med Chem Lett 2016; 26(16): 4127-32.
[http://dx.doi.org/10.1016/j.bmcl.2016.06.045] [PMID: 27353531]

[76] Zhang X, Zhang C, Tang L, *et al.* Synthesis and biological evaluation of piperidyl benzimidazole carboxamide derivatives as potent PARP-1 inhibitors and antitumor agents. Chin Chem Lett 2020; 31: 136-40.
[http://dx.doi.org/10.1016/j.cclet.2019.04.045]

[77] Zhu Q, Wang X, Hu Y, He X, Gong G, Xu Y. Discovery and SAR study of 2-(1-propylpiperidin-4-yl)-3H-imidazo[4,5-c]pyridine-7-carboxamide: A potent inhibitor of poly(ADP-ribose) polymerase-1 (PARP-1) for the treatment of cancer. Bioorg Med Chem 2015; 23(20): 6551-9.
[http://dx.doi.org/10.1016/j.bmc.2015.09.026] [PMID: 26422786]

[78] Ang YLE, Tan DSP. Development of PARP inhibitors in gynecological malignancies. Curr Probl Cancer 2017; 41(4): 273-86.
[http://dx.doi.org/10.1016/j.currproblcancer.2017.02.008] [PMID: 28583748]

[79] Ghorai A, Mahaddalkar T, Thorat R, Dutt S. Sustained inhibition of PARP-1 activity delays glioblastoma recurrence by enhancing radiation-induced senescence. Cancer Lett 2020; 490: 44-53.
[http://dx.doi.org/10.1016/j.canlet.2020.06.023] [PMID: 32645394]

[80]   Jannetti SA, Zeglis BM, Zalutsky MR, Reiner T. Poly(ADP-Ribose)Polymerase (PARP) Inhibitors and Radiation Therapy. Front Pharmacol 2020; 11(170): 170.
[http://dx.doi.org/10.3389/fphar.2020.00170] [PMID: 32194409]

[81]   Mukhopadhyay A, Drew Y, Matheson E, *et al.* Evaluating the potential of kinase inhibitors to suppress DNA repair and sensitise ovarian cancer cells to PARP inhibitors. Biochem Pharmacol 2019; 167: 125-32.
[http://dx.doi.org/10.1016/j.bcp.2018.10.011] [PMID: 30342021]

[82]   Karapetian M, Tsikarishvili S, Kulikova N, Kurdadze A, Zaalishvili G. Genotoxic effects of topoisomerase poisoning and PARP inhibition on zebrafish embryos. DNA Repair (Amst) 2020; 87: 102772.
[http://dx.doi.org/10.1016/j.dnarep.2019.102772] [PMID: 31877465]

[83]   Yuan Z, Chen S, Chen C, *et al.* Design, synthesis and biological evaluation of 4-amidobenzimidazole acridine derivatives as dual PARP and Topo inhibitors for cancer therapy. Eur J Med Chem 2017; 138: 1135-46.
[http://dx.doi.org/10.1016/j.ejmech.2017.07.050] [PMID: 28763648]

[84]   Dai Q, Chen J, Gao C, *et al.* Design, synthesis and biological evaluation of novel phthalazinone acridine derivatives as dual PARP and Topo inhibitors for potential anticancer agents. Chin Chem Lett 2020; 31: 404-8.
[http://dx.doi.org/10.1016/j.cclet.2019.06.019]

[85]   Yuan Z, Chen S, Sun Q, *et al.* Olaparib hydroxamic acid derivatives as dual PARP and HDAC inhibitors for cancer therapy. Bioorg Med Chem 2017; 25(15): 4100-9.
[http://dx.doi.org/10.1016/j.bmc.2017.05.058] [PMID: 28601509]

[86]   Lin S, Zhang L, Zhang X, *et al.* Synthesis of novel dual target inhibitors of PARP and HSP90 and their antitumor activities. Bioorg Med Chem 2020; 28(9): 115434.
[http://dx.doi.org/10.1016/j.bmc.2020.115434] [PMID: 32222339]

[87]   Jiang J, Lu Y, Li Z, *et al.* Ganetespib overcomes resistance to PARP inhibitors in breast cancer by targeting core proteins in the DNA repair machinery. Invest New Drugs 2017; 35(3): 251-9.
[http://dx.doi.org/10.1007/s10637-016-0424-x] [PMID: 28111726]

[88]   Li S, Li XY, Zhang TJ, *et al.* Design, synthesis and biological evaluation of homoerythrina alkaloid derivatives bearing a triazole moiety as PARP-1 inhibitors and as potential antitumor drugs. Bioorg Chem 2020; 94: 103385.
[http://dx.doi.org/10.1016/j.bioorg.2019.103385] [PMID: 31669094]

[89]   Li S, Li XY, Zhang TJ, *et al.* Design, synthesis and biological evaluation of erythrina derivatives bearing a 1,2,3-triazole moiety as PARP-1 inhibitors. Bioorg Chem 2020; 96: 103575.
[http://dx.doi.org/10.1016/j.bioorg.2020.103575] [PMID: 31962202]

[90]   Xie Z, Zhou Y, Zhao W, *et al.* Identification of novel PARP-1 inhibitors: Drug design, synthesis and biological evaluation. Bioorg Med Chem Lett 2015; 25(20): 4557-61.
[http://dx.doi.org/10.1016/j.bmcl.2015.08.060] [PMID: 26342868]

[91]   Guo C, Wang L, Li X, *et al.* Discovery of novel bromophenol-thiosemicarbazone hybrids as potent selective inhibitors of poly(adp-ribose) polymerase-1 (parp-1) for use in cancer. J Med Chem 2019; 62(6): 3051-67.
[http://dx.doi.org/10.1021/acs.jmedchem.8b01946] [PMID: 30844273]

[92]   Guo C, Zhang F, Wu X, *et al.* BTH-8, a novel poly (ADP-ribose) polymerase-1 (PARP-1) inhibitor, causes DNA double-strand breaks and exhibits anticancer activities *in vitro* and *in vivo*. Int J Biol Macromol 2020; 150: 238-45.
[http://dx.doi.org/10.1016/j.ijbiomac.2020.02.069] [PMID: 32057845]

[93]   Yuan B, Ye N, Song SS, *et al.* Poly(ADP-ribose)polymerase (PARP) inhibition and anticancer activity of simmiparib, a new inhibitor undergoing clinical trials. Cancer Lett 2017; 386: 47-56.

[http://dx.doi.org/10.1016/j.canlet.2016.11.010] [PMID: 27847302]

[94]   Xiong Y, Guo Y, Liu Y, *et al.* Pamiparib is a potent and selective PARP inhibitor with unique potential for the treatment of brain tumor. Neoplasia 2020; 22(9): 431-40.
[http://dx.doi.org/10.1016/j.neo.2020.06.009] [PMID: 32652442]

[95]   Li J, Xiao D, Liu L, *et al.* Design, synthesis, and *in vitro* evaluation of the photoactivatable prodrug of the parp inhibitor talazoparib. Molecules 2020; 25(2): 1-14.
[http://dx.doi.org/10.3390/molecules25020407] [PMID: 31963730]

[96]   Baptista SJ, Silva MMC, Moroni E, *et al.* Novel parp-1 inhibitor scaffolds disclosed by a dynamic structure-based pharmacophore approach. PLoS One 2017; 12(1): e0170846.
[http://dx.doi.org/10.1371/journal.pone.0170846] [PMID: 28122037]

[97]   Komirishetty P, Areti A, Yerra VG, *et al.* PARP inhibition attenuates neuroinflammation and oxidative stress in chronic constriction injury induced peripheral neuropathy. Life Sci 2016; 150: 50-60.
[http://dx.doi.org/10.1016/j.lfs.2016.02.085] [PMID: 26921631]

[98]   Gogola E, Duarte AA, de Ruiter JR, *et al.* Selective loss of parg restores parylation and counteracts parp inhibitor-mediated synthetic lethality. Cancer Cell 2018; 33(6): 1078-1093.e12.
[http://dx.doi.org/10.1016/j.ccell.2018.05.008] [PMID: 29894693]

[99]   Reilly SW, Puentes LN, Schmitz A, *et al.* Synthesis and evaluation of an AZD2461 [^{18}F]PET probe in non-human primates reveals the PARP-1 inhibitor to be non-blood-brain barrier penetrant. Bioorg Chem 2019; 83: 242-9.
[http://dx.doi.org/10.1016/j.bioorg.2018.10.015] [PMID: 30390553]

[100] Zakaria EM, El-Bassossy HM, El-Maraghy NN, Ahmed AF, Ali AA. PARP-1 inhibition alleviates diabetic cardiac complications in experimental animals. Eur J Pharmacol 2016; 791: 444-54.
[http://dx.doi.org/10.1016/j.ejphar.2016.09.008] [PMID: 27612628]

[101] Fehr AR, Singh SA, Kerr CM, Mukai S, Higashi H, Aikawa M. The impact of PARPs and ADP-ribosylation on inflammation and host-pathogen interactions. Genes Dev 2020; 34(5-6): 341-59.
[http://dx.doi.org/10.1101/gad.334425.119] [PMID: 32029454]

[102] Wang H, Yang X, Yang Q, Gong L, Xu H, Wu Z. PARP-1 inhibition attenuates cardiac fibrosis induced by myocardial infarction through regulating autophagy. Biochem Biophys Res Commun 2018; 503(3): 1625-32.
[http://dx.doi.org/10.1016/j.bbrc.2018.07.091] [PMID: 30041821]

[103] Curtin N, Bányai K, Thaventhiran J, Le Quesne J, Helyes Z, Bai P. Repositioning PARP inhibitors for SARS-CoV-2 infection(COVID-19); a new multi-pronged therapy for acute respiratory distress syndrome? Br J Pharmacol 2020; 177(16): 3635-45.
[http://dx.doi.org/10.1111/bph.15137] [PMID: 32441764]

[104] Capoluongo E. PARP-inhibitors in a non-oncological indication as COVID-19: Are we aware about its potential role as anti-thrombotic drugs? The discussion is open. Biomed Pharmacother 2020; 130: 110536.
[http://dx.doi.org/10.1016/j.biopha.2020.110536] [PMID: 32688139]

SUBJECT INDEX

A

Abdominal discomfort 55
Ablation 102, 109, 115, 124, 125, 126, 127
    thermal 102
Ablation therapies 102, 111
    locoregional 102
Absorption, intestinal 53
Acid(s) 13, 14, 38, 75, 170
    arachidonic 13
    cannabidiolic 14
    glycine amino 170
    hyaluronic 75
    polyunsaturated fatty 38
Acquired immunodeficiency syndrome 43
Activation 4, 7, 8, 54, 70, 72, 79, 103, 104,
        105, 143, 145, 153, 186
    dependent 8
    immune 70
    macrophage 186
    of caspases 8, 54
Activity 10, 14, 15, 17, 18, 19, 21, 46, 49,
        106, 171, 177, 183, 185
    anti-tumor 106
    antitumoral 19
    antitumorigenic 18, 19
Acute myeloid leukemia (AML) 6, 73, 74, 85
Acute respiratory distress syndrome 121
Adenine nucleotide translocator (ANT) 146
Adipogenesis 174
ADP 168
    ribose subunits 168
    ribosyltransferase 168
Advanced 77, 84, 86, 102
    breast cancer 77
    cholangiocarcinoma 84
    esophageal cancer 86
    hepatocellular carcinoma management 102
Advanced HCC 108, 109, 110, 111, 113, 114,
        115, 118, 119, 120, 121, 122, 123, 124,
        125, 128
    cytologically-confirmed 110

treatment, second-line 111
Agents 16, 42, 49, 77, 80, 106, 108, 110, 118,
        119, 121, 125, 126, 127, 128, 152, 179
    anti-angiogenic 49
    antineoplastic 179
    chemosensitizing 179
    cytotoxic 16, 77, 80, 179
    gadolinium-based 152
    neuroprotective 42
American 109, 112
    association for the study of liver diseases
        (AASLD) 109
    society of clinical oncology (ASCO) 112
Aminoalkylindole scaffold 17
AMP-activated protein kinase 8
Anemia 54, 117, 172, 174
    chronic 54, 174
Angiogenesis 9, 37, 49, 52, 141, 152, 153,
        168, 174
Antiangiogenic action 122
Antibody-dependent cellular cytotoxicity
        (ADCC) 76
Antibody-dependent phagocytosis 116
Anticancer 5, 10, 21, 22, 51, 56, 57, 183
    agents 5, 21, 22, 57, 183
    therapeutics 10
    therapy 51, 56
Anticancer drugs 22, 52, 164, 174, 182
    aggressive 22
    effective 182
Anticancer effects 16, 19, 20, 48
    synergistic 48
Antigen-presenting cells (APCs) 69, 76, 77,
        105
Antigens 46, 77, 78, 79, 80, 81, 82, 84, 87,
        105, 149, 153, 155
    anti-cytotoxic T-lymphocyte 153
    cell surface 81
    human trophoblast cell surface 46
    lymphocyte 77
    overexpressed 87
    safe tumor 80

Atta-ur-Rahman & M. Iqbal Choudhary (Eds.)
All rights reserved-© 2021 Bentham Science Publishers

tumor-associated 84
Anti-inflammatory activities 40
Anti-metastatic activities 46, 51, 52
Antioxidant 37, 38, 39, 40, 42, 43, 57, 75
   activities 42, 43
   and prooxidant nature of curcumin 43
   capacity 75
Antiproliferative 12, 15, 17, 18, 19, 20, 179, 184
   activities 19, 20, 179
   effects 12, 15, 17, 18, 184
   profile 12, 19
Antitumor 9, 52, 70, 80, 128
   drugs 9, 52
   efficacy 128
   immunity 70, 80
Antitumor activity 5, 7, 50, 52, 79, 105
   demonstrated durable 79
   immune 105
Antitumor agents 1, 2, 20, 179
   potential cannabinoids 20
   synergistic 179
Anti-VEGF monoclonal antibody combination 113, 124
Apoptosis 5, 7, 8, 9, 12, 14, 16, 17, 37, 47, 48, 68, 69, 144, 146, 175
   induced 47, 48, 175
Atezolizumab monotherapy 113, 114, 120
Atherosclerosis 42
ATP-dependent helicase 145

B

Base excision repair (BER) 165, 173
BER 166
   mechanism 166
   pathway 166
   system 166
Biocatalysis 13
Bone tumors 4
Bowel cancer, large 52
Brain and colon cancer 74
BRCA168, 174, 181
   mutated breast cancer 168

mutated metastatic breast cancers 174
mutated ovarian cancer 174
protein 181
Breast 6, 14, 18, 20
   adenocarcinoma 6, 14
   carcinoma 20
   malignacies 18
Breast cancer 4, 16, 17, 18, 19, 44, 46, 47, 51, 54, 74, 75, 77, 164, 165, 168, 174, 175
   cell growth 46
   metastatic 18
   treatment 4
   triple-negative 17, 19
Breast tumors 6, 77
   diverse 6
   receptor-negative 6
Burkitt's lymphoma 19

C

Calcium/calmodulin-dependent protein kinase 8
Camrelizumab 118, 119, 122, 123, 127
   monotherapy 119, 123
Cancer(s) 1, 2, 5, 6, 9, 11, 12, 14, 21, 37, 39, 40, 43, 46, 49, 50, 52, 53, 54, 57, 68, 69, 70, 73, 74, 75, 76, 82, 84, 85, 102, 122, 145, 147, 164, 165, 185
   angiogenesis 52
   brain 73
   chemoprevention 53
   chemotherapy 2
   esophagogastric 122
   growth 9
   immunotherapy principles 70
   infection-related 102
   nasopharyngeal 84
   pathology 2
   physiopathology 11, 14
   progression 11, 37, 39, 46, 70
   receptors 40
   regulation 147
   risk 37
   suppression 49

tissues 5, 12, 21, 50, 74, 145, 185
    signaling pathways 49
Cancer cell(s) 2, 5, 6, 7, 8, 9, 11, 12, 13, 16,
    18, 39, 46, 47, 48, 49, 50, 51, 52, 68, 69,
    70, 73, 74, 105
    bladder 46
    cervical 47
    colon 18
    colorectal 16
    cycle 5
    hepatic 7
    human breast 11, 12
    non-small-cell lung 46
    ovarian 47, 74
    proliferation 7
    prostate 12, 13, 48
    survival 2
Cancer immunotherapy 76, 77, 78, 84, 103
    next-generation 84
Cancer pain 3, 4
    bone 4
    management of 3, 4
    metastatic bone 4
Cancer stem cell 80, 85
    based immunotherapy 80
Cannabinoid(s) 1, 2, 3, 4, 5, 7, 9, 10, 12, 21
    anticancer strategies 21
    antitumor actions 7
    based drugs 7
    efficacy 3
    peripherally-restricted 4
    treatments 4, 5
Carcinogenesis 39
Carcinoma 6, 17, 44, 45, 76, 113
    cell lung 76, 113
    gastric 6
    renal 17
    squamous skin cell 6
Cardiac dysfunction 186
Cell adhesion molecules (CAMs) 50
Cell cycle 8, 17, 76, 148
    arrest 8, 17, 76
    regulation 148
Cell death 7, 8, 9, 39, 46, 49, 75, 76, 77, 87,
    106, 146, 164, 165, 168, 187

apoptotic 146
autophagic 46
cannabinoid-induced 7, 8
cannabinoid-induced cancer 7
endometrial cancer 7
immunogenic 106
programmed 7, 39
Cell proliferation 5, 7, 16, 37, 46, 48, 49, 51,
    70, 72, 143, 149
    proteins 51
Cellular 57, 82, 87
    immune responses 82, 87
    targets 57
Central nervous system (CNS) 3, 141, 176
Cerebral ischemia 72
Cerebrospinal fluid 143
Cervical Cancer 44, 47
Chemoresistance, cancer cell 39
Chemotherapeutic 4, 15, 17, 46, 51, 52, 57,
    164, 169, 171, 181, 188
    agents 4, 15, 17, 164, 169, 171, 181, 188
    chemicals 52
    drug combinations 57
    drug cytarabine 51
    drug gefitinib 46
Chemotherapy 1, 4, 37, 39, 52, 53, 69, 75, 76,
    80, 81, 83, 141, 142, 179, 188
    conventional 76
    cytotoxicity 188
    induced peripheral neuropathy 4
    perioperative 69
Cirrhosis 102, 109
Cisplatin-induced 4, 16
    nephrotoxicity 4
    neuropathy 4, 16
Colon cancer 18, 19, 20, 43, 45, 49, 52, 54,
    55, 74, 82
Colorectal cancer 6, 16, 56, 76, 79, 112, 171
    advanced 76
    colitis-associated 6
Colorectal carcinoma 13, 14
Cryoablation 102, 125
Curcuma longa 37, 38
Curcumin 37, 40, 41, 42, 43, 44, 45, 46, 47,
    48, 49, 50, 51, 52, 53, 54, 55, 56, 57

and metformin combination 44
and paclitaxel combination 44
chemical constituent 37
inhibitory effects of 46, 48
nanoparticles, polymeric 52
oil 54
phosphor lipid complexes 54
prooxidant nature of 43, 47
Cyclooxygenase 50

D

Deaths 68, 69, 107, 109, 110, 111, 114, 127,
    164
cancer-related 165
damage-induced 80
Dendritic cell (DC) 68, 76, 77, 78, 81, 82, 83,
    87, 103, 105
Diarrhea 80, 107, 110, 112, 119, 120, 121,
    124, 172
Disease(s) 12, 37, 38, 39, 42, 50, 57, 68, 69,
    72, 102, 107, 108, 109, 110, 111, 112,
    113, 114, 115, 117, 118, 119, 120, 122,
    123, 127, 165, 186, 188
acute coronary heart 42
chronic obstructive pulmonary 42
coronavirus 186
control rate (DCR) 107, 108, 109, 110, 111,
    112, 113, 114, 115, 117, 118, 119, 120,
    122, 123
immune 42
inflammatory 42
liver 42, 102
malignant 50
pandemic 186
progression 127
urinary 42
DNA 19, 143, 166, 177, 184
alkylating agents 184
dependent pathways 177
glycosylase 166
integrity 166
methyltransferase 143
topoisomerase II enzyme 19

DNA lesions 165, 166, 168, 173, 187
helix-distorting 166
Downregulated expression 44
Downstream signaling 76
Duration of response (DoR) 107, 117, 125,
    126, 127
Durvalumab monotherapy 119, 124, 125
Durvalumab therapy 125
Dyslipidemia 42

E

Effects 12, 16, 46, 49, 105, 106, 146, 153,
    154, 173, 177, 187
anti-apoptotic 154
anti-telomerase 49
anti-thrombotic 187
anti-tumor 153
apoptotic 12, 16, 146
chemosensitizing 46
immune-activating 106
immunosuppressive 105
radio-sensitization 173
toxic 177
Efficacy 3, 4, 49, 78, 79, 80, 101, 107, 110,
    114, 115, 117, 119, 120, 122, 123, 124
immunomodulating 49
immunotherapeutic 80
Encephalomyelitis 42
Endocannabinoid 1, 2, 6, 20
action 6
biodegradation 20
system 1, 2
Endometrial sarcoma 6
Enzymes 2, 9, 21, 40, 107, 166, 169, 171, 176,
    177, 182, 183
endonuclease 166
extracellular 9
hepatic 107
kinase 177
metabolic 2, 21
Epidermal 46, 71, 76, 77, 143, 152
growth factor receptor (EGFR) 46, 76, 77,
    143, 152

stem cells (ESC) 71
Epithelial cancer 5
Erythropoiesis 168
Esophageal 45, 115
    cancer 45
    varices 115
Extracellular regulated kinase (ERK) 8, 52

F

Fallopian tube cancers 173
Fatigue 80, 107, 110, 112, 116, 118, 119, 120,
    121, 124, 171
Fatty acid amide hydrolase (FAAH) 2, 6
Food and drug administration (FDA) 3, 76,
    77, 103, 110, 115, 121, 122, 168, 173,
    174

G

Ganetespib 181
Gastric cancer 16, 17, 45, 49, 50, 56, 122
Gastrointestinal 42, 43, 71, 108, 141, 142,
    144, 149, 150, 153, 154, 155
    cancer 43, 108
    disorders 42
    stem cells (GSCs) 71, 141, 142, 144, 149,
        150, 153, 154, 155
Gemicitabine 53
Genes 72, 82, 110, 143, 145, 146, 148, 149,
    150, 151, 152, 154, 155, 165, 168
    apoptosis-resistance 82
    cancer susceptibility 165
    lymphocyte-activation 110
    tumor suppressor 148, 168
    tyrosine kinase 149
Gingival hemorrhage 124
Glioblastoma 1, 6, 10, 11, 14, 19, 20, 43, 86,
    145, 149, 152
    stem cells 149
G-protein coupled receptors (GPCRs) 2, 21
Gynecologic disorders 173

H

Hand-foot syndrome 122
HBV infection 107, 118
Headache 172
Head and neck cancer 45, 48, 55, 74, 84
Heat shock protein-70 154
Hematopoietic stem cells (HSC) 71
Hepatic artery infusion chemotherapy (HAIC)
    124
Hepatitis 114
HER2-positive breast cancer 85
Histone deacetylases 179
Human 16, 43, 79
    immunodeficiency virus 43
    papillomavirus 79
    prostate carcinoma androgen 16
Humanized monoclonal antibody toripalimab
    119
Hypofractionated radiotherapy 126

I

Immune 2, 49, 69, 76, 77, 82, 101, 103, 104,
    106, 107, 110, 116, 126, 128
    checkpoint inhibitors (ICIs) 101, 103, 106,
        107, 110, 116, 126, 128
    system 2, 49, 69, 76, 77, 82, 103, 104, 116
Immunomodulatory 43, 106
    activities 43
    effects, distinct 106
Immunotherapeutic approaches 87
Inhibiting JNK signaling pathway 48
Inhibition 44, 76, 149
    of cell proliferation and invasion 149
    of EGFR signaling by mAb binding 76
    of JNK signaling pathway 44

J

JNK signaling pathway 44

L

Lenvatinib monotherapy 121
Leukapheresis 78
Leukemia 6, 15, 18, 51, 73, 74, 85
  acute myeloid 6, 73, 74, 85
Lewis lung adenocarcinoma growth 5
Lipase 2, 107
  monoacylglycerol 2
Liver 120, 121, 123, 173
  enzymes 120, 173
  failure 121, 123
Low-density lipoprotein (LDL) 42
Lung 5, 53, 175, 186
  adenocarcinoma 175
  cancer stem cells 53
  carcinomas 5
  fibrosis 186
Lymphocytes 2, 79, 105, 106, 186
  tumor-infiltrating 79, 105
Lymphoma 5, 14, 51

M

Magnetic resonance spectroscopic imaging
  (MRSI) 151, 152
Malignancies 13, 15, 21, 80, 84, 105, 110,
  112, 113, 114, 152
  gynecological 84
  hematological 80
Malignant 6, 53, 74
  astrocytomas 6
  brain tumor 53
  insulinoma cells 74
MAPK pathway 15
Mesenchymal stem cells (MSCs) 71
Metabolic disorders 179
Metastasis 2, 4, 7, 9, 11, 15, 16, 49, 68, 69, 70,
  73, 74, 75, 82, 148, 150
  and relapses 68, 69
  lymphatic 11
  preventing lung 82
Metastatic 79, 86
  cholangiocarcinoma 79

colorectal cancer 86
Metformin combination 44
Middle carotid artery occlusion (MCAO) 72
Myeloid-derived suppressor cells (MDSCs) 50
Myeloma 14, 15, 17, 21, 56
Myocardial infarction 186

N

Nausea 1, 2, 80, 119, 171
Negative allosteric modulator (NAM) 2
Neural stem cells (NSCs) 71
Neurodegenerative disorders 186
Neuroprotective action 42
Neurosphere formation 150
Non-alcoholic fatty liver disease (NAFLD)
  102
Non-FDA approved immunotherapy 116
Non-homologous end-joining (NHEJ) 165,
  166, 173
Nuclear 13, 50, 166, 187
  enzyme 166, 187
  factor (NF) 13, 50

O

Objective response rate (ORR) 107, 108, 109,
  110, 112, 113, 114, 116, 117, 118, 119,
  122, 123, 125, 126
Oral 48, 74, 82
  cancers 74
  carcinomas 82
  mucositis 48
  squamous cell carcinoma (OSCC) 74
Ovarian cancer 15, 17, 44, 47, 164, 172, 187
Oxidative carboxylation 145

P

Pancreatic 11, 14, 43, 45, 49, 55, 71, 82, 169,
  174
  cancer 11, 14, 43, 45, 55, 82, 169, 174
  ductal adenocarcinoma cells (PDAC) 49
  stem cells (PSCs) 71

Pathways 7, 8, 9, 49, 50, 52, 70, 73, 76, 104,
    141, 142, 143, 146, 147, 177
  anti-apoptotic 52
  death receptor 49
  histone-dependent 177
  inflammatory 50
  mediated autophagy 7, 8
  metabolic 141, 142
  mitochondrial apoptosis 146
  protein kinase 49
  tumor suppressor 49
Pembrolizumab 101, 104, 105, 110, 111, 112,
    116, 118, 120, 121, 126, 127
  efficacy of 110, 111
Peptides 77, 78
  exogenous tumor 78
Phosphorylation 8, 52, 149
  tyrosine kinase 149
Phytochemistry of curcumin 40
Platelet derived growth factor receptor
    (PDGFR) 122
Platinum-sensitive ovarian cancer 174
Poly-ADP-ribose polymerase (PARP) 144,
    164, 166, 183
Portal vein tumor thrombosis (PVTT) 123
Positron emission tomography (PET) 151
Pro-angiogenic cytokine 9
Processes 4, 39, 145, 166
  anti-inflammatory 4
  catalysis 145
  metabolic 39
  oncogenesis 166
Prognosis 68, 73, 142, 146, 150, 151, 152
Prognostic 144, 145, 147, 148, 149, 150, 151,
    152, 154
  biomarker 144, 150, 151, 154
  cell cycle progression 148
Progression-free survival (PFS) 109, 110, 111,
    114, 116, 117, 121, 122, 123, 125, 126,
    127, 142, 144, 149
Proliferation 14, 16, 46, 48, 49, 68, 69, 73, 81,
    84, 141, 143, 145, 147, 148, 149, 152
  cellular 152
  inhibited 81
  membrane 152

Properties 12, 13, 14, 20, 22, 38, 39, 41, 42,
    52, 69
  anti-angiogenic 52
  anti-inflammatory 39, 42
  antimetastatic 13
  antimutagenic 39
  antiproliferative 13, 14
  proapoptotic 20
  tumor-suppressing 69
Prostate cancer 16, 17, 19, 44, 48, 55, 74
  diverse 16
Prostate carcinoma 16, 20
Protein(s) 7, 41, 47, 48, 49, 51, 75, 77, 80,
    104, 142, 143, 144, 145, 146, 150, 153,
    154, 166, 168
  anti-apoptotic 75, 80, 146
  caveolae-associated 154
  immune-related chaperone 154
  kinases 51
  mismatch repair 143, 144
  oxidative stress sensor 47
  programmed cell death 77, 104, 153
  stress-regulated 7
  targeting bioactive 49
  tumor suppressor 145

R

Radiation therapy 102, 142, 165
  selective internal 102
Radiofrequency ablation 106
Reactive oxygen species (ROS) 15, 16, 19, 37,
    43, 44, 47, 75, 145, 165
Receptors 2, 20, 21, 50, 76, 77, 153
  growth factor 50
  induced TNF 77
  ionotropic 2
  motif chemokine 153
  nuclear 21
  putative cannabinoid 20
  tyrosine kinase 76
Recurrence-free survival (RFS) 109, 111, 115,
    124, 126, 127
Redox reactions 43

Reduction 18, 44, 45, 47, 48, 69, 75, 143
  cancer cells viability 18
  pharmacologic 75
Regulation 11, 47, 51, 69, 83, 106, 164, 168
  abnormal endocannabinoidome 11
  of T-cell activation 106
  telomerase 164
Relapses 63, 68, 69, 83
  systemic 83
Relative cerebral blood volume, measuring
    151
Repair 71, 72, 164, 165, 166, 168, 173, 187
  genomic 164
  homologs recombination 168
  nucleotide excision 165
  of single-strand DNA breaks 166, 168, 187
  single-strand break 165
Resistant cancer cells 81
RNA expression data 48
ROS 19, 75
  production 19
  scavengers 75

S

Selective internal radiation therapy (SIRT)
    102
Severe combined immune-deficient (SCID) 73
Signaling pathways 7, 8, 37, 39, 51, 81
Signal 49, 50, 76, 166, 168, 173, 187
  transducer 50
  transduction 49, 76
  strand DNA breaks 166, 168, 173, 187
Skin 5, 9, 38, 42, 56, 80
  burns 38
  carcinomas 5, 9
  exfoliation 80
  lesions 56
  problems 42
  rash 80
Solid 73, 85, 86, 121
  malignancies 121
  tumors 73, 85, 86
Spermatogenesis 174

Stem cells 46, 71, 84, 87
  bladder cancer 46
  epidermal 71
  gastrointestinal 71
  hepatic 71
  mesenchymal 71
  neural 71
  pancreatic 71
  resistant cancer 87
  targeting cancer 84, 87
Stereotactic body radiotherapy 111, 113
Stress-related transcription factors ATF4 7
Suppression 7, 9, 45, 46, 52, 77, 80
  cannabinoid-evoked angiogenesis 9
  of yes-associated proteins 45
Synergistic antitumor effects 180
Synthesis 7, 54, 171
  repressing hepcidin 54
Synthetic 1, 2, 11, 17, 18, 19, 20, 21, 22
  aminoalkylindole 18
  cannabinergic molecules 17
  cannabinoids 1, 2, 11, 17, 20, 21, 22
  chromenopyrazole scaffold 19
Systemic lupus erythematosus (SLE) 42

T

TACE 106, 113, 124, 126
  and hepatic artery infusion chemotherapy
    124
  and radiofrequency ablation 106
  progression 113, 126
Target proteins 50, 168
  targeting multiple cancer 50
Taxane-induced peripheral neuropathy 4
T cell receptor (TCR) 76, 79, 80, 84
TCR gene transfer 80
Testicular cancer 17
Therapy 1, 39, 50, 52, 57, 74, 75, 79, 103,
    114, 125, 142, 165
  cannabinoid-based antitumor 1
  chimeric antigen receptor T-cell 103
  endocrine 165
  gene 142

immuno 39
  photodynamic 52, 57
Thrombocytopenia 173
Thyroid carcinomas 9
Tissues 2, 3, 5, 11, 70, 71, 72, 73, 78
  adipose 2, 3
  damage repair 72
  healthy 11
  homeostasis 71
  lysate 78
  non-tumor 5
  regeneration 72
Topoisomerases 179
Transition metals 41
Transmucosal absorption 48
Treg 50, 105, 106
  downregulation 106
  proliferation 105
  and myeloid-derived suppressor cells 50
Tremelimumab 120, 125, 126
  efficacy of 125, 126
  monotherapy 120, 125
Tumoral heterogeneity 73
Tumor(s) 5, 6, 7, 9, 10, 12, 14, 45, 48, 49, 50,
    52, 68, 69, 70, 72, 73, 74, 75, 76, 78, 79,
    80, 83, 84, 101, 104, 105, 141, 142, 143,
    145, 149, 150, 151, 152, 153, 154
  angiogenesis 7, 14, 52
  associated antigens (TAA) 84
  growth inhibition 12, 83
  Infiltrating Lymphocytes (TILs) 79, 105
  lysis 70
  malignant 83
  mass 68, 69, 75
  microenvironment 69, 76, 80, 101, 105
  necrosis factor (TNF) 45, 48, 50, 150
  progression 7, 9, 10, 14, 49, 69, 73
  proliferation 104
  protein 145
  relapse 10, 80
  resistant 52
  RNA 78
  suppression 149
Tumor growth 1, 5, 9, 10, 12, 13, 14, 15, 17,
    19, 20, 21, 52, 82, 84, 149, 152

inhibited 82, 84
  modulate 1
  reducing 52
  suppressing vascular 9
Tumorigenesis 6, 7, 69, 70
Tyrosine kinase inhibitors (TKIs) 103, 117,
    121, 122, 128

U

Ulcerative esophagitis 110
UV irradiation 185

V

Vaccines 68, 77
  dendritic cell 68
  dendritic cell-based therapeutic 77
Vascular adhesiveness 5
Vascular endothelial growth factor (VEGF) 9,
    51, 52, 80, 101, 104, 106, 113, 127
  receptor (VEGFR) 80
Voltage-dependent anion channel (VDAC)
    146
Vomiting 1, 2, 3, 9, 171

W

World health organization 101, 143
Wounds, external 38

X

Xenograft study 144

Y

Yes-associated proteins (YAP) 44, 45, 47, 49

www.ingramcontent.com/pod-product-compliance
Lightning Source LLC
Chambersburg PA
CBHW080019240326

41598CB00075B/426